Automated Image Detection of RETINAL PATHOLOGY

Edited by
HERBERT F. JELINEK
MICHAEL J. CREE

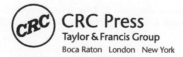

CRC Press
Taylor & Francis Group
Boca Raton   London   New York

CRC Press is an imprint of the
Taylor & Francis Group, an **informa** business

CRC Press
Taylor & Francis Group
6000 Broken Sound Parkway NW, Suite 300
Boca Raton, FL 33487-2742

First issued in paperback 2017

© 2010 by Taylor and Francis Group, LLC
CRC Press is an imprint of Taylor & Francis Group, an Informa business

No claim to original U.S. Government works

ISBN 13: 978-1-138-11449-4 (pbk)
ISBN 13: 978-0-8493-7556-9 (hbk)

Library of Congress Cataloging-in-Publication Data

Automated image detection of retinal pathology / editors, Herbert Jelinek, Michael J. Cree.
    p. ; cm.
Includes bibliographical references and index.
ISBN 978-0-8493-7556-9 (hardcover : alk. paper)
    1. Retina--Diseases--Imaging--Data processing. 2. Image processing--Digital techniques. 3. Diabetic retinopathy--Imaging--Data processing. I. Jelinek, Herbert. II. Cree, Michael J.
    [DNLM: 1. Retinal Diseases--diagnosis. 2. Diagnosis, Computer-Assisted. 3. Diagnostic Imaging--methods. 4. Retina--pathology. WW 270 A939 2010]

RE551.A98 2010
617.7'350754--dc22   2009025019

Visit the Taylor & Francis Web site at
http://www.taylorandfrancis.com

and the CRC Press Web site at
http://www.crcpress.com

Contents

Preface xiii

Contributors xvii

1 Introduction 1
H. F. Jelinek and M. J. Cree
 1.1 Why Automated Image Detection of Retinal Pathology? 1
  1.1.1 The general clinical need 2
  1.1.2 Diabetes: A global problem 2
  1.1.3 Diabetic retinopathy 2
  1.1.4 Eye-screening for diabetic retinopathy 3
  1.1.5 Other retinal pathologies 5
  1.1.6 The retina as an indicator for disease elsewhere 6
  1.1.7 Research needs in automated retinopathy detection 6
  1.1.8 The engineering opportunity 7
 1.2 Automated Assessment of Retinal Eye Disease 7
  1.2.1 Automated microaneurysm detection in diabetic retinopathy 8
  1.2.2 Hemorrhages 9
  1.2.3 White lesion segmentation 9
  1.2.4 Localization of important markers 10
  1.2.5 Retinal vessel diameter changes in disease 11
  1.2.6 Retinal blood vessel segmentation 11
  1.2.7 Mathematical analysis of vessel patterns 12
 1.3 The Contribution of This Book 13

2 Diabetic Retinopathy and Public Health 27
D. Worsley and D. Simmons
 2.1 Introduction 27
 2.2 The Pandemic of Diabetes and Its Complications 28
 2.3 Retinal Structure and Function 29
 2.4 Definition and Description 35
 2.5 Classification of Diabetic Retinopathy 40
 2.6 Differential Diagnosis of Diabetic Retinopathy 40
 2.7 Systemic Associations of Diabetic Retinopathy 42
  2.7.1 Duration of diabetes 42
  2.7.2 Type of diabetes 42
  2.7.3 Blood glucose control 42
  2.7.4 Blood pressure 42

	2.7.5	Serum lipids	43
	2.7.6	Renal disease	43
	2.7.7	Anemia	43
	2.7.8	Pregnancy	43
	2.7.9	Smoking	43
2.8	Pathogenesis		43
	2.8.1	Hyperglycemia	43
	2.8.2	Hematological abnormalities	44
	2.8.3	Leukostasis and inflammation	44
	2.8.4	Growth factors	44
	2.8.5	Neurodegeneration	45
2.9	Treatment		45
	2.9.1	Management of systemic associations	45
	2.9.2	Ocular treatments	45
	2.9.3	Investigational treatments	46
2.10	Screening		48
	2.10.1	Methods of screening	48
	2.10.2	Frequency of screening	54
	2.10.3	Cost effectiveness of screening	54
	2.10.4	Access to care and screening	54
2.11	Conclusion		55

3 Detecting Retinal Pathology Automatically with Special Emphasis on Diabetic Retinopathy   67
M. D. Abràmoff and M. Niemeijer

3.1	Historical Aside	67
3.2	Approaches to Computer (Aided) Diagnosis	68
3.3	Detection of Diabetic Retinopathy Lesions	70
3.4	Detection of Lesions and Segmentation of Retinal Anatomy	71
3.5	Detection and Staging of Diabetic Retinopathy: Pixel to Patient	71
3.6	Directions for Research	72

4 Finding a Role for Computer-Aided Early Diagnosis of Diabetic Retinopathy   79
L. B. Bäcklund

4.1	Mass Examinations of Eyes in Diabetes		79
	4.1.1	Motive for accurate early diagnosis of retinopathy	80
	4.1.2	Definition of screening	81
	4.1.3	Practical importance of the concept of screening	81
	4.1.4	Coverage and timely re-examination	81
4.2	Developing and Defending a Risk Reduction Program		82
	4.2.1	Explaining why retinopathy is suitable for screening	82
	4.2.2	Understanding reasons for possible criticism	83
	4.2.3	Fulfilling criteria for screening tests	83
	4.2.4	Setting quality assurance standards	84

4.2.5   Training and assessment   84
4.3   Assessing Accuracy of a Diagnostic Test   84
    4.3.1   Predictive value, estimation, power   85
    4.3.2   Receiver operating characteristic curve   87
    4.3.3   Area under curve   89
    4.3.4   Covariates   90
4.4   Improving Detection of Diabetic Retinopathy   90
    4.4.1   Improving work environment   91
    4.4.2   Going digital   91
    4.4.3   Obtaining clear images   91
    4.4.4   Avoiding loss of information   92
    4.4.5   Viewing images   92
    4.4.6   Ensuring accurate grading   93
    4.4.7   Organizing for success   93
4.5   Measuring Outcomes of Risk Reduction Programs   93
    4.5.1   Reducing new blindness and visual impairment   94
    4.5.2   Counting people who lost vision   94
    4.5.3   Understanding the importance of visual impairment   95
4.6   User Experiences of Computer-Aided Diagnosis   96
    4.6.1   Perceived accuracy of lesion detection   97
    4.6.2   Finding and reading evaluations of software for retinopathy
          diagnosis   101
    4.6.3   Opportunities and challenges for programmers   102
4.7   Planning a Study to Evaluate Accuracy   103
    4.7.1   Getting help from a statistician   103
    4.7.2   Choosing a measurement scale   103
    4.7.3   Optimizing design   104
    4.7.4   Carrying out different phases of research   108
    4.7.5   An example from another field   109
4.8   Conclusion   110
4.A   Appendix: Measures of Binary Test Performance   120

5   Retinal Markers for Early Detection of Eye Disease   **121**
    A. Osareh
5.1   Abstract   121
5.2   Introduction   122
5.3   Nonproliferative Diabetic Retinopathy   123
5.4   Chapter Overview   124
5.5   Related Works on Identification of Retinal Exudates and the Optic
    Disc   128
    5.5.1   Exudate identification and classification   128
    5.5.2   Optic disc detection   130
5.6   Preprocessing   132
5.7   Pixel-Level Exudate Recognition   134

5.8   Application of Pixel-Level Exudate Recognition on the Whole
        Retinal Image   137
5.9   Locating the Optic Disc in Retinal Images   139
        5.9.1   Template matching   141
        5.9.2   Color morphology preprocessing   141
        5.9.3   Accurate localization of the optic disc-based snakes   144
        5.9.4   Optic disc localization results   146
5.10   Conclusion   148

6   Automated Microaneurysm Detection for Screening   155
      M. J. Cree
6.1   Characteristics of Microaneurysms and Dot-Hemorrhages   155
6.2   History of Automated Microaneurysm Detection   156
        6.2.1   Early morphological approaches   156
        6.2.2   The "standard approach" to automated microaneurysm
                  detection   157
        6.2.3   Extensions of the standard approach   159
        6.2.4   Other approaches   162
        6.2.5   General red lesion detection   164
6.3   Microaneurysm Detection in Color Retinal Images   165
6.4   The Waikato Automated Microaneurysm Detector   167
        6.4.1   Further comments on the use of color   171
6.5   Issues for Microaneurysm Detection   172
        6.5.1   Image quality assessment   172
        6.5.2   Image compression implications   173
        6.5.3   Optic disc detection   175
        6.5.4   Meaningful comparisons of implementations   175
6.6   Research Application of Microaneurysm Detection   177
6.7   Conclusion   178

**7   Retinal Vascular Changes as Biomarkers of Systemic Cardiovascular
      Diseases   185**
      N. Cheung, T. Y. Wong, and L. Hodgson
7.1   Introduction   185
7.2   Early Description of Retinal Vascular Changes   186
7.3   Retinal Vascular Imaging   187
        7.3.1   Assessment of retinal vascular signs from retinal photographs   187
        7.3.2   Limitations in current retinal vascular imaging techniques .   187
7.4   Retinal Vascular Changes and Cardiovascular Disease   189
        7.4.1   Hypertension   189
        7.4.2   Stroke and cerebrovascular disease   191
        7.4.3   Coronary heart disease and congestive heart failure   193
7.5   Retinal Vascular Changes and Metabolic Diseases   194
        7.5.1   Diabetes mellitus   196
        7.5.2   The metabolic syndrome   196

	7.5.3	Overweight and obesity	197
7.6		Retinal Vascular Changes and Other Systemic Diseases	197
	7.6.1	Renal disease	197
	7.6.2	Atherosclerosis	198
	7.6.3	Inflammation and endothelial dysfunction	198
	7.6.4	Subclinical cardiac morphology	200
7.7		Genetic Associations of Retinal Vascular Changes	200
7.8		Conclusion	201
7.A		Appendix: Retinal Vessel Caliber Grading Protocol	201
	7.A.1	Grading an image	202
	7.A.2	Example of the grading process	204
	7.A.3	Obtaining results	205
	7.A.4	Saving data	206

8 Segmentation of Retinal Vasculature Using Wavelets and Supervised Classification: Theory and Implementation 221

J. V. B. Soares and R. M. Cesar Jr.

8.1		Introduction	221
8.2		Theoretical Background	224
	8.2.1	The 1-D CWT	224
	8.2.2	The 2-D CWT	225
	8.2.3	The 2-D Gabor wavelet	228
	8.2.4	Supervised classification	229
	8.2.5	Bayesian decision theory	231
	8.2.6	Bayesian Gaussian mixture model classifier	231
	8.2.7	k-nearest neighbor classifier	233
	8.2.8	Linear minimum squared error classifier	234
8.3		Segmentation Using the 2-D Gabor Wavelet and Supervised Classification	235
	8.3.1	Preprocessing	235
	8.3.2	2-D Gabor wavelet features	237
	8.3.3	Feature normalization	238
	8.3.4	Supervised pixel classification	239
	8.3.5	Public image databases	240
	8.3.6	Experiments and settings	241
	8.3.7	ROC analysis	242
8.4		Implementation and Graphical User Interface	245
	8.4.1	Overview	245
	8.4.2	Installation	246
	8.4.3	Command line interface	246
	8.4.4	Graphical user interface	247
8.5		Experimental Results	249
8.6		Conclusion	258
	8.6.1	Summary	258
	8.6.2	Future work	258

9 Determining Retinal Vessel Widths and Detection of Width Changes 269
K. H. Fritzsche, C. V. Stewart, and B. Roysam

9.1 Identifying Blood Vessels 270
9.2 Vessel Models 270
9.3 Vessel Extraction Methods 271
9.4 Can's Vessel Extraction Algorithm 271
    9.4.1 Improving Can's algorithm 272
    9.4.2 Limitations of the modified Can algorithm 275
9.5 Measuring Vessel Width 276
9.6 Precise Boundary Detection 278
9.7 Continuous Vessel Models with Spline-Based Ribbons 279
    9.7.1 Spline representation of vessels 279
    9.7.2 B-spline ribbons 284
9.8 Estimation of Vessel Boundaries Using Snakes 288
    9.8.1 Snakes 288
    9.8.2 Ribbon snakes 289
    9.8.3 B-spline ribbon snake 289
    9.8.4 Cross section-based B-spline snakes 292
    9.8.5 B-spline ribbon snakes comparison 293
9.9 Vessel Width Change Detection 294
    9.9.1 Methodology 294
    9.9.2 Change detection via hypothesis test 296
    9.9.3 Summary 298
9.10 Conclusion 298

10 Geometrical and Topological Analysis of Vascular Branches from Fundus Retinal Images 305
N. W. Witt, M. E. Martínez-Pérez, K. H. Parker, S. A. McG. Thom, and A. D. Hughes

10.1 Introduction 305
10.2 Geometry of Vessel Segments and Bifurcations 306
    10.2.1 Arterial to venous diameter ratio 306
    10.2.2 Bifurcation geometry 308
    10.2.3 Vessel length to diameter ratios 311
    10.2.4 Tortuosity 312
10.3 Vessel Diameter Measurements from Retinal Images 312
    10.3.1 The half-height method 313
    10.3.2 Double Gaussian fitting 314
    10.3.3 The sliding linear regression filter (SLRF) 314
10.4 Clinical Findings from Retinal Vascular Geometry 315
10.5 Topology of the Vascular Tree 318
    10.5.1 Strahler branching ratio 321
    10.5.2 Path length 321
    10.5.3 Number of edges 321
    10.5.4 Tree asymmetry index 322

10.6   Automated Segmentation and Analysis of Retinal Fundus Images   323
    10.6.1   Feature extraction   324
    10.6.2   Region growing   326
    10.6.3   Analysis of binary images   327
10.7   Clinical Findings from Retinal Vascular Topology   328
10.8   Conclusion   329

11   Tele-Diabetic Retinopathy Screening and Image-Based Clinical Decision Support   339
K. Yogesan, F. Reinholz, and I. J. Constable
11.1   Introduction   339
11.2   Telemedicine   339
    11.2.1   Image capture   340
    11.2.2   Image resolution   341
    11.2.3   Image transmission   342
    11.2.4   Image compression   342
11.3   Telemedicine Screening for Diabetic Retinopathy   344
11.4   Image-Based Clinical Decision Support Systems   346
11.5   Conclusion   347

Index   351

Preface

With the start of the 21st century, digital image processing and analysis is coming of age. Advances in hardware for capturing the minute detail in biological tissues such as the retina, and the unrelenting improvement in computational power in accordance with Moore's law, have provided the basis for mathematicians, computer scientists, and engineers to apply pattern recognition and image analysis in medical and biological applications. A better understanding of disease processes, which incorporate preclinical markers that identify people at risk combined with medical advances in diagnosis and treatment pave the way for improvement in health care generally and specifically for people with retinal disease such as that found in diabetes.

Globally the prevalence of diabetes mellitus is on the rise and with it the associated complications including retinopathy, heart disease, and peripheral vascular disease. Early detection of features often not directly discernible by clinical investigation has the potential to reduce the global burden of diabetes and cardiovascular disease. Although there are good public health reasons for screening certain populations or sub-populations, several factors need to be considered as outlined by the World Health Organization. These include the following: the disease is an important health problem, the natural history of the disease needs to be understood, there should be a detectable early stage, and treatment at the early stage should be more beneficial than treatment at later stages of disease. Diabetes and cardiovascular disease meet these criteria.

Diabetic retinopathy (DR) and heart disease are associated with changes in the characteristics of the blood vessels either in the retina, heart, or in the peripheral circulation. The retina is a tissue that is easily accessible and investigated. Signs of developing or current diabetic retinopathy and heart disease include changes in vessel diameter, occurrence of vessel tortuosity, new vessel growth, small enlargements of retinal capillaries referred to as microaneurysms, small and large hemorrhages and lipid exudates. Changes in either venule or arteriolar diameter have been associated with an increased risk of diabetes, hypertension, cardiovascular disease, and stroke. Even small increases in blood sugar levels, being below the accepted concentration for the diagnosis of diabetes, can affect the retina and lead to the presence of microaneurysms. To assess an appropriate number of people in the community, screening methods have to be economical, accurate, and easily performed. Therefore, automated assessment of preclinical or clinical signs associated with diabetic retinopathy and cardiovascular disease has been of great interest.

Engineering tools such as digital image processing combined with advanced machine learning allow identification and automated classification of features, lesions, and retinal changes in digital images of the retina. Objective diagnostic criteria for diabetic retinopathy progression have been available for 30 years, with the Early

Treatment Diabetic Retinopathy Study providing a robust tool in 1991. Various permutations of this classification system have been proposed but essentially the grading system includes: minimal, mild, moderate, and severe nonproliferative retinopathy and proliferative retinopathy, both with or without macular involvement. Each of these stages is associated with the presence of particular pathological features. By combining different branches of engineering and medicine it has become possible to utilize today's technology and to contribute to the needs of physicians in providing optimal health care.

For any computer-based classification system to be successful the images need to be of adequate quality and resolution. The resolution of digital images can now exceed 10 megapixels and arguably surpasses the 35 mm photographic standard. There has been work carried out in image preprocessing that addresses uneven retinal illumination, poor focus, or differences in background epithelium hue. The optic disc is the main feature in the retinal fundus. Numerous methods in image analysis such as using the measure of pixel intensity variance of a window size equal to the optic disc for locating the optic disc to applying the Hough transform and snake-based algorithms for identification of the boundary of the optic disk have been proposed. Automated microaneurysm segmentation was first applied to fluorescein-labeled images in the early 1990s and recently extended to nonmydriatic color retinal images. The latter is well suited for large population screening as it is noninvasive and economical. The literature on retinal vessel segmentation is numerous and varied. More work is needed, not only to characterize and compare algorithms, but also to improve algorithms to achieve better reliability in segmenting vessels. Segmentation of the vascular tree allows the determination of length, diameter, and coverage. It is also required to allow identification of lesions associated with diabetic retinopathy progression by removing the vessels as a confounder. Matched filters, local operators such as wavelet transforms, local gradients in the form of the first and second derivatives, neural networks that sweep over the whole image, vessel tracking algorithms, and many other approaches have been proposed. Local variation in vessel widths and vessel branching patterns can then be used to identify venous beading, vessel nicking, and the arteriolar-venous ratio.

Advances in automated image detection of retinal pathology require interaction and dialogue between practitioners from diverse fields. In this spirit, the contributors to this book include engineers, physicists, computer scientists, and physicians to provide a nexus between these fields. Each contributor is a recognized expert and has made significant contributions to the development of automated analysis of retinal images. There is much that has been discovered and proved to be effective in research institutes but has failed to make the transition to general clinical practice. Therefore many problems are yet to be solved.

This book is intended for researchers in the diverse fields of engineering, mathematics, and physics, as well as biologists and physicians. It discusses the epidemiology of disease, screening protocols, algorithm development, image processing, and feature analysis applied to the retina. Hopefully it inspires readers that automated analysis of retinal images is an exciting field, both for the physician and nonphysician alike, and one in which many developments have been made, but much more needs to be done if the products of our labor are to benefit the health of the community.

Chapter 1, by Jelinek and Cree, presents the general argument for automated image detection of retinal pathology. The field of diabetic retinopathy in terms of pathologies that affect the retina and those that are possibly identifiable by automated processing is emphasized. Prevalence and incidence of diabetic retinopathy are discussed with respect to the need for automated assessment. The chapter further outlines the use of automated retinal assessment as an indicator for disease elsewhere such as cardiovascular disease and peripheral vascular disease. A brief overview of work to date of automated image assessment of retinal disease is presented and opportunities for further development are highlighted.

Before embarking on applying image analysis techniques to retinal images, one needs to be aware of the clinical context. Chapter 2, by Worsley and Simmons, focuses on the pandemic of diabetes that is spurred by the reduction in physical activity and increases in energy-dense foods leading to an increase in obesity, insulin resistance, and Type 2 diabetes. The chapter discusses the importance of diabetic retinopathy and its contribution to blindness as well as its utility in providing a window on the natural history of diabetes in the population. The main focus is on how diabetic retinopathy is defined and classified, the disease process, the population distribution, and its prevention and screening for early changes.

Chapter 3, by Abràmoff and Niemeijer, addresses optimization of retinal image digitization and detection of retinopathy. There are several approaches one can take, that is, decide whether there is disease / no disease or decide on progression. The chapter focuses on the frequency of occurrence of disease indicators in relation to a typical screening population and how research emphasis needs to focus on making automated detection methods more robust for clinical practice.

Chapter 4, by Bäcklund, concentrates on outlining the reasons why well-designed retinopathy risk-reduction programs need to be implemented on a large scale. Considerable efforts are required to address the importance and difficulty of achieving reliable early diagnosis of DR at a reasonable cost and to evaluate computer-aided diagnosis. Observations of a practitioner who has some experience with computer-aided diagnosis on why systems for automated detection of retinal lesions have made little impact to date, are presented.

Chapter 5, by Osareh, is the first to provide an application of the nexus between engineering and medicine. The chapter concentrates on detection of the optic disc and retinal exudate identification. Color retinal images are classified to exudate and nonexudate classes following some preprocessing steps. The authors investigate K nearest neighbor, Gaussian quadratic, and Gaussian mixture model classifiers. The optic disc detection is based on color mathematical morphology and active contours. Implications for screening are discussed.

Cree, in Chapter 6, outlines the differences between microaneurysms and dot hemorrhages as part of the disease process and how their presentation can be used for automated detection and classification. Microaneurysms are usually the first sign of diabetic retinopathy and a positive correlation between the number of microaneurysms and disease progression has been reported. A historical background to automated detection of microaneurysms is followed by an overview of the standard approach to microaneurysm detection and extensions of this standard approach including application for population screening of color digital images.

Certain subtle vascular changes in retinal images are believed to predict the risk of disease elsewhere in the body. In Chapter 7, Cheung, Wong and Hodgson, develop the case that the arteriolar-venous ratio measured from retinal images is a good predictor of risk of diabetes, cardiovascular disease, and stroke as well as hypertension.

To automate measurement of features, such as the arteriolar-venous ratio, one must first reliably segment the blood vessels of the retina. In Chapter 8, Soares and Cesar, focus on the use of wavelet transforms to segment retinal blood vessels, discussing first the theoretical background of 1-D, 2-D continuous wavelet transforms, and the 2-D Gabor wavelet as a specific application that is suitable for blood vessel segmentation. Pixels are classified as either belonging to the vessel or not using a Bayesian Gaussian mixture model.

Chapters 9 (by Fritzsche et al.) and 10 (by Witt et al.) set the scene for analysis of the blood vessels including vessel diameter and branching angle, which can be indicators of pathology. Fritzsche et al. concentrate on how vessels can be detected using diverse models such as edge detectors, cross-sectional models, as well as algorithms that use intensity measures combined with thresholding, relaxation, morphological operators or affine convex sets to identify ridges and valleys. Following consideration of vessel segmentation the measure of vessel width is considered. Two potential issues arise, one being the orientation in which the width is measured and determination of the points at which to begin and end the measurement. Witt and co-workers concentrate on feature parameters associated with the geometry of vessel segments and bifurcations. One of the first parameters describing vascular geometry was the ratio of arterial to venous diameters. The geometry of bifurcating vessels may have a significant impact on hemodynamics of the vessel network and include the bifurcation angle, junction exponent, and tortuosity. These parameters are then discussed in the context of clinical findings such as hypertension, peripheral vascular disease, and ischemic heart disease.

The last chapter, by Yogesan et al., investigates the use of teleophthalmology in clinical practice. The chapter focuses on issues of image size and quality, health care costs, and early detection of diabetic retinopathy; and continues by considering combining teleophthalmology with automated assessment.

Contributors

Michael D. Abràmoff
University of Iowa
Iowa City, Iowa

Lars B. Bäcklund
Karolinska Institutet and Uppsala Universitet
Stockholm, Sweden

Roberto M. Cesar Jr.
University of São Paulo
São Paulo, Brazil

Ning Cheung
Centre for Eye Research Australia
Springfield, Australia

Ian J. Constable
The Lions Eye Institute
Nedlands, Australia

Michael J. Cree
University of Waikato
Hamilton, New Zealand

Kenneth H. Fritzsche
United States Military Academy
Springfield, Virginia

Lauren Hodgson
Centre for Eye Research Australia
Springfield, Australia

Alun D. Hughes
Imperial College
London, United Kingdom

Herbert F. Jelinek
Charles Sturt University
Albury, Australia

M. Elena Martínez-Pérez
National Autonomous University of Mexico
Mexico City, Mexico

Meindert Niemeijer
University of Iowa
Iowa City, Iowa

Alireza Osareh
Shahid Chamran University of Ahvaz
Ahvaz, Iran

Kim H. Parker
Imperial College
London, United Kingdom

Fred Reinholz
The Lions Eye Institute
Nedlands, Australia

Bardrinath Roysam
Rensselaer Polytechnic Institute
Troy, New York

David Simmons
Waikato Clinical School
Hamilton, New Zealand

João V. B. Soares
University of São Paulo
São Paulo, Brazil

Charles V. Stewart
Rensselaer Polytechnic Institute
Troy, New York

Simon A. McG. Thom
Imperial College
London, United Kingdom

Nicholas W. Witt
Imperial College
London, United Kingdom

David Worsley
Waikato Health Ltd.
Hamilton, New Zealand

Tien Y. Wong
Centre for Eye Research Australia
Springfield, Australia

Kanagasingam Yogesan
The Lions Eye Institute
Nedlands, Australia

1

Introduction

Herbert F. Jelinek and Michael J. Cree

CONTENTS

1.1 Why Automated Image Detection of Retinal Pathology? 1
1.2 Automated Assessment of Retinal Eye Disease 7
1.3 The Contribution of This Book 13
    References 13

1.1 Why Automated Image Detection of Retinal Pathology?

Indeed, why? What are the driving forces that are leading to the development of automated computer detection and quantification of retinal lesions? Why is there a multi-disciplinary approach involving medical specialists, health professionals, medical physicists, biomedical engineers, and computer scientists to develop systems capable of automated detection of retinal pathology?

In this section we examine the reasons why a number of research groups have embarked on developing methodology and computer software for automated image detection of retinal pathology. We shall see (1) that there is a need in clinical practice to find better and cheaper ways of identifying, managing, and treating retinal disease; (2) that in the research community there is a desire to better understand the underlying causes and progression of disease that requires the detailed analysis of large cohorts of retinal images; (3) that the recent advances in computer hardware and computing power, coupled with increasingly sophisticated image analysis and machine learning techniques, provide opportunities to meet the needs of clinical practice and the eye research community; and, finally, that images of the retina are both a gold mine and a minefield for the application of digital image processing and machine learning techniques, that can both reward the recent graduate and test to exasperation the most competent and innovative engineer.

We begin with the impetus arising from the medical community for new, cheaper, and more efficient means of detecting and managing retinal disease. The impetus arises from a number of quarters and we consider each in turn.

1.1.1   The general clinical need

With an increase in the aged population worldwide there is increasing eye disease, therefore there is a relative decrease in ophthalmic services, especially in rural areas and developing countries. The World Health Organization has launched "Vision 2020," a global initiative for the prevention of avoidable visual impairment by the year 2020 [1]. Eye health encompasses several approaches such as expanding efforts to raise awareness about eye health, early detection of disease, accurate diagnosis, and targeted prevention to improve outcomes. Recent data suggest that there are 37 million blind people and 124 million with low vision worldwide, excluding those with uncorrected refractive errors. The main causes of global blindness are cataract, glaucoma, corneal scarring, age-related macular degeneration, and diabetic retinopathy. The global Vision 2020 initiative is having an impact to reduce avoidable blindness particularly from ocular infections, but more needs to be done to address cataract, glaucoma, and diabetic retinopathy [2]. It is diabetic retinopathy that represents the most pressing problem and it is to this that most work on automated detection has been directed.

1.1.2   Diabetes: A global problem

Diabetes is a metabolic disorder that leads to complications including cardiovascular, renal, and eye disease. It has been identified as a significant and growing global public health problem with the expected worldwide prevalence of 300 million by the year 2025 [3–6]. Current prevalence of diabetes in the United States is 6.3% with greater prevalence in certain ethnic groups and socioeconomic classes [6–8]. The New Zealand situation is similar [3]. In Australia approximately one million people (5%) are affected by diabetes and health care costs associated with treatment of complications amounts to approximately AUS\$7 billion dollars [9]. Diabetes is a significant and costly heath problem in the Western world, and is growing in incidence at almost epidemic levels. New and innovative ways of identification, diagnosis, treatment and follow-up are needed to manage this growing problem.

1.1.3   Diabetic retinopathy

Increase in blood sugar levels associated with diabetes is the known cause of diabetic retinopathy (DR), a progressive degenerative disease of the retina that has an asymptomatic stage that can start long before the onset of recognized diabetes.

Diabetic retinopathy is divided into various stages. The earliest signs of DR are microaneurysms, small hemorrhages, cotton wool spots, and exudates that result from abnormal permeability and nonperfusion of capillaries. These early signs are known as nonproliferative diabetic retinopathy (NPDR). There may even be earlier indications of diabetic retinopathy [10–12]. Fluid leaking from the retinal capillaries indicates a further progression of the disease. This may lead to sight threatening diabetic retinopathy (STDR) if the leakage is located in the area of most acute vision (the macula) [13–15]. Diabetic macular edema is the most common cause of vision loss in diabetes. Proliferative diabetic retinopathy (PDR) develops from occluded capillaries that lead to retinal ischemia and formation of new vessels on the surface of the retina either near the optic disc or in the retinal periphery.

With an increase in diabetes prevalence, the prevalence and incidence of diabetic retinopathy are also increasing [16]. Early studies suggested that some form of diabetic eye disease is present in up to 60% of people with type 2 (insulin independent) diabetes [17]. More recent evidence suggests that 40% to 45% of the diabetic population have some DR with 10% to 14% having STDR [18]. In type 1 (insulin dependent) diabetes other investigators reported a baseline prevalence of any retinopathy, PDR, and STDR of 45.7%, 3.7%, and 16.4% respectively [15]. In type 2 diabetes, the baseline prevalence of any retinopathy, PDR, and STDR was 25.3%, 0.5%, and 6.0% respectively. Diabetic retinopathy that preceded diagnosis of diabetes in 20.8% of the Wisconsin diabetes study subjects [19] remains an important cause of preventable blindness and visual impairment [19–22]. In other words, one-fifth of people with diabetes (in the Wisconsin study) developed DR before diabetes was diagnosed.

Diabetic retinopathy is characterized by a number of features that are recognizable by the trained observer. The features of DR are described in detail in Chapter 2, but it is worth noting here in advance that certain lesions indicating DR, such as the number of microaneurysms and dot hemorrhages, have been demonstrated to correlate with disease severity and likely progression of the disease, at least for its early stages [23; 24]. Such lesions have a reasonably well defined appearance and represent useful targets for automated image detection, and the detection of them provides useful information.

It is also important that DR is a treatable disease throughout disease progression commencing from the preclinical stage. If detected early and treated then significant saving in cost and reduction in the progression of eyesight loss is possible. The detection, management, and treatment of DR are huge resource drains on governments and health systems worldwide [22]. As the disease is treatable, detection and monitoring of the disease via fundus photography is beneficial, and more efficient detection and monitoring saves costs, it would seem that automated image detection of diabetic retinopathy is an engineering solution to a growing need.

1.1.4 Eye-screening for diabetic retinopathy

Screening is generally considered effective if a number of criteria are met. These criteria include but are not limited to identification of disease at an early, preferably preclinical, stage and that the disease in its early or late stage is amenable to treatment. Screening for DR and monitoring progression, especially in the early asymptomatic stage, has been shown to be effective in the prevention of vision loss and reducing cost associated with disease progression and treatment [25–28]. Estimates of the rate of annual eye examinations are generally fairly low, from 40% to 65% depending on the country.

Various methods of screening have been shown to be sufficiently sensitive and specific for the detection of sight-threatening eye disease at justifiable costs [18; 29–31]. There still remains potential for reduction in costs, increased effectiveness and timeliness, and extension of eye-screening to remote areas that are not serviced by ophthalmologists. Automated assessment of retinal images may be a key ingredient to achieving these benefits. We further explore these claims in the following.

The U.S. "Healthy People 2010" project aims at increasing the number of people with diabetes screened annually for diabetic retinopathy from the current 46% to 75%. To achieve or improve on this goal, several different screening models for diabetic eye disease have been proposed for diverse health care professionals from ophthalmology to rural community screening by health technicians [32]. The Australian National Health and Medical Research Council as well as other health departments including those of the United States and United Kingdom have established guidelines for screening of diabetic retinopathy [26; 33; 34]. National screening programs have the potential to be not only cost effective but also improve health care outcomes and quality of life for individuals with DR.

In rural and remote areas as well as in developing countries regular assessment for diabetic eye disease is difficult. Any method that simplifies the process, increases efficiency, and reduces costs of retinal screening will have significant health benefits [35; 36]. In terms of method, retinal photography has shown to be the screening test of choice [37]. Retinal photography using 35 mm slides, color photography, or Polaroid films has now been extended to digital photography that has additional advantages such as low technical failure, good sensitivity and specificity, as well as being cost effective [38; 39]. The original seven-field criterion for diabetic retinopathy classification using photography has also been reduced to two-field and one-field retinal image analysis for screening purposes [40; 41].

Several field studies illustrate the utility of retinal vascular imaging. A study in the Goulburn and La Trobe Valleys in Victoria, Australia, using nonmydriatic (i.e., nondilated pupil) retinal photography reported 60% of participants with no abnormality, 18% with diabetic retinopathy, 9% with other fundus pathology, 3% reduced acuity alone, and 10% of photographs were ungradeable and 29% had never had a fundus examination [42]. Reducing the number that had never had an eye examination is critical in improving community health and quality of life as early identification leads to effective treatment and a reduction in sight threatening diabetic retinopathy [32; 43]. A community-based screening of diabetic patients in rural Western Australia using retinal photography found that 28% of subjects had retinopathy [44]. Rates increased by approximately 20% every 10 years (e.g., 42% had retinopathy by 15 years duration). Vision threatening retinopathy was present in 13% of patients.

Waikato Regional Mobile Diabetic Retinopathy Photoscreening Programme attended over 200 sites between 1993 and 2003 and screened 79% of the expected number of patients [45]. The study concluded that mobile retinal photoscreening is practical in a large rural area, and its implementation has been associated with a reduction in presentations with vision-threatening retinopathy within the total community [46]. These data lead to the conclusion that effective screening increases detection of early DR and therefore better treatment outcomes [29; 44].

Targeting screening incorporating automated detection of retinal pathology has the potential to improve identification and follow-up of diabetic retinopathy by increas-

Table 1.1: List of Pathologies That Affect the Retina and the Possibility of Automated Detection Leading to Early Treatment

Retinal Pathology Screening Possible	Automated Detection Possible	Early Treatment Possible
Diabetic retinopathy	Yes	Yes
Refractive error in preschool children	Yes	Yes
Newborns for gonococcal eye disease (swab)		Yes
Retinopathy of prematurity	Yes	Yes
Hydroxychloroquine medication for retinopathy	Yes	Yes
Glaucoma	Yes	Yes
Age-related macular degeneration	Yes	Yes
Systemic atherosclerotic disease/systemic hypertension	Yes	Yes

ing the availability of this screening method and reducing cost either by combining it with teleophthalmology [47–50], or for use in rural and remote health by community health centers and primary care practitioners. Freeing up ophthalmologists, who otherwise read the retinal images of the screening program, allows them to focus on primary health care. By combining screening programs with health nurses, a larger population can be screened. Furthermore, automated assessment enables immediate feedback to patients [38; 47; 49; 51–54].

1.1.5 Other retinal pathologies

Other retinal diseases that can also be considered for automated image analysis are listed in Table 1.1. Here we highlight three.

Age-related macular degeneration (AMD) is the most common cause of legal blindness among industrialized nations in the population aged 50 years and above. It is characterized by the presence of drusen, choroidal neovascularization, and detachments of the retinal pigment epithelium and geographic atrophy (GA) of retinal pigment epithelium (RPE). Age-related macular degeneration is now treatable and therefore worth detecting and monitoring. Choroidal neovascularization and geographic atrophy is amenable to automated computer-based identification algorithms. There are two forms of AMD including dry (also called atrophic, nonneovascular, or nonexudative) and wet (also called exudative). Dry AMD is the more common form of the disease and accounts for 90% of all AMD. The key identifier for dry AMD is small, round, white-yellow deposits called drusen that build up in the macula. Automated segmentation of drusen can be reliably performed and can be added to efforts in community screening to reduce the progression of disease by early identification and treatment options now available.

Macular edema and other eye pathology either related or not related to diabetes can also lead to blindness. Four techniques are most often used for identification and quantification of macular edema including ultrasound, optical coherence tomography, retinal thickness analyzer, and scanning laser ophthalmology. These techniques vary in resolution and sensitivity with the optical techniques providing the best results. At this stage the cost of the equipment and technology for optical coherence tomography and the retinal thickness analyzer is too excessive for use in routine community screening. However, digital biomicroscopy combined with visual acuity testing is economically viable and can be automated, for instance, by detection of the grey patches associated with clinical significant macular edema.

The shape and appearance of the optic nerve head region are sensitive to changes associated with glaucoma and diabetes that may be otherwise asymptomatic. Initial screening for the presence of glaucoma and tracking disease progression are currently under intense investigation by characterizing the optic disc. Glaucoma is associated with an inadequate fluid flow from the drainage canals of the eye. Crystallization of the fluid in the cornea and iris region is a consequence of this blockage and also provides an opportunity to automatically compute this accretion. A semi-automated algorithm for quantitative representation of the optic disc and cup contours by computing accumulated disparities in the disc and cup regions from stereo fundus image pairs has also been developed using advanced digital image analysis methodologies. A 3-D visualization of the disc and cup is achieved assuming camera geometry.

1.1.6   The retina as an indicator for disease elsewhere

Retinal morphology and the associated blood vessel pattern can also provide an indication of the risk of hypertension, cardiovascular, and cerebrovascular disease as well as diabetes [55–58]. Early identification of people at risk of morbidity and mortality due to diverse disease processes allows preventative measures to be commenced with the greatest efficacy. As such, preclinical signs are not easily recognized and often appear as signs or symptoms that are not specific for a particular disease. Using the retina and its blood vessel characteristics can provide a window into several disease processes. The identification of increased risk of disease progression is based on the change in the venous or arterial vessel diameter especially in proximity to the optic disc. This morphological characteristic allows the application of image analysis and automated classification in risk assessment of cardiovascular and cerebrovascular disease as well as diabetes [59–61].

1.1.7   Research needs in automated retinopathy detection

The underlying causes and mechanisms of retinopathy, such as diabetic retinopathy, are not fully understood and further research is needed. Getting data to help guide hypothesis and model formation and testing is a mammoth task. Obtaining information by dismembering eyes and fundus tissues for assays and microscopic studies is usually not an option. Data result therefore mostly from close examination of the progression of the clinical signs of retinopathy. The acquisition of such data requires careful and fine grading of retinal images of large cohorts over an extended period of time. This has historically required time-consuming and mind-numbing manual grading of large numbers of retinal images. Consequently, such studies are few in number and only pursued by a number of centers (Wisconsin most notable) that have huge financial resources at hand. There is also evidence that preclinical signs, such as arteriolar and venule caliber changes that are not easily determined with manual grading, may be important factors. Such features are so subtle that this evidence can only be gained, in practice, with assisted computer analysis of the retinal images.

There is therefore a need for automated image detection and analysis of retinal pathologies and features to make the grading of large numbers of images practicable and cost-effective [55]. There is also a need for measurement of features that are not easily observable with the human eye. These are much more demanding tasks than that of eye-screening for diabetic retinopathy, as a much finer quantitative analysis of the retina is needed. Therefore a greater effort is required to develop computer-based programs for detection of the more difficult aspects of retinopathy.

1.1.8 The engineering opportunity

Retinal images are a rich, varied, and fascinating set of interesting images to work with. Even in healthy images there are a number of key features that for automated detection require varied and ingenious image processing and pattern recognition techniques. With retinal pathology comes an even richer field of patterns and features to target. Some are quite distinctive; others bear similarity to one another and prove to be a challenging task for current algorithms to reliably distinguish. Engineers and scientists expert in pattern recognition and image processing will find retinal images exciting, challenging, and rewarding to work with. There remain quite a number of problems in automated retinal analysis that need to be solved before automated pathology detection systems can be rolled out for general clinical use.

1.2 Automated Assessment of Retinal Eye Disease

Use of computer-based systems has been shown to be valuable for the diagnosis of visual function loss in people with diverse retinal diseases. One of the most successful clinical areas is the application of computer-based automated assessment of diabetic retinopathy. Several countries including Scotland are implementing or considering automated assessment as part of a national diabetes retinopathy screening program. Detection of microaneurysms, cotton wool spots, soft exudates, and small hemorrhages indicate nonproliferative retinopathy, whereas ischemic areas in the retina, loss of vessels, and vessel proliferation are indicators for proliferative retinopathy and identifiable by automated assessment protocols based on digital image analysis and expert systems [62–68]. Some of the diseases mentioned in Table 1.1 are now amenable to automated identification and assessment. In addition, retinal blood vessel pattern and characteristics can also provide information on the presence or risk of developing hypertension, cardio- and cerebrovascular disease, and diabetes.

In the following we give a summary of some the work on automated retinal analysis. Our aim is to give a few examples to give a feel for the breadth and depth of the field, and to highlight some areas requiring further research. The reader should also consult the literature including useful review papers [48; 69].

1.2.1   Automated microaneurysm detection in diabetic retinopathy

Early attempts at computerized detection of lesions in retinal images date back to the 1980s but it is only in the late 1990s that useable and somewhat reliable results began to be achieved [70]. The first reliable system capable of detecting microaneurysms in fluorescein angiographic images was reported by the Aberdeen group [71; 72]. Work to transfer this technology to red-free and color retinal images is ongoing and has been discussed by several laboratories. The significance of microaneurysm counts in diabetic retinopathy and their close correlation to the severity of the disease is well documented [23; 24]. Microaneurysm formation is a dynamic process [73–75] and there are indications that turnover is an early indicator of retinopathy progression [24; 75]. Therefore detecting microaneurysms should form an important component in an automated diabetic retinopathy screening tool. Hipwell et al. [76] applied automated microaneurysm detection in directly digitized images as a screening tool. Despite that fewer microaneurysms are visible in red-free images than in fluorescein angiography, they achieved 85% sensitivity and 76% specificity for the detection of patients with any retinopathy. They suggest that their system could be useful in eliminating 50% or more of the screening population who have no retinopathy thereby halving the number of images that trained experts need to examine.

It is because of the established clinical implications of microaneurysm counts, the distinctive appearance of microaneurysms, and the advances in high resolution, sensitive and affordable digital camera technology that quite a few algorithms for automated microaneurysm detection have been proposed. As these are summarized in Chapter 6 we restrict ourselves to making some general observations here.

High sensitivities have been achieved in automated detection of microaneurysms but the number of false positive reports tends to still exceed that of trained manual observers. Some automated microaneurysm detection systems are developed with the express aim of screening for diabetic retinopathy and when used for this purpose the sensitivity for detecting microaneurysms can be lowered as only one microaneurysm per image needs to be detected to identify images with microaneurysms. The British Diabetic Retinopathy Working Group recommended a minimum sensitivity of 80% and minimum specificity of 95% for the screening of diabetic retinopathy [77]. Many automated screening projects based on microaneurysm detection (as described above and in Chapter 6) achieve the required sensitivity, but none achieve the required specificity. Achieving high specificity is a major difficulty in developing automated screening systems. Another important difficulty is when severe lesions are not accompanied by microaneurysms or distort the image in such a way that detecting microaneurysms fails. Reporting only sensitivities and specificities can mask the failure of the system to report such rare, but very important, cases.

Also glossed over in the above is the problem of actually establishing the sensitivity and specificity of an automated lesion detection system. Testing methodologies and test image datasets used in papers on automated microaneurysm detection are almost as numerous as the total number of algorithms reported! This makes comparing systems difficult. This issue is picked up and expanded upon by the authors of Chapters 4 and 6, for example.

Automated microaneurysm detection, of itself, is not sufficient for completely automating eye screening for diabetic retinopathy. An automated eye-screening system will also need to be able to detect the quality of the image and the eye field including locations of the optic disc and macula (if present), and integrate results from analyses of multiple images of the same patient. Work on these aspects of automated eye screening has only just started to be reported [78]. Furthermore, integration with automated detection of other lesions will be important. It is to this we now turn attention.

1.2.2 Hemorrhages

Hemorrhages are one of the first signs of diabetic retinopathy and are also prominent in other ocular disease. They take on a range of size, color and texture from the small round dot hemorrhages that are related to microaneurysms and indistinguishable from microaneuryoms in color fundus images, through the flame shaped and blotch (cluster) hemorrhages whose names describe their appearance, to the larger boat shaped hemorrhages. It may well be that a multifaceted pattern recognition approach is needed to reliably detect hemorrhages of all descriptions.

Automated detection of hemorrhages is not as well described in the literature as automated microaneurysm detection, except for dot-hemorrhages, which, by default, are detected by automated detection of microaneurysms working on color fundus images due to the close simularity in appearance with microaneurysms. Reports of automated detection of the larger hemorrhages include a "spider-net" approach [79], neural networks [80], segmentation of dark lesions with classification [64], and mathematical morphology [81; 82].

1.2.3 White lesion segmentation

The so called white lesions consist of exudate, cotton wool spots, and drusen. They are characterized by a white to yellow appearance brighter than the surrounding retina and are typically medium sized lesions but that is as far as there similarity goes. We consider them together because the simplest feature to detect them (high intensity in the green plane) is effective in segmenting these lesions, but insufficient to distinguish them from each other and from other bright features such as the optic disc, light artifacts and laser photocoagulation scars. Indeed the earliest automated exudate detectors were based on thresholding of red-free images [83].

To distinguish the white lesions from each another and from other confounding bright features requires a more sophisticated algorithm. Of some interest is the detection of exudates, without confusion with cotton wool spots and bright light artifacts, to aid in diabetic retinopathy eye screening. Features that can be used are the yellowish color of exudates, their sharp edges, their rougher texture, and the clustering of exudates together and in circles about areas of leakage.

Exudate detection, which has some robustness against confusion with other white lesions or bright artifacts, has been performed with neural networks [80; 84], fuzzy C-means clustering [85; 86], mathematical morphology [87] coupled with region growing [82; 88], region growing coupled with classification [64], clustering techniques coupled with color and vessel analysis [89], and the work reported in Chapter 5 herein. High sensitivities near or above 95% are regularly reported for detecting exudates, however specificity is typically lower. Maybe one of the most significant studies on exudate detection, at least in terms of the large number of images used in testing, is that of Fleming et al. [88]. They achieved 95% sensitivity for a specificity of 85% for detecting images with exudates on a test set of 13 219 images, of which 300 contained exudates.

Because of the low incidence of exudates (and other white lesions) in retinal images (only 2.2% for the study mentioned above) it can be difficult to acquire enough images containing exudates and other white features to be able to sufficiently test a proposed algorithm. Many reported studies test with fewer than 30 images, and sometimes do not even include images with other white features. The reported sensitivities and specificities are therefore likely to be inflated, and give no indication how the algorithm performs on rare, but nevertheless important, difficult cases. Since automated microaneurysm detection can be performed with greater than 80% sensitivity and good specificity for detecting images with diabetic retinopathy, an included automated exudate detector stage must be able to reliably detect the rare and more difficult to analyze cases to effect an improvement in detecting images with diabetic retinopathy.

Less attention has been given to automated detection of other white lesions. Automated detection of cotton wool spots has usually been performed in association with detection of exudates [64; 90; 91]. Drusen occur in age-related macular degeneration and there has been some interest in automated detection [92–97]. Many of the approaches are similar to those used for exudate and cotton wool spot detection.

1.2.4   Localization of important markers

It is important to not only detect and quantify lesions but also to know their location with respect to one another and to the eye. Retinal images normally cover from 35° to 50° field of view of the retina, and multiple images (typically seven) are required to create a substantial picture of the retina. The macula (central point of vision) and the optic disc (entry point of the nervous and blood system to the retina) provide important markers for location. The flow of blood vessels from the optic disc enable one to establish the retinal field and whether it is the right or left eye. The location of lesions, for example the proximity of exudates to the macula, has important clinical implications. It is therefore important that automated detection of the optic disc, macula, and field of view be developed.

In fluorescein angiographic images the macula can often be detected by the absence of flouresence in the foveal avascular zone (a zone at the center of the macula devoid of retinal vessels). A correlation of the gross background fluoresence with a standardized model often enables accurate localization of the macula [98], though abnormal maculae prove problematic to detect. This method is less effective for color fundus images. A refinement is to search the expected location of the fovea based on prior detection of the optic disc [99–101].

The optic disc is a very distinctive feature of the eye. It is often the brightest object, ranging from white to yellow, is circular and of reasonably consistent size from patient to patient, and the retinal vasculature radiates out from its center. Strategies for automated detection of the optic disc include those based on locating the area of maximal intensity and image variance [99; 102; 103], detecting the circular edge of the optic disc [104], whether by fitting snakes to the edge [105; 106], or Hough transform [101] and by using vessel convergence and orientation [107; 108]. Reported sensitivities for detection of the optic disc range from 85% to 98%. Abnormal optic discs present problems for most methods.

1.2.5 Retinal vessel diameter changes in disease

Retinal vessel dilatation is a well known phenomenon in diabetes and significant dilatation and elongation of retinal arterioles, venules, and their macular branches have been shown to occur in the development of diabetic macular edema that can be linked to hydrostatic pressure changes [11; 109]. These vessel changes are not limited to diabetic associated changes and as Wong and collaborators reported can be associated with risk of cardiovascular and cerebrovascular disease as well [55; 110]. Retinal microvascular abnormalities, such as generalized and focal arteriolar narrowing, arteriovenous nicking and retinopathy, reflect cumulative vascular damage from hypertension, ageing, and other processes. Epidemiological studies indicate that these abnormalities can be observed in 2% to 15% of the nondiabetic general population and are strongly and consistently associated with elevated blood pressure. Generalized arteriolar narrowing and arteriovenous nicking also appear to be irreversible long-term markers of hypertension, related not only to current but past blood pressure levels as well [60; 111].

1.2.6 Retinal blood vessel segmentation

The literature on computer algorithms to delineate the vessel network in fluorescein retinal images [99; 112; 113] and color fundus images [62; 114; 115] is extensive and we can not do justice to the field in an introduction such as this. Approaches to automated vessel detection include matched filtering [116] coupled with threshold probing [117], mathematical morphology [118; 119], scale-space analysis with region growing [120], multi-threshold probing [121], pixel classification [122], and wavelet analysis [62], among many others [123–126]. A fundamentally different approach is vessel tracking in which one starts from an initial seed point on a vessel and makes small steps in the direction of the vessel from determinations of the direction of the vessel in the local region [127–132].

The public availability of the STARE [117] and DRIVE [123] databases of retinal images, with accompanying manually produced annotations of locations of the vessel, has provided a test set of images that has enabled quantitative and fair comparisons between vessel detection algorithms. Studies have been published comparing various vessel detection algorithms with the STARE and DRIVE dataset [122; 133] and any new algorithms should be tested on these datasets.

It should be noted that the reasons for detecting blood vessels are varied, ranging from a need to identify vessel locations to aid in reducing false-detections of other lesions, to detecting the vessel networks to establish their geometrical relationships or identifying the field-of-view of the retina, through to accurate delineation of the vessels for quantitative measurement of various vessel parameters (width, branching ratios, and tortuousity) and for identifying vessel features such as venous dilatation and arteriolar narrowing.

1.2.7   Mathematical analysis of vessel patterns

Blood vessels in the optic fundus are a complex network of branches that spread out from the optic disc to provide nutrients and oxygen to the fundus. In proliferative diabetic retinopathy new blood vessels are formed that emerge from the area of the optic disc and spread towards the macula or emerge from peripheral vessels [134]. Automated procedures are not required to identify the smallest vessels that are seen by visual inspection, but new vessel growth and small vessel leakage that is clinically significant require attention. The most important attribute of the automated vessel identification and classification system is that it provides clinically relevant data [65; 135; 136]. Segmented blood vessels can be analyzed for branching patterns, bifurcation points, diameters and other physical attributes associated with disease such as venous beading or tortuosity. Furthermore a pool of morphological descriptors that identify several different attributes important in identifying blood vessels include edge detection and to detect the blood vessels with different diameters while leaving undesirable artifacts such as noise out [137].

Branching patterns have been analyzed using mathematical techniques such as fractal and local fractal dimension. These techniques are able to quantify complex branching patterns including blood vessels [138–142]. Initial studies of the optic fundus that concentrated on the analysis of optic fundus blood vessel patterns used hand-drawn vessel patterns to obtain the fractal dimension. These studies demonstrated that blood vessels in the optic fundus are fractal and that vessel occlusion and neovascularization could be identified [143–149]. These authors demonstrated the fractal nature of the retinal blood vessel network and that the fractal dimension can be used to identify pathology.

1.3   The Contribution of This Book

Computer and camera technology have substantially improved over the last decade to provide effective, fast and afforable systems for fundus image analysis. Software development in the field has developed to the point that automated image detection of retinal pathology is coming of age. This chapter has introduced the field, outlined some of the successes, and brought attention to some of the remaining problems. In the following chapters the reader shall find descriptions of retinal image analysis as practiced by experts in the field.

Chapter 2 is a brief introduction to diabetes, diabetic retinopathy, and ophthalmic terminology, to give the reader new to the field the necessary medical and ophthalmic knowledge. The authors of Chapters 3 and 4 write primarily as users of automated image analysis software, and outline some of the successes and opportunities for automated image detection of retinal pathology and the reasons why automated systems have failed to be embraced in clinical practice.

The engineering description of automated image detection of retinal pathology begins in Chapter 5 with the automated detection of exudates and the optic disc, and continued in Chapter 6 with the automated detection of microaneurysms. Detection of blood vessels and quantification of various vessel parameters is an important field and it is in Chapter 7 that the clinical impetus is outlined. Segmentation of blood vessels is the subject of Chapter 8 and the quantification of vessel parameters is the focus of Chapters 9 and 10. In this day of the Internet and the potential for easy and fast transmission of digital data, it seems appropriate that in Chapter 11 the potential for teleophthalmology is explored.

References

[1] Thylefors, B., A global initiative for the elimination of avoidable blindness, *American Journal of Ophthalmology*, 125(1), 90, 1998.

[2] Foster, A. and Resnikoff, S., The impact of Vision 2020 on global blindness, *Eye*, 19(10), 1133, 2005.

[3] Joshy, G. and Simmons, D., Epidemiology of diabetes in New Zealand: revisit to a changing landscape, *The New Zealand Medical Journal*, 119(1235), 2006.

[4] Colagiuri, S., Colagiuri, R., and Ward, J., *National Diabetes Strategy and Implementation Plan.*, Diabetes Australia, Paragon Printers, Canberra, 1998.

[5] King, H., Aubert, R.E., and Herman, W.H., Global burden of diabetes, 1995–2025: prevalence, numerical estimates and projections, *Diabetes Care*, 21, 1414, 1998.

[6] Wild, S., Roglic, G., Green, A., et al., Globel prevalence of diabetes: estimates for the year 2000 and projections for 2030, *Diabetes Care*, 27(10), 2569, 2004.

[7] Centers for Disease Control and Prevention, National diabetes fact sheet: general information and national estimates on diabetes in the United States, Technical report, U.S. Department of Health and Human Services, Centers for Disease Control and Prevention, 2003.

[8] The Eye Diseases Prevalence Research Group, The prevalence of diabetic retinopathy among adults in the United States, *Archives of Ophthalmology*, 122(4), 552, 2004.

[9] Mathers, C. and Penm, R., Health system costs of cardiovascular diseases and diabetes in Australia 1993–94, Technical Report HWE 11, Australian Institute of Health and Welfare, 1999.

[10] Engerman, R., Pathogenesis of diabetic retinopathy, *Diabetes*, 38, 1203, 1989.

[11] Kristinsson, J.K., Gottfredsdottir, M.S., and Stefansson, E., Retinal vessel dilatation and elongation precedes diabetic macular oedema, *Br J Ophthalmol*, 81(4), 274, 1997.

[12] Wong, T.Y., Klein, R., Sharrett, A.R., et al., Retinal arteriolar narrowing and risk of diabetes mellitus in middle-aged persons, *Journal of the American Medical Association*, 287(19), 2528, 2002.

[13] Cockburn, D., Diabetic retinopathy: classification, description and optometric management, *Clinical and Experimental Optometry*, 82(2-3), 59, 1999.

[14] Ciulla, T., Amador, A., and Zinman, B., Diabetic retinopathy and diabetic macular edema: pathophysiology, screening, and novel therapies, *Diabetes Care*, 26(9), 2653, 2003.

[15] Younis, N., Broadbent, D., Harding, S., et al., Prevalence of diabetic eye disease in patients entering a systematic primary care-based eye screening programme, *Diabetic Medicine*, 19, 1014, 2002.

[16] Williams, R., Airey, M., Baxter, H., et al., Epidemiology of diabetic retinopathy and macular oedema: a systematic review, *Eye*, 18, 963, 2004.

[17] Klein, R., Klein, B.E., Moss, S.E., et al., The Wisconsin Epidemiologic Study of Diabetic Retinopathy. III. Prevalence and risk of diabetic retinopathy when age at diagnosis is 30 or more years, *Arch Ophthalmol*, 102(4), 527, 1984.

[18] Harding, S.P., Broadbent, D.M., Neoh, C., et al., Sensitivity and specificity

of photography and direct ophthalmology in screening for sight threatening eye disease: the Liverpool Diabetic Eye Study, *British Medical Journal*, 311, 1131, 1995.

[19] Betz-Brown, J., Pedula, K., and Summers, K., Diabetic retinopathy — contemporary prevalence in a well-controlled population, *Diabetes Care*, 26(9), 2637, 2003.

[20] Icks, A., Trautner, C., Haastert, B., et al., Blindness due to diabetes: population-based age- and sex-specific incidence rates, *Diabetic Medicine*, 14, 571, 1997.

[21] Cunha-Vaz, J., Lowering the risk of visual impairment and blindness, *Diabetic Medicine*, 15(S4), S47, 1998.

[22] Taylor, H.R., Vu, H.T.V., McCarty, C.A., et al., The need for routine eye examinations, *Investigative Ophthalmology and Visual Science*, 45(8), 2539, 2004.

[23] Kohner, E. and Sleightholm, M., Does microaneurysm count reflect the severity of early diabetic retinopathy? *Ophthalmology*, 93, 586, 1986.

[24] Klein, R., Meuer, S.M., Moss, S.E., et al., Retinal microaneurysm counts and 10-year progression of diabetic retinopathy, *Archives of Ophthalmology*, 113(11), 1386, 1995.

[25] Mazze, R. and Simonson, G., Staged diabetes management: a systematic evidence-based approach to the prevention and treatment of diabetes and its co-morbidities, *Practical Diabetes International*, 18(7), S1, 2001.

[26] National Health and Medical Research Council, Management of diabetic retinopathy clinical practice guidelines, Technical report, Australian Government Publishing Service, 1997.

[27] Lee, S.J., McCarty, C.A., Taylor, H.R., et al., Costs of mobile screening for diabetic retinopathy: a practical framework for rural populations, *Australian Journal of Rural Health*, 9, 186, 2001.

[28] Facey, K., Cummins, E., Macpherson, K., et al., Organisation of services for diabetic retinopathy screening, Technical Report 1, Health Technology Board for Scotland, 2002.

[29] Lee, S., McCarty, C., Taylor, H.R., et al., Costs of mobile screening for diabetic retinopathy: a practical framework for rural populations, *Australian Journal of Rural Health*, 9, 186, 2001a.

[30] James, M., Turner, D., Broadbent, D., et al., Cost-effectiveness analysis of screening for sight threatening diabetic eye disease, *British Medical Journal*, 320, 1627, 2000.

[31] Leese, G., Tesfaye, S., Dengler-Harles, M., et al., Screening for diabetic eye disease by optometrists using slit lamps, *Journal of Royal College of Physi-*

cians London, 31, 65, 1997.

[32] Hutchinson, A., McIntosh, A., Peters, J., et al., Effectiveness of screening and montitoring tests for diabetic retinopathy — a systematic review, *Diabetic Medicine*, 17, 495, 2000.

[33] UK National Screening Committee, Essential elements in developing a diabetic retinopathy screening programme, Technical report, 2004.

[34] American Diabetic Association, Screening for type 2 diabetes: American Diabetes Association position statement, *Diabetes Care*, 26(Suppl 1), S21, 2003.

[35] Lee, V., Kingsley, R., and Lee, E., The diagnosis of diabetic retinopathy. Ophthalmology versus fundus photography, *Ophthalmology*, 100., 1504, 1993.

[36] Taylor, H.R. and Keeffe, J.E., World blindness: a 21st century perspective, *British Journal of Ophthalmology*, 85, 261, 2001.

[37] Bachmann, M.O. and Nelson, S., Impact of diabetic retinopathy screening on a British district population: case detection and blindess prevention in an evidence-based model, *Journal of Epidemiology and Community Health*, 52, 45, 1998.

[38] Sharp, P.F., Olsen, J., Strachan, F.M., et al., The value of digital imaging in diabetic retinopathy, Technical Report 7(30), Health Technology Assessment, 2003.

[39] Phiri, R., Keeffe, J.E., Harper, C.A., et al., Comparative study of the Polaroid and digital non-mydriatic cameras in the detection of referrable diabetic retinopathy in Australia, *Diabetic Medicine*, 23(8), 867, 2006.

[40] Bursell, S.E., Caverallerano, J., Caverallerano, A., et al., Joslin Vision Network Research Team: Stereo nonmydriatic digital-video color retinal imaging compared with early treatment diabetic retinopathy study seven standard field 35mm stereo color photos for determining level of diabetic retinopathy, *Ophthalmology*, 108, 572, 2001.

[41] Olson, J.A., Strachan, F.M., Hipwell, J.H., et al., A comparative evaluation of digital imaging, retinal photography and optometrist examination in screening for diabetic retinopathy, *Diabetic Medicine*, 20(7), 528, 2003.

[42] Harper, C.A., Livingston, P.M., Wood, C., et al., Screening for diabetic retinopathy using a non-mydriatic camera in rural Victoria, *Australian and New Zealand Journal of Ophthalmology*, 28, 135, 1998.

[43] Sussman, E., Tsiaras, W., and Soper, K., Diagnosis of diabetic eye disease, *JAMA*, 247, 3231, 1982.

[44] Howsam, G., The Albury-Wodonga syndrome: A tale of two cities, *Australian and New Zealand Journal of Opthalmololgy*, 23, 135, 1995.

[45] Lawrenson, R., Dunn, P., Worsley, D., et al., Discover diabetes: a community

based screening programme for diabetic eye disease, *The New Zealand Medical Journal*, 107, 172, 1994.

[46] Reda, E., Dunn, P., Straker, C., et al., Screening for diabetic retinopathy using the mobile retinal camera: the Waikato experience, *The New Zealand Medical Journal*, 116(1180), 562, 2003.

[47] Yogesan, K., Constable, I.J., Barry, C.J., et al., Telemedicine screening of diabetic retinopathy using a hand-held fundus camera, *Telemedicine Journal*, 6(2), 219, 2000.

[48] Patton, N., Aslam, T.M., MacGillivray, T., et al., Retinal image analysis: concepts, applications and potential, *Progress in Retinal and Eye Research*, 25, 99, 2006.

[49] Whited, J.D., Accuracy and reliability of teleophthalmology for diagnosing diabetic retinopathy and macular edema: A review of the literature, *Diabetes Technology and Therapeutics*, 8(1), 102, 2006.

[50] Constable, I.J., Yogesan, K., Eikelboom, R.H., et al., Fred Hollows lecture: Digital screening for eye disease, *Clinical and Experimental Ophthalmology*, 28, 129, 2000.

[51] Lin, D., Blumenkranz, M., Brothers, R., et al., The sensitivity and specificity of single-field nonmydriatic monochromatic digital fundus photography with remote images interpretation for diabetic retinopathy screening: a comparison with ophthalmology and standardized mydriatic color photography, *American Journal of Ophthalmology*, 134, 204, 2002.

[52] Davis, R., Fowler, S., Bellis, K., et al., Telemedicine improves eye examination rates in individuals with diabetes, *Diabetes Care*, 26(8), 2476, 2003.

[53] Lee, S., Sicari, C., Harper, C., et al., Program for the early detection of diabetic retinopathy: a two-year follow-up, *Clinical and Experimental Ophthalmology*, 29, 12, 2001b.

[54] Madden, A.C., Simmons, D., McCarty, C.A., et al., Eye health in rural Australia, *Clinical and Experimental Ophthalmology*, 30(5), 316, 2002.

[55] Wong, T.Y., Shankar, A., Klein, R., et al., Retinal arteriolar narrowing, hypertension and subsequent risk of diabetes mellitus, *Archives of Internal Medicine*, 165(9), 1060, 2005.

[56] Li, H., Hsu, W., Lee, M.L., et al., Automated grading of retinal vessel caliber, *IEEE Transactions on Biomedical Engineering*, 52(7), 1352, 2005.

[57] Witt, N., Wong, T.Y., Hughes, A.D., et al., Abnormalities of retinal microvascular structure and risk of mortality from ischemic heart disease and stroke, *Hypertension*, 47, 345, 2000.

[58] Forracchia, M., Grisan, E., and Ruggeri, A., Extraction and quantitative

description of vessel features in hypertensive retinopathy fundus images, in *CAFIA2001*, 2001, 6.

[59] Sherry, L.M., Wang, J.J., Rochtchina, E., et al., Reliability of computer-assisted retinal vessel measurement in a population, *Clinical & Experimental Ophthalmology*, 30, 179, 2002.

[60] Wang, J.J., Mitchell, P., Sherry, L.M., et al., Generalized retinal arteriolar narrowing predicts 5-year cardiovascular and cerebro-vascular mortality: findings from the Blue Mountains Eye Study, *Investigative Ophthalmology and Visual Science*, 43, 2002.

[61] Klein, R., Klein, B.E., Moss, S.E., et al., The relation of retinal vessel caliber to the incidence and progression of diabetic retinopathy: XIX: The Wisconsin Epidemiologic Study of Diabetic Retinopathy, *Archives of Ophthalmology*, 122(1), 76, 2004.

[62] Soares, J.V.B., Leandro, J.J.G., Cesar, Jr, R.M., et al., Retinal vessel segmentation using the 2-D Gabor wavelet and supervised classification, *IEEE Transactions on Medical Imaging*, 25(9), 1214, 2006.

[63] Lee, S.C., Lee, E.T., Wang, Y., et al., Computer classification of nonproliferative diabetic retinopathy, *Archives of Ophthalmology*, 123, 759, 2005.

[64] Ege, B.M., Hejlesen, O.K., Larsen, O.V., et al., Screening for diabetic retinopathy using computer based image analysis and statistical classification, *Computer Methods and Programs in Biomedicine*, 62(3), 165, 2000.

[65] Osareh, A., Mirmehdi, M., Thomas, B., et al., Classification and localisation of diabetic-related eye disease, in *7th European Conference on Computer Vision (ECCV2002)*, 2002, vol. 2353 of *Lecture Notes in Computer Science*, 502–516.

[66] Goldbaum, M.H., Sample, P.A., Chan, K., et al., Comparing machine learning classifiers for diagnosing glaucoma from standard automated perimetry, *Investigative Ophthalmology and Visual Science*, 43(1), 162, 2002.

[67] Frame, A.J., Undrill, P.E., Cree, M.J., et al., A comparison of computer based classification methods applied to the detection of microaneurysms in ophthalmic fluorescein angiograms, *Computers in Biology and Medicine*, 28, 225, 1998.

[68] Niemeijer, M., van Ginneken, B., Staal, J., et al., Automatic detection of red lesions in digital color fundus photographs, *IEEE Transactions on Medical Imaging*, 24(5), 584, 2005.

[69] Teng, T., Lefley, M., and Claremont, D., Progress towards automated diabetic ocular screening: a review of image analysis and intelligent systems for diabetic retinopathy, *Medical and Biological Engineering and Computing*, 40, 2, 2002.

[70] Baudoin, C.E., Lay, B.J., and Klein, J.C., Automatic detection of microaneurysms in diabetic fluorescein angiography, *Revue d Epidemiologie et de Sante Publique*, 32(3-4), 254, 1984.

[71] Spencer, T., Olson, J., McHardy, K., et al., Image-processing strategy for the segmentation and quantification of microaneurysms in fluorescein angiograms of the ocular fundus, *Computers and Biomedical Research*, 29, 284, 1996.

[72] Cree, M.J., Olson, J.A., McHardy, K.C., et al., A fully automated comparative microaneurysm digital detection system, *Eye*, 11, 622, 1997.

[73] Kohner, E.M. and Dollery, C.T., The rate of formation and disapearance of microaneurysms in diabetic retinopathy, *European Journal of Clinical Investigation*, 1(3), 167, 1970.

[74] Hellstedt, T. and Immonen, I., Disappearance and formation rates of microaneurysms in early diabetic retinopathy, *British Journal of Ophthalmology*, 80(2), 135, 1996.

[75] Goatman, K.A., Cree, M.J., Olson, J.A., et al., Automated measurement of microaneurysm turnover, *Investigative Ophthalmology and Visual Science*, 44, 5335, 2003.

[76] Hipwell, J., Strachan, F., Olson, J., et al., Automated detection of microaneurysms in digital red-free photographs: a diabetic retinopathy screening tool, *Diabetic Medicine*, 17, 588, 2000.

[77] British Diabetic Association, Retinal photography screening for diabetic eye disease, 1994.

[78] Fleming, A.D., Philip, S., Goatman, K.A., et al., Automated assessment of diabetic retinal image quality based on clarity and field definition, *Investigative Ophthalmology and Visual Science*, 47(1120-1125), 2006.

[79] Lee, S.C., Wang, Y., and Lee, E.T., Computer algorithm for automated detection and quantification of microaneurysms and hemorrhages (HMAs) in color retinal images, in *Medical Imaging 1999: Image Perception and Performance*, 1999, vol. 3663 of *Proceedings of the SPIE*, 61–71.

[80] Gardner, G., Keating, D., Williamson, T., et al., Automatic detection of diabetic retinopathy using an artificial neural network: a screening tool, *British Journal of Ophthalmology*, 80, 940, 1996.

[81] Luo, G., Chutatape, O., Li, H., et al., Abnormality detection in automated mass screening system of diabetic retinopathy, in *14th IEEE Symposium on Computer-Based Medical Systems 2001*, 2001, 332.

[82] Sinthanayothin, C., Boyce, J.F., Williamson, T.H., et al., Automated detection of diabetic retinopathy on digital fundus images, *Diabet Med*, 19(2), 105, 2002.

[83] Phillips, R., Forrester, J., and Sharp, P., Automated detection and quantification of retinal exudates, *Graefes Arch Clin Exp Ophthalmol*, 231(2), 90, 1993.

[84] Hunter, A., Lowell, J., Owen, J., et al., Quantification of diabetic retinopathy using neural networks and sensitivity analysis, Technical Report SCET9901, University of Sunderland, 2000.

[85] Osareh, A., Mirmehdi, M., Thomas, B., et al., Automatic recognition of exudative maculopathy using fuzzy C-means clustering and neural networks, in *Proceedings of the Medical Image Understanding and Analysis Conference*, 2001, 49–52.

[86] Osareh, A., Mirmehdi, M., Thomas, B., et al., Automated identification of diabetic retinal exudates in digital colour images, *British Journal of Ophthalmology*, 87, 1220, 2003.

[87] Walter, T., Klein, J.C., Massin, P., et al., A contribution of image processing to the diagnosis of diabetic retinopathy — detection of exudates in color fundus images of the human retina, *IEEE Transactions on Medical Imaging*, 21(10), 1236, 2002.

[88] Fleming, A.D., Philip, S., Goatman, K.A., et al., Automated detection of exudates for diabetic retinopathy screening, *Physics in Medicine and Biology*, 52, 7385, 2007.

[89] Hsu, W., Pallawala, P.M.D.S., Lee, M.L., et al., The role of domain knowledge in the detection of retinal hard exudates, in *2001 IEEE Computer Society Conference on Computer Vision and Pattern Recognition (CVPR'01)*, 2001, vol. 2, 246–251.

[90] Xiaohui, Z. and Chutatape, O., Detection and classification of bright lesions in color fundus images, in *International Conference on Image Processing (ICIP'04)*, 2004, vol. 1, 139–142.

[91] Lee, S.C., Lee, E.T., Kingsley, R.M., et al., Comparison of diagnosis of early retinal lesions of diabetic retinopathy between a computer system and human experts, *Archives of Ophthalmology*, 119(4), 509, 2001.

[92] Barthes, A., Conrath, J., Rasigni, M., et al., Mathematical morphology in computerized analysis of angiograms in age-related macular degeneration, *Medical Physics*, 28(12), 2410, 2001.

[93] ben Sbeh, Z., Cohen, L.D., Mimoun, G., et al., A new approach of geodesic reconstruction for drusen segmentation in eye fundus images, *IEEE Transactions on Medical Imaging*, 20(12), 1321, 2001.

[94] Brandon, L. and Hoover, A., Drusen detection in a retinal image using multilevel analysis, in *Medical Image Computing and Computer-Assisted Intervention (MICCAI 2003)*, 2003, vol. 2878 of *Lecture Notes in Computer Science*, 618–625.

[95] Shin, D.S., Javornik, N.B., and Berger, J.W., Computer-assisted, interactive fundus image processing for macular drusen quantitation, *Ophthalmology*, 106(6), 1119, 1999.

[96] Sivagnanavel, V., Smith, R.T., Lau, G.B., et al., An interinstitutional comparative study and validation of computer aided drusen detection, *British Journal of Ophthalmology*, 89, 554, 2005.

[97] Smith, R.T., Chan, J.K., Nagasaki, T., et al., Automated detection of macular drusen using geometric background leveling and threshold selection, *Archives of Ophthalmology*, 123(2), 200, 2005.

[98] Cree, M.J., Olson, J.A., McHardy, K.C., et al., Automated microaneurysm detection, in *International Conference on Image Processing*, Lausanne, Switzerland, 1996, vol. 3, 699–702.

[99] Sinthanayothin, C., Boyce, J., Cook, H., et al., Automated localisation of the optic disc, fovea and retinal blood vessels from digital colour fundus images, *British Journal of Ophthalmology*, 83(8), 902, 1999.

[100] Li, H.Q. and Chutatape, O., Automated feature extraction in color retinal images by a model based approach, *IEEE Transactions on Biomedical Engineering*, 51(2), 246, 2004.

[101] Pinz, A., Bernogger, S., Datlinger, P., et al., Mapping the human retina, *IEEE Transactions on Medical Imaging*, 17(4), 606, 1998.

[102] Li, H.Q. and Chutatape, O., Automatic detection and boundary estimation of the optic disk in retinal images using a model-based approach, *Journal of Electronic Imaging*, 12(1), 97, 2003.

[103] Lowell, J., Hunter, A., Steel, D., et al., Optic nerve head segmentation, *IEEE Transactions on Medical Imaging*, 23(2), 256, 2004.

[104] Abdel-Ghafara, R.A., Morrisa, Ritchingsb, T.T., et al., Detection and characterisation of the optic disk in glaucoma and diabetic retinopathy, 2005.

[105] Chanwimaluang, T. and Fan, G., An efficient algorithm for extraction of anatomical structures in retinal images, in *2003 International Conference on Image Processing*, 2003, vol. 1, 1093–1096.

[106] Osareh, A., Mirmehdi, M., Thomas, B., et al., Colour morphology and snakes for optic disc localisation, in *Proceedings of the Medical Image Underestanding and Analysis Conference (MIUA 2002)*, Portsmouth, UK, 2002, 21–24.

[107] Hoover, A. and Goldbaum, M., Locating the optic nerve in a retinal image using the fuzzy convergence of the blood vessels, *IEEE Transactions on Medical Imaging*, 22(8), 951, 2003.

[108] Foracchia, M., Grisan, E., and Ruggeri, A., Detection of optic disc in retinal images by means of a geometrical model of vessel structure, *IEEE Transac-*

tions on Medical Imaging, 23(10), 1189, 2004.

[109] Guan, K., Hudson, C., Wong, T.Y., et al., Retinal hemodynamics in early diabetic macular edema, *Diabetes*, 55(3), 813, 2006.

[110] Wong, T., Shankar, A., Klein, R., et al., Prospective cohort study of retinal vessel diameters and risk of hypertension, *British Medical Journal*, 329, 79, 2004.

[111] Wong, T.Y., Klein, R., Klein, B.E., et al., Retinal microvascular abnormalities and their relationship with hypertension, cardiovascular disease, and mortality, *Survey of Ophthalmology*, 46(1), 59, 2001.

[112] Lin, T.S. and Zheng, Y.B., Experimental study of automated diameter measurement of retinal blood vessel, *Journal of Information and Computational Science*, 2(1), 81, 2005.

[113] Leandro, J.J.G., Cesar-Jr, R.M., and Jelinek, H.F., Blood vessels segmentation in retina: preliminary assessment of the mathematical morphology and of the wavelet transform techniques, in *XIV Brazilian Symposium on Computer Graphics and Image Processing (SIBGRAPI-01)*, Florianopólis, Brazil, 2001, 84–90.

[114] Cesar, Jr, R.M. and Jelinek, H., Segmentation of retinal fundus vasculature in nonmydriatic camera images using wavelets, in *Angiography and plaque imaging*, J. Suri and S. Laxminarayan, eds., CRC Press, London, 193–224, 2003.

[115] Leandro, J.J.G., Soares, J.V.B., Cesar, J., R., et al., Blood vessel segmentation of non-mydriatic images using wavelets and statistical classifiers, in *16th Brazilian Symposium on Computer Graphics and Image Processing (SIBGRAPI03)*, Sao Carlos, Brazil, 2003, 262–269.

[116] Chaudhuri, S., Chatterjee, S., Katz, N., et al., Detection of blood vessels in retinal images using two-dimensional matched filters, *IEEE Transactions on Medical Imaging*, 8(3), 263, 1989.

[117] Hoover, A., Kouznetsova, V., and Goldbaum, M., Locating blood vessels in retinal images by piecewise threshold probing of a matched filter response, *IEEE Transactions on Medical Imaging*, 19(3), 203, 2000.

[118] Zana, F. and Klein, J.C., A multimodal registration algorithm of eye fundus images using vessels detection and hough transform, *IEEE Transactions on Medical Imaging*, 18(5), 419, 1999.

[119] Zana, F. and Klein, J.C., Segmentation of vessel-like patterns using mathematical morphology and curvature evaluation, *IEEE Transactions on Image Processing*, 10(7), 1010, 2001.

[120] Martínez-Pérez, M.E., Hughes, A.D., Stanton, A.V., et al., Segmentation of retinal blood vessels based on the second directional derivative and region

growing, in *IEEE International Conference in Image Processing (ICIP'99)*, Kobe, Japan, 1999, 173–176.

[121] Jiang, X. and Mojon, D., Adaptive local thresholding by verification-based multithreshold probing with application to vessel detection in retinal images, *IEEE Transactions on Pattern Analysis and Machine Intelligence*, 25(1), 131, 2003.

[122] Niemeijer, M., Staal, J., van Ginneken, B., et al., Comparative study of retinal vessel segmentation methods on a new publicly available database, *Proceedings of the SPIE*, 5370, 648, 2004.

[123] Staal, J., Abramoff, M., Niemeijer, M., et al., Ridge-based vessel segmentation in color images of the retina, *IEEE Transactions on Medical Imaging*, 23(4), 501, 2004.

[124] Hongqing, Z., Huazhong, S., and Limin, L., Blood vessels segmentation in retina via wavelet transforms using steerable filters, in *Proceedings of the 17th IEEE Symposium on Computer-Based Medical Systems (CBMS'04)*, 2004, 316–321.

[125] Mendonca, A. and Campilho, A., Segmentation of retinal blood vessels by combining the detection of centerlines and morphological reconstruction, *IEEE Transactions on Medical Imaging*, 25(9), 1200, 2006.

[126] Fritzsche, K., Computer vision algorithms for retinal vessel width change detection and quantification, 2005.

[127] Kochner, B., Schuhmann, D., Michaelis, M., et al., Course tracking and contour extraction of retinal vessels from color fundus photographs: most efficient use of steerable filters for model-based image analysis, *Proceedings of the SPIE*, 3338, 755, 1998.

[128] Tamura, S., Okamoto, Y., and Yanashima, K., Zero-crossing interval correction in tracing eye-fundus blood vessels, *Pattern Recognition*, 21, 227, 1988.

[129] Tolias, Y.A. and Panas, S.M., A fuzzy vessel tracking algorithm for retinal images based on fuzzy clustering, *IEEE Transactions on Medical Imaging*, 17(2), 263, 1998.

[130] Gao, X., Bharath, A., Stanton, A., et al., A method of vessel tracking for vessel diameter measurement on retinal images, in *Proceedings of the International Conference on Image Processing (ICIP'01)*, 2001, vol. 2, 881–884.

[131] Kirbas, C. and Quek, F., A review of vessel extraction techniques and algorithms, *ACM Computing Surveys*, 36(2), 81, 2004.

[132] Cree, M.J., Cornforth, D.J., and Jelinek, H.F., Vessel segmentation and tracking using a two-dimensional model, in *Image and Vision Computing New Zealand*, Dunedin, New Zealand, 2005, 345–350.

[133] Cree, M.J., Leandro, J.J.G., Soares, J.V.B., et al., Comparison of various methods to delineate blood vessels in retinal images, in *Proceedings of the 16th National Congress of the Australian Institute of Physics*, Canbera, Australia, 2005.

[134] Kanski, J., *Clinical Ophthalmology: A systematic approach*, Butterworth-Heinemann, London, 1989.

[135] Martínez-Pérez, M.E., Hughes, A.D., Stanton, A.V., et al., Retinal vascular tree morphology: a semi-automatic quantification, *IEEE Transactions on Biomedical Engineering*, 49(8), 912, 2002.

[136] Gao, X., Bharath, A., Stanton, A., et al., Quantification and characterisation of arteries in retinal images, *Computer Methods and Programs in Biomedicine*, 63(2), 133, 2000.

[137] Antoine, J.P., Barache, D., Cesar, Jr., R.M., et al., Shape characterization with the wavelet transform, *Signal Processing*, 62(3), 265, 1997.

[138] Fernandez, E. and Jelinek, H., Use of fractal theory in neuroscience: methods, advantages, and potential problems, *Methods*, 24, 309, 2001.

[139] Landini, G., Murray, P.I., and Misson, G.P., Local connected fractal dimension and lacunarity analysis of 60 degree fluorescein angiograms, *Investigative Ophthalmology and Visual Science*, 36, 2749, 1995.

[140] Losa, G., Merlini, D., Nonnenmacher, T.F., et al., *Fractals in Biology and Medicine*, Birkhäuser, Basel, 2nd ed., 1997.

[141] Sernetz, M., Wubbeke, J., and Wiezek, P., Three-dimensional image analysis and fractal characterization of kidney arterial vessels, *Physica A*, 191, 13, 1992.

[142] Avakian, A., Kalina, R.E., Sage, H.E., et al., Fractal analysis of region-based vascular change in the normal and non-proliferativediabetic retina, *Current Eye Research*, 24(4), 274, 2002.

[143] Daxer, A., The fractal geometry of proliferative diabetic retinopathy: implications for the diagnosis and the process of retinal vasculogenesis, *Current Eye Research*, 12, 1103, 1993.

[144] Masters, B., Fractal analysis of the vascular tree in the human retina, *Annual Review of Biomedical Engineering*, 6, 427, 2004.

[145] Family, F., Masters, B.R., and Platt, D., Fractal pattern formation in human retinal vessels, *Physica D*, 38, 98, 1989.

[146] Landini, G., Applications of fractal geometry in pathology, in *Fractal geometry in biological systems*, P. Iannaccone and M. Khokha, eds., CRC Press, Amsterdam, 205–245, 1996.

[147] Luckie, A.P., Jelinek, H.F., Cree, M.J., et al., Identification and follow-up

of diabetic retinopathy in rural Australia: an automated screening model, in *AVRO*, Ft. Lauderdale, FL, 2004, 5245/B569.

[148] McQuellin, C., Jelinek, H., and Joss, G., Characterisation of fluorescein angiograms of retinal fundus using mathematical morphology: a pilot study., in *5th International Conference on Ophthalmic Photography*, Adelaide, 2002, 83.

[149] Stošić, T. and Stošić, B.D., Multifractal analysis of human retinal vessels, *IEEE Transactions on Medical Imaging*, 25(8), 1101, 2006.

2

Diabetic Retinopathy and Public Health

David Worsley and David Simmons

CONTENTS

2.1	Introduction	27
2.2	The Pandemic of Diabetes and Its Complications	28
2.3	Retinal Structure and Function	29
2.4	Definition and Description	35
2.5	Classification of Diabetic Retinopathy	40
2.6	Differential Diagnosis of Diabetic Retinopathy	40
2.7	Systemic Associations of Diabetic Retinopathy	42
2.8	Pathogenesis	43
2.9	Treatment	45
2.10	Screening	48
2.11	Conclusion	55
	References	55

2.1 Introduction

Diabetic retinopathy (DR) is the commonest complication of diabetes and is one of the leading causes of blindness [1]. Recent research has given a better understanding of the disease processes and is opening up new avenues for prevention and treatment. Very effective treatments are available and are optimally used when retinopathy is detected early, well before the patient is aware of symptoms. For this reason screening programs for early detection of retinopathy are an essential part of diabetes care and are in widespread use. Several screening modalities have been used, however, digital retinal photography is now considered the preferred screening tool. There is potential for automated image analysis to manage the large volume of images generated from screening the ever-increasing number of people with diabetes.

2.2 The Pandemic of Diabetes and Its Complications

Diabetes mellitus is considered one of the major diseases of the 21st century, indeed it has been said that "What AIDS was in the last 20 years of the 20th century, diabetes is going to be in the first 20 years of this century" [2; 3]. Much of this growth is due to the increasing prevalence of type 2 diabetes, where insulin secretion from the beta cells of the pancreas is inadequate for daily demands [4]. Such demand depends upon a complex balance between various hormones, existing energy stores (e.g. as adipose tissue), physical activity, and resistance to insulin action in muscle, liver, and adipose tissue. Contemporary life in both the developed and developing world increasingly involves reductions in physical activity and increases in energy dense food, with a resulting energy imbalance leading to greater obesity, insulin resistance, and type 2 diabetes. There is now good evidence that the progression from lesser degrees of glucose intolerance (i.e., impaired fasting glucose and impaired glucose tolerance) to type 2 diabetes can be prevented, or at least delayed, through lifestyle change providing that substantial support is provided [5–7]. The other major group of patients have type 1 diabetes, where there is destruction of the beta cells through either auto-immune or other mechanisms. Type 1 diabetes is also increasing in prevalence [8]. Other rarer forms of diabetes mellitus exist including Maturity Onset Diabetes of Youth (MODY) and other inherited forms [9].

The epidemic of type 2 diabetes is not only associated with an increasing number of people with diabetes within a given age group, the mean age at which it is diagnosed (and presumably commences) is becoming younger [10]. Type 2 diabetes in youth and children is becoming more prevalent with type 2 diabetes now becoming as common as type 1 diabetes in pediatric diabetes clinics [11]. Of great concern is the growth in the number of women of child-bearing age with type 2 diabetes who become pregnant with poor glucose control with both immediate and long term teratogenic effects—the latter increasing the risk of diabetes in the offspring [12; 13].

Diabetes is associated with a range of acute and chronic complications, although the prevalence of these varies by ethnicity, country, and over time [14; 15]. Both type 1 and type 2 diabetes are associated with long term macrovascular complications such as ischemic heart disease, stroke, peripheral vascular disease, and heart failure, and microvascular complications such as nephropathy, neuropathy, and retinopathy. Other complications also continue to occur due to glycation such as cataract and cheiroarthropathy or with combined causes such as the diabetic foot.

The biochemical criteria for diabetes were originally defined by their ability to predict microvascular disease, particularly diabetic retinopathy, over time [16]. Indeed, diabetic retinopathy was considered such a specific diabetes-related complication that studies predicted the length of time between development and diagnosis of diabetes by backward linear regression [17]. In the first AusDiab study, however, using linear regression between duration and prevalence of retinopathy, the clinical diagnosis of diabetes was thought to have been made at the same time as diabetes developed [18]. AusDiab also showed that retinopathy (defined as the presence of at least one definite retinal hemorrhage and/or microaneurysm) was present before overt diabetes was detected: 6.7% (5.3% to 8.4%) in impaired fasting glucose and impaired glucose tolerance with a comparable prevalence in newly diagnosed diabetes 6.2% (4.0% to 9.2%) and in those without diabetes 5.8% (3.7% to 8.5%) [18]. Similar prevalences were found in the Blue Mountains Eye Study [19].

Diabetic retinopathy is a leading cause of visual loss in working-age adults worldwide [20]. Severe vision loss is primarily from diabetic macular edema (DME) and proliferative diabetic retinopathy (PDR). As DME is more common than PDR in type 2 diabetes, and 90% of diabetics are type 2, DME is the leading cause of visual loss in diabetic retinopathy [21].

The prevalence of diabetic retinopathy has recently been thoroughly reviewed by Williams et al. [22]. Tables 2.1a, 2.1b, 2.2a, 2.2b, and 2.2c show the prevalence and incidence respectively of diabetic retinopathy by retinopathy grade and type of diabetes (type 1, type 2 diabetes, and mixtures of both) across countries, ethnic groups, and over time. There are clearly major differences in prevalence and incidence between studies depending on when and where they were undertaken and depending on the methods used for assessing retinopathy. There are likely to be ethnic differences in diabetic retinopathy as there are in nephropathy, but these remain inconsistent [22].

The most significant predictor of the prevalence of DR is duration of diabetes. In view of the importance of diabetic retinopathy and its contribution to blindness, as well as its utility in providing a window on the natural history of diabetes in individuals and populations, this chapter will focus on how diabetic retinopathy is defined and classified, the pathophysiology, the epidemiology, its prevention through optimizing metabolic control and associated health care issues, and screening for early changes.

2.3 Retinal Structure and Function

The retina is a transparent layer of vascularized neural tissue lining the inner layer of the back wall of the eye, between the retinal pigment epithelium on the outer and the vitreous on the inner side. The retina captures photons and converts these to photochemical and electrical energy, integrates the signals, and transmits the resultant signal to the visual cortex of the brain via the optic nerve, tracts, and radiations.

The retinal architecture is lamellar. Within this there are major cell types performing sensory, nutritional, regulatory, immunomodulatory, and structural functions. The retina is uniquely partitioned from the vascular system by the blood-retinal barrier and blood-aqueous barrier. The blood supply is dual; to the inner retina it is by the retinal circulation lying within the inner retina (the inner blood-retinal barrier) and to the outer retina it is by the choroidal circulation, a thick vascular layer lying outside of the retinal pigment epithelium (the outer blood-retinal barrier). The retinal pigment epithelium and the choroid are critical to retinal function.

Table 2.1a: Summary of the Range of Global Prevalence Estimates in Type 1, Type 2, and Mixed Cohort Diabetic Patients

Population	Grade Retinopathy	Type 1	Type 2	Mixed Cohort
United States	Any DR	0–84% (97.5% 415 years DM duration)	7–55%	37–61.1%
	PDR	3.8–25% (70% 430 years DM duration)	0.9–5%	
	CSMO	6%	2–4%	
United Kingdom	Any DR	33.6–36.7%	21–52%	16.5–41%
	PDR	1.1–2.0%	1.1–4%	1.1–8%
	CSMO	2.3–6.4%		6.4–6.8%
Australian	Any DR	42%	13–59.7%	29.1% (10% at 5 years and 80% 435 years DM duration)
	PDR			1.6–7%
	CSMO			4.3–10%
European	Any DR	16.6–76.5%	32.6–61.8%	26.2%
	PDR	7.3–17%	3.1–15.9%	1.8%
	CSMO		5.4%	
Scandinavian	Any DR	10.8–68.3% (90% 420 years DM duration)	18.8–65.9%	13.8–75.1%
	PDR	2.6–28.4%	4.2–14.5%	1.7–2.4%
	CSMO	16%	0.6–26.1%	8%
	Blindness	1.4%		
African American	Any DR	63.9%	26.5–31.4%	28.5%
	PDR	18.9%	0.9–1.5%	0.9%
	CSMO		8.6%	8.6%
	Blindness	3.1%		
Hispanic American	Any DR		33.4–45%	48%
	PDR		5.6–6.0%	
	CSMO			
American Indian	Any DR	19.7–20.9%	19–49.3%	1.7% (total pop.)
	PDR		5.1–7%	
	CSMO			

CSMO, clinically significant macular edema; DM, diabetes mellitus, DR, diabetic retinopathy; PDR, proliferative DR.
Adapted from Williams et al., *Eye*, 18, 963, 2004, Ref. [22]. With permission.

Table 2.1b: Summary of the Range of Global Prevalence Estimates in Type 1, Type 2, and Mixed Cohort Diabetic Patients (continued)

Population	Grade Retinopathy	Type 1	Type 2	Mixed Cohort
NZ European	Any DR		37.3%	
	PDR		2.7%	
	CSMO		8.7%	
NZ Maori	Any DR		40.7%	
	PDR		5.0%	
	CSMO		8.6%	
NZ Pacific	Any DR		43.8%	
	PDR		6.2%	
	CSMO		13.0%	
South Asia	Any DR	13.6%	6.7–34.1%	
	PDR	1.9%	0.7–10.3%	
	CSMO		6.4–13.3%	
	Blindness		4.1%	
UK South Asians	Any DR		11.6%	
	PDR			
	CSMO			
Japanese	Any DR		31.6–38%	
	PDR		2.8–10%	
	CSMO			
	Blindness		2.9%	
Chinese	Any DR		19–42%	28–45.2%
	PDR		0.4–12.7%	2.2%
	CSMO		2.7%	
	Blindness		0.3%	
African	Any DR	26–43%	30.5–43%	12.7–42.4%
	PDR			12.8%
	CSMO			
South American	Any DR		54–51.2%	
	PDR		3.4–5.5%	
	CSMO		4.7–8.2%	

CSMO, clinically significant macular edema; DM, diabetes mellitus, DR, diabetic retinopathy; PDR, proliferative DR.
Adapted from Williams et al., *Eye*, 18, 963, 2004, Ref. [22]. With permission.
NZ data from ref. [23]

Table 2.2a: Summary of the Range of Global Incidence Estimates in Type 1, Type 2, and Mixed Cohort Diabetic Patients

Population	Retinopathy grade	Type 1	Type 2	Mixed Cohort
United States	No DR to DR	33% > 2 yrs[1]	76.1/1000PY	17.4/1000PY
		89.3% > 10 yrs	66.9% > 10 yrs	
	DR to PDR	37% > 4 yrs	53–69% > 10 yrs	1.6/1000PY
	Two-step progression	76% > 10 yrs	10–24% > 10 yrs	
	CSMO	20.1% > 10 yrs	13.9% > 10 yrs	
	Blindness	1.8% > 10 yrs	4.8% > 10 yrs	
		2.4% > 14 yrs		
United Kingdom	No DR to DR		60/1000PY	
			22% > 6 yrs	
	No DR to PDR		7/1000PY	15.0/1000PY
	Non-PDR to PDR			42.1/1000PY
	Two-step progression		29% > 6 yrs	
	CSMO			
	Blindness			64/100 000 PY
Australian	No DR to DR			8% per year
	DR to PDR			7% per year
	CSMO			7% per year

[1]Diabetes duration. CSMO, clinically significant macular edema; DR, diabetic retinopathy; FPG fasting plasma glucose; PDR, proliferative DR; PY, person–years.
Adapted from Williams et al., *Eye*, 18, 963, 2004, Ref. [22]. With permission.

Table 2.2b: Summary of the Range of Global Incidence Estimates in Type 1, Type 2, and Mixed Cohort Diabetic Patients (continued)

Population	Retinopathy grade	Type 1	Type 2	Mixed cohort
European	No DR to DR	56% > 7 yrs[1] 47% > 5 yrs		
	DR to PDR	9% > 5 yrs		
	CSMO			
	Blindness	60.5/100 000/year for DM population		
Scandinavian	No DR to DR	85% > 15 yrs 38% > 4 yrs		
	No DR to PDR	13% > 10 yrs 16% > 20 yrs		
	CSMO	3.4% > 4 yrs		
	Blindness	0.23–1.1/10 000 yrs	0.6% > 5 yrs	
		0.5% > 5 yrs		
African American	No DR to DR			
	DR to PDR	2% > 4 yrs		
	Two-step progression	19% > 4 yrs		
	CSMO			
Hispanic American	No DR to DR		58.3/1000PY	
	DR to PDR			
	Two-step progression	24.1% > 4 yrs		
	CSMO			

[1]Diabetes duration. CSMO, clinically significant macular edema; DR, diabetic retinopathy; FPG fasting plasma glucose; PDR, proliferative DR; PY, person–years.
Adapted from Williams et al., *Eye*, 18, 963, 2004, Ref. [22]. With permission.

Table 2.2c: Summary of the Range of Global Incidence Estimates in Type 1, Type 2, and Mixed Cohort Diabetic Patients (continued)

Population	Retinopathy grade	Type 1	Type 2	Mixed Cohort
American Indian	No DR to DR		72.3% > 12.8 yrs	
	No DR to PDR		12/1000PY	
	CSMO			
Japanese	No DR to DR	70% at 29 years	39.8/1000PY, 48.1/1000PY	FPG <125 mg/dl: 3/1000PY
	DR to PDR		57.7/1000PY	FPG 126–139 mg/dl: 6.9/1000 PY
				FPG 4140 mg/dl: 13.9/1000 PY
Chinese	No DR to DR		19.2% > 4 yrs,	
			44.4/1000 PY	
	DR to PDR		5.8% > 4 yrs	
			37.5/1000 PY	
	CSMO			
South American	No DR to DR	6.6/100 PY		
	DR to PDR			
	CSMO			

CSMO, clinically significant macular edema; DR, diabetic retinopathy; FPG fasting plasma glucose; PDR, proliferative DR; PY, person–years. Adapted from Williams et al., *Eye*, 18, 963, 2004, Ref. [22]. With permission.

The macula is the central approximately 6 mm diameter area of retina. It is responsible for the fine central vision. The retina beyond the macula is termed the peripheral retina.

2.4 Definition and Description

Diabetic retinopathy is defined as a clinical diagnosis, characterized by the presence of one or more of several retinal lesions in a patient with diabetes mellitus (Table 2.3).

Table 2.3: Diabetic Retinopathy Lesions

Microaneurysms ($< 60 \, \mu m$)
Dot-hemorrhages
Hard exudates
Blotchy hemorrhages
Intraretinal microvascular abnormalities (IRMAs)
Venous beading
Cotton wool spots
New vessels on or within one disc diameter of the disc (NVD)
New vessels elsewhere (NVE)
Fibrous proliferation
Preretinal hemorrhage
Vitreous hemorrhage
Traction retinal detachment
Rhegmatogenous retinal detachment
Macular retinal thickening (edema)
Clinically significant macular edema (CSME)

Diabetic retinopathy is a progressive disease. It begins as mild nonproliferative retinopathy characterized by clinical features secondary to capillary changes with increased permeability. It may progress to moderate and severe nonproliferative retinopathy characterized by clinical features secondary to capillary closure as well as increased capillary permeability. Disease progression continues to proliferative retinopathy characterized by growth of new blood vessels, in and on the retina and even on the iris. Diabetic macular edema characterized by intraretinal accumulation of fluid and lipid within the macula can occur at any stage of the disease progression.

The pathology of diabetic retinopathy is a progressive microangiopathy of the retinal capillaries. Early changes are a loss of retinal capillary pericytes, thickening of the basement membrane, and the characteristic appearance of microaneurysms (saccular outpouchings of the capillary wall). There are changes in retinal blood flow. The inner blood-retinal barrier breaks down manifesting as increased retinal capillary permeability and intraretinal hemorrhage. Retinal capillaries and arterioles close (retinal nonperfusion). Later there is proliferation of blood vessels (termed "new vessels"), first within the retina and then on the retinal surface and onto the posterior surface of the vitreous. Accompanying vessel proliferation is fibrous tissue proliferation on the retinal surface and along the posterior vitreous surface. Contraction of fibrous tissue leads to complications such as vitreous hemorrhage and traction retinal detachment. In advanced disease new vessels proliferate on the iris.

Microaneurysms are almost always the first clinical sign of diabetic retinopathy, and are seen as intraretinal deep red spots 15 to 60 µm in diameter. There is a continuous turnover of microaneurysms; individual microaneurysms may persist for long time periods before eventually disappearing. Rupture of microaneurysms and increased capillary permeability give rise to intraretinal hemorrhage. Small pinpoint intraretinal (dot) hemorrhages are typical of diabetic retinopathy. They may be difficult to distinguish clinically from microaneurysms. Distinguishing between microaneurysms and dot-hemorrhages is of little clinical importance and therefore small intraretinal red lesions can be classified together as "hemorrhages and microaneurysms" (Figure 2.1).

Increased capillary permeability gives rise to intraretinal accumulation of fluid (edema) clinically termed "retinal thickening," and lipid, seen as yellow-white well-defined intraretinal accumulations termed "hard exudate" (Figure 2.2).

Patches of capillary closure develop and coalesce as areas of nonperfused retina. Capillary closure is not visible clinically without fluorescein angiography. Adjacent to areas of nonperfusion tortuous vessels termed "intraretinal microvascular abnormalities" (IRMA) may arise. It is not clear whether IRMA are new vessel proliferation or abnormal preexisting vessels. Other features associated with capillary closure include large intraretinal hemorrhages ("blotchy hemorrhages"), segmental vein dilatation ("venous beading") and a halt in axoplasmic flow in the nerve fiber layer seen as fluffy white patches in the innermost retina ("cotton wool spots") — see Figure 2.2(b)).

Nonperfused retina releases vascular endothelial growth factors (VEGFs). These are a family of peptides produced by a single gene. VEGF isoforms act specifically on vascular endothelial cells leading to new vessel proliferation and increased vessel permeability. VEGF expression, synthesis and release are enhanced by hypoxia from areas of nonperfusion [24]. VEGF diffuses throughout the eye and results in the growth of new vessels on the retinal surface and eventually on the iris. This is termed "proliferative diabetic retinopathy" (PDR) while all retinopathy prior to new vessel formation is "nonproliferative diabetic retinopathy" (NPDR). This is the basis of the classification of diabetic retinopathy discussed later. The presence of severe NPDR (three of the following four in at least two quadrants of the retina: IRMA, cotton wool spots, venous beading, extensive retinal hemorrhages, or microaneurysms) is a predictor of the development of PDR; about 50% will develop PDR within 15 months [25]. However, these features are not universally found with early new vessels. Cotton wool spots are transient; IRMA and retinal hemorrhages may not be seen with more extensive capillary closure.

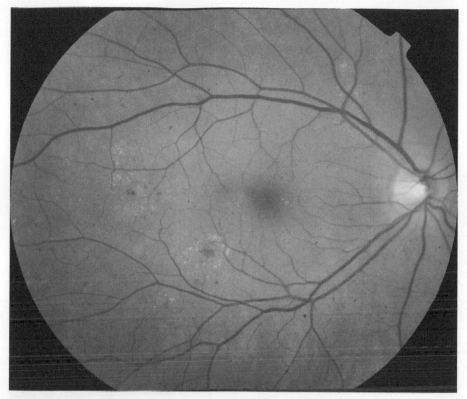

FIGURE 2.1
Moderate nonproliferative diabetic retinopathy with moderate diabetic macular edema. **(See color insert following page 174.)**

New vessels are usually first evident within 45 degrees of the optic disc, 15% on or within one disc diameter of the optic disc, termed "new vessels disc" (NVD); 40% only outside of this area termed "new vessels elsewhere" (NVE); and 45% had vessels in both areas [26].

Early NVD are loops or networks of fine vessels on the optic disc. As they grow the vessel complex extends outside the optic disc margin and the vessel caliber increases. NVE begin as small loops or networks usually near a retinal vein. As they grow they form networks that distinctively pass across the underlying retinal veins and arterioles. The new vessels grow into the scaffold of the posterior vitreous surface. New vessels are fragile and highly permeable. Vitreous traction on these fragile new vessels may lead to preretinal and vitreous hemorrhage (Figure 2.3).

With time fibroglial tissue develops adjacent to the new vessels and within the new vessel complexes. The combination of fibrous and vascular tissue is termed fibrovascular tissue. As the fibrovascular tissue grows, the proportion of the fibrous component increases. Eventually new vessels may regress. Fibrovascular tissue is

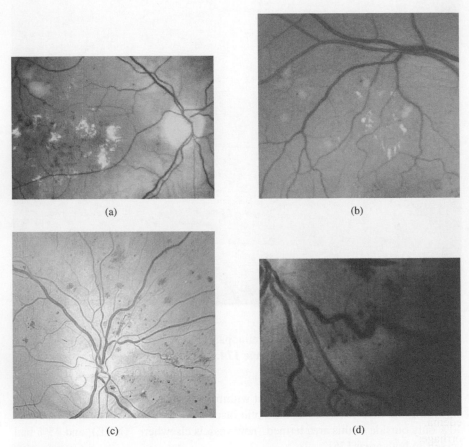

(a)

(b)

(c)

(d)

FIGURE 2.2

Nonproliferative diabetic retinopathy (NPDR). (a) Moderate NPDR and severe diabetic macular edema; hard exudates involve the center of the macula. (b) Moderate NPDR; microaneurysms/dot hemorrhages, hard exudate (ring) and cotton wool spots. (c) Severe NPDR; > 20 intraretinal hemorrhages in four quadrants (three shown here) and IRMA (possibly NVE). Biomicroscopy showed the latter lesion to be intraretinal, hence it is IRMA. (d) Venous beading. **(See color insert.)**

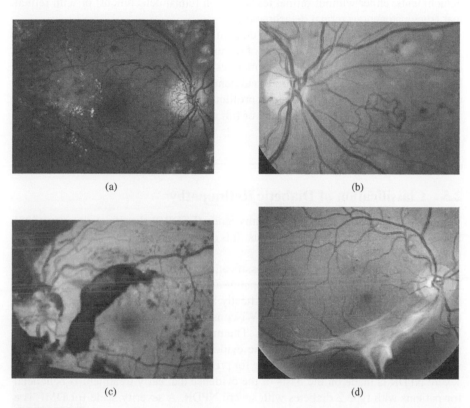

(a)   (b)

(c)   (d)

FIGURE 2.3
Proliferative diabetic retinopathy (PDR). (a) PDR with moderate diabetic macular edema. There are new vessels disc, new vessels elsewhere, IRMA, blotchy hemorrhages, microaneurysms/dot-hemorrhages, and hard exudates. Hard exudate approach the center of the macula. Pan retinal photocoagulation scars are seen in the top left and top and bottom far right. (b) New vessels elsewhere. (c) PDR with preretinal hemorrhage. Hemorrhage is contained within the space between the retina and the posterior vitreous face. The hemorrhage obscures the retinal new vessels. (d) Fibrous proliferation with traction macular detachment. PDR has regressed. Regressed fibro-vascular tissue along the inferior temporal vascular arcade has contracted causing traction macular detachment. Traction lines can be seen extending into the central macula. **(See color insert.)**

adherent to both the retina and the posterior vitreous surface. In many eyes the fibrovascular tissue contracts, and via these adhesions exerts traction on the retina. Traction may cause retinal edema, striation, and heterotropia (dragging), and retinal detachments; either without retinal tear (traction retinal detachment) or with retinal tear (rhegmatogenous retinal detachment).

Diabetic macular edema (DME) is defined as intraretinal accumulation of fluid within two disc diameters of the center of the macula. DME may develop at any stage of diabetic retinopathy. Macular abnormalities found in diabetic retinopathy include DME, capillary nonperfusion, intraretinal hemorrhage, preretinal hemorrhage, macular surface traction from fibrovascular proliferation, preretinal membrane (avascular fibrous tissue proliferation) and partial or full thickness macular hole.

2.5   Classification of Diabetic Retinopathy

The Early Treatment Diabetic Retinopathy Study (ETDRS) classification system [25] is the gold standard used in clinical trials. It is complex and not easy to use in clinical practice.

Proposed to replace the ETDRS classification for use in clinical practice are the International Clinical Diabetic Retinopathy and Diabetic Macular Edema Disease Severity Scales [27]. These are scientifically based and practical classification systems derived from the ETDRS and the Wisconsin Epidemiological Study of Diabetic Retinopathy study (WESDR) [28; 29]. The major modifications to previous classification systems are based on scientific evidence. IRMA and venous beading are included as they are the most predictive for progression to PDR. A separate stage for severe NPDR is made on the basis of the evidence that early treatment is beneficial for patients with type 2 diabetes with severe NPDR. A severity scale for DME is a new and important addition. Included are the factors that determine if macular edema is sight threatening; the location and area of retinal thickening and hard exudates.

2.6   Differential Diagnosis of Diabetic Retinopathy

A number of retinal vascular diseases share many of the clinical signs seen in diabetic retinopathy; these include central retinal vein occlusion, branch retinal vein occlusion, hypertensive retinopathy, ocular ischemic syndrome (hypoperfusion retinopathy), the retinopathies of blood dyscrasias such as anemia and leukemia, parafoveal telangiectasis and other retinal telangiectases, sickle cell retinopathy, and radiation retinopathy.

One of the more common of these diseases such as branch retinal vein occlusion or central retinal vein occlusion may well be seen concurrently with diabetic retinopathy and may be difficult to differentiate. If suspected from the clinical features, ocular

Table 2.4: International Clinical Diabetic Retinopathy Disease Severity Scale

Disease Severity Level	Findings
No apparent retinopathy	No abnormalities
Mild nonproliferative diabetic retinopathy	Microaneurysms only
Moderate nonproliferative diabetic retinopathy	More than just microaneurysms but less than severe nonproliferative diabetic retinopathy
Severe nonproliferative diabetic retinopathy	Any of the following: • > 20 intraretinal hemorrhages in each of four quadrants • Venous beading in two or more quadrants • Intraretinal microvascular abnormalities in one or more quadrants and no signs of proliferative retinopathy
Proliferative diabetic retinopathy	One or both of the following: • Neovascularization • Vitreous/preretinal hemorrhage

Table 2.5: International Clinical Diabetic Macular Edema Disease Severity Scale

Disease Severity Level	Findings
Diabetic macular edema apparently absent	No apparent retinal thickening or hard exudates in posterior pole
Diabetic macular edema apparently present	Some apparent retinal thickening or hard exudates in posterior pole
If diabetic macular edema present then:	
Mild diabetic macular edema	Some retinal thickening or hard exudate in the posterior retina but distant from the center of the macula
Moderate diabetic macular edema	Retinal thickening or hard exudate near but not involving the center of the macula
Severe diabetic macular edema	Retinal thickening or hard exudate in the center of the macula

investigations such as fluorescein angiography or optical coherence tomography and systemic investigations may be needed to distinguish from diabetic retinopathy.

2.7 Systemic Associations of Diabetic Retinopathy

Coexistent systemic factors can have a significant bearing on the development and progression of diabetic retinopathy.

2.7.1 Duration of diabetes

The most significant predictor of the development and progression of diabetic retinopathy is duration of diabetes. For type 1 diabetes, diabetic retinopathy is rare before 5 years duration, 8% for 3 years, 25% for 5 years, 60% for 10 years and 80% for 15 years. PDR has 0% prevalence at 3 years and 25% at 15 years [30]. In type 2 diabetes prevalence is 23% 11 to 13 years after diagnosis and 60% after 16 years or more [31].

2.7.2 Type of diabetes

Some data suggest that diabetes type is important in some aspects of treatment of diabetic retinopathy. Type 2 diabetes with severe nonproliferative retinopathy may benefit from pan-retinal photocoagulation according to reanalysis of data from the ETDRS [20]. The Diabetic Retinopathy Study found a similar trend.

The Diabetic Vitrectomy Study found early vitrectomy for vitreous hemorrhage beneficial for type 1 diabetes but not for type 2 [32]. However this study is some 20 years old and more modern vitrectomy techniques put this conclusion in question.

2.7.3 Blood glucose control

The Diabetes Control and Complications Trial and the United Kingdom Prospective Diabetes Study demonstrate the benefit of intensive glycemic control on delaying the development and slowing progression of diabetic retinopathy in both type 1 and type 2 diabetes [33–35].

2.7.4 Blood pressure

High blood pressure can produce a retinopathy characterized by microaneurysms, intraretinal hemorrhages, cotton wool spots, hard exudates, and optic nerve swelling, which is related to the level of systolic blood pressure. Coexistent hypertension is seen in 25% of type 1 diabetics after 10 years [36] and 38–68% of type 2 diabetics [37]. Studies show hypertension to be a risk factor for development and progression of diabetic retinopathy [20; 36; 38].

2.7.5 Serum lipids

The relationship between serum lipids and diabetic retinopathy is unclear. The ETDRS found an association with faster development of hard exudate [20]. Hard exudate is associated with an increased risk of moderate visual loss [20]. The WESDR found no association between diabetic retinopathy and serum lipids [20].

2.7.6 Renal disease

Renal disease secondary to diabetes predicts diabetic retinopathy [28; 39] and conversely diabetic retinopathy predicts renal disease [40; 41]. The nature of the interrelationship is not defined and probably complex. Concurrence could represent the influence of common risk factors such as hyperglycemia, duration of diabetes, and systemic hypertension [28; 42–44]

2.7.7 Anemia

Several studies link anemia with development and progression of diabetic retinopathy [20].

2.7.8 Pregnancy

Pregnancy may be associated with a rapid progression of diabetic retinopathy [45; 46], but this is generally temporary so that long-term risk is unchanged [47]. Postulated reasons include progesterone-induced upregulation of VEGF [48] and altered hemodynamics [49; 50].

2.7.9 Smoking

Any association between smoking and diabetic retinopathy is unclear [51], however smoking is a risk factor for cardiovascular disease, hypertension, and renal disease in diabetics [52].

2.8 Pathogenesis

The exact mechanism by which diabetes causes retinopathy is unknown. There are numerous pieces of evidence that could explain some aspects of the disease.

2.8.1 Hyperglycemia

In NPDR chronic hyperglycemia induces oxidative stress, mitochondria dysfunction, and ultimately cell death (apoptosis). Hyperglycemia activates enzymes that may initiate apoptosis [53]. Retinal capillary cells (pericytes and endothelial cells) and

Muller cells are damaged and may undergo apoptosis [54]. Pericyte damage leads to altered hemodynamics with abnormal autoregulation of retinal blood flow and reduced blood flow velocity [55; 56].

Excess glucose enters the polyol pathway to be converted into sorbitol [57]. This causes disruption of cell osmotic balance leading to retinal capillary pericyte damage [58], in turn leading to microaneurysm formation.

Advanced glycation end products (AGEs) are produced from nonenzymatic interaction of the excess glucose with proteins [59; 60]. AGEs may lead to oxidative stress, microvascular disease with altered hemodynamics and endothelial cell damage, stimulation of inflammation and thrombosis [61; 62].

Excess glucose also forms diacylglycerol (DAG). This activates protein kinase C (PKC) [63; 64]. PKC may also be increased after oxidative stress to endothelial cells [65; 66]. PKC, particularly the beta form, is associated with increased retinal capillary permeability and increased VEGF activity [67; 68].

Reactive oxygen species (ROS) could derive from glucose oxidation, an unregulated polyol pathway, and protein glycation. ROS may activate PKC and increase AGEs and DAG levels [65; 69].

2.8.2   Hematological abnormalities

There are a number of hematological abnormalities seen in diabetes that could lead to reduction of blood flow and have a role in retinal capillary damage and occlusion [70]. The abnormalities include increased plasma viscosity [71], decreased red erythrocyte deformability [72], increased erythrocyte and platelet aggregation [73; 74], and leukocyte abnormalities (discussed below).

2.8.3   Leukostasis and inflammation

Leukocytes are large, rigid white blood cells that have a normal tendency to adhere to endothelial cells lining blood vessels (leukostasis). They then produce superoxide radicals and proteolytic enzymes [75]. There is increased leukostasis in diabetes and the leukocytes are less deformable and more activated. This causes endothelial cell dysfunction, reduced capillary perfusion, occlusion, altered permeability, and angiogenesis [75].

There is evidence linking a role for inflammation induced by hyperglycemia [76]. Findings in DR in common with inflammation include leukostasis, capillary occlusion, increased vascular permeability, increased inducible nitric oxide (iNOS), cytokines, and nuclear factor kappa B (NF-B) [77].

2.8.4   Growth factors

Vascular endothelial growth factor (VEGF) is a cytokine promoting angiogenesis and is considered the major growth factor in ocular angiogenesis and for neovascularization in diabetic retinopathy [78]. VEGF not only promotes growth of new vessels but maintains the endothelial cells until they have pericyte coverage. VEGF also promotes endothelial cell migration, increased permeability, and vasodilatation. Cell stress resulting from reduced oxygen tension is the key stimulus for VEGF release. In diabetic retinopathy retinal nonperfusion is considered the initiator of excess VEGF release [79].

The insulin-like growth factor system comprises IGF-1 and -2 plus at least six IGF binding proteins. These factors have many functions. Research indicates an important role of these factors in diabetic retinopathy [76].

2.8.5 Neurodegeneration

The retina is a neural tissue. Diabetic retinopathy may be a neurodegenerative disorder as well as a vascular disorder. Glucose-induced glutamate elevation may lead to oxidative stress causing neuronal and glial cell toxicity [80]. Retinal ganglion cell apoptosis appears very early in diabetic retinopathy and progresses throughout the disease course [54]. Retinal glial cell dysfunction leads to endothelial cell dysfunction [80].

2.9 Treatment

The care of a patient with diabetic retinopathy involves determining the stage of retinopathy and macular edema, promptly giving any indicated ocular treatments, managing any associated systemic conditions, and arranging appropriately-timed follow-up examination. The risks of disease progression based on baseline retinopathy determine the management recommendations.

2.9.1 Management of systemic associations

Attention to the modifiable systemic associations can delay development and slow the progression of diabetic retinopathy. Rigorous maintenance of blood glucose at near to normal levels significantly reduces the development and progression of diabetic retinopathy in both type 1 diabetes [33] and type 2 diabetes [35]. Tight control of blood pressure in type 1 and 2 diabetes reduces progression of diabetic retinopathy [33; 38; 81; 82]. There is an association between development of hard exudate and higher serum lipid levels. As hard exudate accumulation is associated with visual loss, control of serum lipid may reduce the risk of visual loss [83].

2.9.2 Ocular treatments

2.9.2.1 Laser photocoagulation

Laser photocoagulation of the retina is the mainstay treatment for diabetic retinopathy. Pan retinal laser where the peripheral retina outside of the macula is covered with spaced laser burns is used for PDR. The rationale is that ablation of a significant proportion of retina reduces the load of angiogenic factors (including VEGF) produced by a nonperfused retina. The Diabetic Retinopathy Study demonstrated that pan-retinal laser significantly reduces severe vision loss (visual acuity $< 5/200$) in eyes with PDR [82; 84; 85]. Treatment should also be considered for severe NPDR, especially for type 2 diabetes [86]. Early pan retinal laser may also be considered in at-risk situations such as pregnancy or renal failure.

DME is treated with laser to the macula. The mechanisms by which macular laser may work are not fully understood. Laser may directly close leaking microaneurysms, alter retinal blood flow, or work via changes in the retinal pigment epithelium [87]. The ETDRS demonstrated a greater than 50% reduction in moderate visual loss using macular laser for DME with defined at-risk characteristics [88; 89] termed clinically significant diabetic macular edema (CSDME). These are: (1) Retinal thickening at or within 500 microns of the macular center. (2) Hard exudate at or within 500 microns of the macular center associated with adjacent retinal thickening; and (3) A zone(s) of retinal thickening ≥ 1 disc diameter, any part of which is within 1 disc diameter of the macular center [88].

Laser technology has advanced since these studies were performed. Indirect laser deliver systems allow treatment to far peripheral retina and through media opacity such as cataract and vitreous hemorrhage. New technologies and techniques aim to reduce the degree of thermal retinal damage as a consequence of treatment. Subthreshold micropulse laser delivery techniques are being investigated for treatment of PDR and DME [90; 91].

2.9.2.2 Vitreoretinal surgery

Vitreoretinal microsurgery can be used to remove media opacity and relieve vitreoretinal traction. It is indicated for advanced diabetic retinopathy with certain complications including vitreous hemorrhage, severe new vessel proliferation, traction macular detachment, and rhegmatogenous retinal detachment [92; 93]. Our understanding of disease processes and the instrumentation and techniques for vitreous surgery have advanced significantly since these studies were published. More complex pathology can now be treated and surgical complications are less frequent and better managed. Consequently, the surgical results have improved dramatically. The indications for surgery have widened to include earlier stages of disease, including certain subsets of DME [94]. In eyes with DME and vitreous traction, vitrectomy with or without peeling of the internal limiting membrane may reduce macular edema. Submacular hard exudates can be removed using vitrectomy techniques [95; 96].

2.9.3 Investigational treatments

2.9.3.1 Corticosteroids

Corticosteroids reduce vasopermeability, stabilize the blood-retinal barrier, downregulate VEGF, and are anti-inflammatory.

Triamcinolone acetonide injected into the subtenon's space adjacent to the eye reduces macular edema and improves visual acuity in eyes with DME [97–99]. Intravitreal triamcinolone has been found to be more effective than subtenon injection. The main problem is the short duration of efficacy, measured in months [100; 101]. This necessitates multiple treatments that increase the risk of complications, which include endophthalmitis, cataract, retinal detachment, and glaucoma [99].

Sustained-release corticosteroid intraocular implants *Retisert* (fluocinolone acetonide; Bausch & Lomb; Rochester, New York) and *Posurdex* (dexamethasone; Allergan, Inc.; Irvine, California) are being evaluated for the treatment of DME.

2.9.3.2 Angiogenesis inhibitors

Vascular endothelial growth factor (VEGF) is a potent stimulus for both retinal neovascularization and macular edema in diabetic retinopathy [102]. Several molecules that block VEGF activity are under investigation for the treatment of diabetic retinopathy. Pegaptanib (Macugen, Eyetech) is a VEGF aptamer and ranibizumab (lucentis, Genentech) and bevacizumab (Avastin, Genetech) are anti-VEGF monoclonal antibodies. These agents lead to regression of retinal and iris neovascularization and macular edema [103–106]. The apparent effectiveness of these drugs has led to widespread clinical use for the treatment of DME and PDR without completed clinical trials.

2.9.3.3 Protein kinase C inhibitors

Ruboxistaurin is a specific inhibitor of protein kinase C beta taken as a daily oral medication. It has shown promising effects in animal models [107] and on human diabetic retinal blood flow abnormalities [108]. Inconclusive effects have been demonstrated for reducing visual loss from nonproliferative retinopathy [109] and on DME [110]. Further studies are ongoing.

2.9.3.4 Other agents

A number of other agents including angiotensin converting enzyme inhibitors, angiotensin II receptor blockers, growth hormone inhibitors, cycloxgenase-2 inhibitor, pigment epithelium-derived factor, and interferon-alpha 2a are under investigation for treatment of diabetic retinopathy.

2.9.3.5 Surgical adjuncts

Investigational surgical adjuncts include hyaluronidase and plasmin. Hyaluronidase breaks down vitreous structure thereby liquefying the vitreous. Intravitreal injection of purified ovine hyaluronidase (Vitrase, ISTA Pharmaceuticals) is under study for treatment of vitreous hemorrhage [111; 112]. Plasmin is a protease that can cleave the vitreoretinal junction and potentially allow a relatively atraumatic separation of the vitreous from the retina [113; 114].

2.10   Screening

Screening is the systematic evaluation of apparently healthy people with a significant risk of having a specific disease with consequences that can be prevented by medical intervention. Screening is offered to a defined group within the population. Those found to have a positive screening test are referred for further diagnostic evaluation.

Diabetic retinopathy has few if any symptoms until the advanced stages of disease, either the development of macular edema or complications of proliferative retinopathy. Because treatment is aimed at preventing vision loss rather than restoring lost vision and treatable retinopathy is frequently asymptomatic, it is important to identify patients at an early stage of retinal disease. Then regular re-examination is needed to detect progression of retinopathy to a threshold level for initiating treatment. The benefits of early detection of retinopathy, regular examination, and timely treatment in reducing vision loss and costs to society have been shown [115; 116].

Diabetic retinopathy satisfies all the criteria for screening: it has (1) significant morbidity, (2) a high prevalence in the diabetic population, (3) diagnosis by definite and simple criteria, (4) acceptable, readily available, and effective treatment, (5) treatment that is more beneficial if initiated at an earlier time than is usual for diagnosis (while still asymptomatic), and (6) an acceptable, economic, reliable, and valid screening test. Validity is measured by the sensitivity (ability of a test to correctly identify disease) and specificity (ability to correctly identify nondisease). A test with 95% sensitivity will correctly identify 95 of 100 cases of disease. 95% specificity means the test will be negative in 95 of 100 normals. A good screening test should have both an acceptably high sensitivity and specificity.

2.10.1   Methods of screening

There are a variety of methods for detection of diabetic retinopathy (Table 2.6). Diabetic retinopathy screening has employed a number of these methods; direct or indirect ophthalmoscopy, mydriatic or nonmydriatic, color or monochromatic, film or digital photography.

2.10.1.1   Retinal photography

Retinal photography is a widely utilized method of screening. The United Kingdom Screening Committee has put digital retinal photography as the preferred modality for newly established screening programs [117].

Seven standard field stereoscopic color photography as defined by the ETDRS is the gold standard for detecting and classifying diabetic retinopathy [25]. It serves as the benchmark to which other screening techniques can be compared. Although very accurate this is logistically demanding on the scale required for screening [118]. To emulate the ETDRS either seven 30°, three 60°, or nine overlapping 45° fields can be used [119; 120]. This is difficult to do for a large number of patients in a screening

Table 2.6: Examination Methods for Diabetic Retinopathy

Direct/indirect ophthalmoscopy
Contact lens/ noncontact lens biomicroscopy
Retinal photography:
    mydriatic 7-standard field (gold standard)
    mydriatic/nonmydriatic film/digital (1 or more fields)

program because of the need for a highly experienced photographer, the long time taken to accurately obtain the required views, the logistics of handling and storing the large number of images generated and of the input from highly skilled image readers. In addition, the pupil needs to be dilated, which adds to the time taken and the cost, and introduces compliance issues.

Nonstereoscopic photographic screening is logistically easier than stereoscopic photography and is a valid simplification for screening. By definition the detection of DME requires identification of retinal thickening, which is not possible with nonstereoscopic photography. Other indicators of the presence of DME can be substituted. Visual acuity is one other easily obtained indication of macular status. The presence of microaneurysms, hemorrhages, or hard exudate in the macula is accepted as a good indicator of DME. Nonstereoscopic photography has comparable sensitivity and specificity with the ETDRS seven standard field images for grading of retinopathy and achieves a fair to moderate comparison for DME [121; 122]. Despite the poorer validity for determining DME, nonstereoscopic photography is considered a good screening method [122; 123].

Nonstereoscopic photography permits nonmydriasis (nondilation of the pupil) and thereby a simplification of the screening method. Nonmydriasis has the advantages of technically easier screening with greater patient compliance but with the disadvantages of lower image quality and sensitivity [118]. There is a significant incidence of ungradable images in the elderly due to lens opacity, however, most become gradable after mydriasis [124].

There has been considerable discussion on the minimum area of image fields required for screening. It is essential to have a field including the macula and a minimum field is considered to be 45 degrees horizontal and 40 degrees vertical. A single field including the macula may be sufficient [118] although multiple field photography does give greater coverage and increased sensitivity [122–125]. Nasal retinopathy has been shown to be accompanied by referable retinopathy in the macular field, and an argument can be made that this obviates the need for the second nasal field. The advantage of single field screening is the lower technical failure rate; the difficulty of multiple field photography is that it is more technically challenging, needs a skilled photographer, mydriasis, increased time for taking and reading images, more storage, and with all these, cost. However, the argument for a single field is not widely accepted in practice.

In the United Kingdom a Minimum Camera Specification for screening has been proposed. Nonmydriatic digital cameras are preferred even when mydriasis is routinely undertaken.

The recommendations are that [126]:

- Image file formats should not result in the loss of any clinically significant information.

- Camera resolution of the original images, as output by the camera, should be a minimum of 20 pixels per degree of retinal image, both horizontally and vertically.

- The field of view, as permanently recorded, should be a minimum of 45° horizontally and 40° vertically.

Images must be reviewed by a skilled reader. This is a significant cost of photographic screening [127]. Digital image capture allows for transmission to a reading center. This is valid for finding vision threatening retinopathy but not for detection of DME [123; 128]. Another study found a high validity for reading 45° digital images sent via the Internet [129]. Internet transmission has created interest in telemedicine for screening. Telemedicine is an accurate method for remote grading and assessing the need for referral for treatment [122].

2.10.1.2   Ophthalmoscopy

Ophthalmoscopy is relatively easy to apply as a method of screening. It is quick to master and can be performed by nonophthalmologists with no specialized equipment. Ophthalmoscopy performed by an experienced examiner such as an ophthalmologist has a high sensitivity and has a greater than 85% correlation with photographic grading [130]. However, nonophthalmologists only achieve a sensitivity of 63% for any retinopathy [131] and about 50% for the detection of PDR [132].

There are limitations to the use of ophthalmoscopy for screening. Although it is possible to have very high sensitivity and specificity, even ophthalmoscopy by ophthalmologists is not as sensitive as photography for detecting the earliest signs of retinopathy and DME [133; 134]. In addition, the resource of experienced ophthalmologists is limited and expensive.

2.10.1.3   Automated image analysis

Digital photographic retinopathy screening programs generate very large numbers of retinal images for manual reading. Acquiring, processing, and reading these images is labor intensive, time consuming, and expensive.

As diabetic retinopathy is diagnosed and classified solely on analysis of visible retinal lesions, automated computer image analysis is an attractive option but until relatively recently has only been of academic interest. The perceived benefits of automated analysis would be rapid, accurate, quantified, and cost-effective processing of large numbers of images. Additionally, there is the potential for "instant" analysis at the time of image capture so a point-of-service screening program is possible. This could be a mobile system that captures, processes, and analyzes the images to give an accurate diagnosis, all at the time of the patient's examination. This would then allow for the immediate arrangement of any referral for treatment or rescheduling for future screening.

A valid automated analysis system will need to perform above the 80% sensitivity and 95% specificity set by the World Health Organization for diabetic retinopathy [135]. In a typical screening program 78% of screenings have no diabetic retinopathy [136], and these could be identified and eliminated from the need for manual image reading by an automated analysis system that detects any diabetic retinopathy [137]. To this end a microaneurysm detector has been shown to be effective [137; 138]. More advanced image analysis would need to identify each of the important clinical lesions; microaneurysms/dot hemorrhages, hard exudates, venous beading, blotchy hemorrhages, and new vessels. This would then make automated classification of retinopathy possible. The critical end points would be severe nonproliferative retinopathy, proliferative retinopathy and, at any point, the presence of macular edema. Distinguishing severe nonproliferative retinopathy requires the definition of blotchy hemorrhages, venous beading, IRMA, and their number and distribution in the four retinal quadrants. For proliferative retinopathy new vessels must be defined. Automated detection of DME is more problematic. Ideally this requires identification of retinal thickening by stereoscopic examination. Photographic screening programs would be unlikely to include stereoscopic macular photography. However, as discussed earlier, for screening purposes the presence of microaneurysms, intraretinal hemorrhages, or hard exudate in the macula is accepted as an indicator of likely DME. Hard exudate is particularly associated with intraretinal edema/retinal thickening. Additionally, retinal thickening may be associated with geometric distributions of lesions, rings and clusters of hard exudate, clusters of microaneurysms, or intraretinal hemorrhages. Such geometric features could be detected by image analysis as an indicator of likely DME.

Alternatively or additionally to photographic methods for defining DME, optical coherence tomography (OCT) could be employed in diabetic retinopathy screening to detect retinal thickening. OCT is an imaging modality using the measurement of time delay and intensity of back-scattered light incident upon the retina to provide high resolution (1–15 µm) cross-sectional images of the retina. The images show the layered structural anatomy of the retina (see Figure 2.4). OCT allows accurate detection and quantification of DME and may be more sensitive than biomicroscopy for detecting mild degrees of macular thickening. Its reproducibility would allow for detection of any change in retinal thickness with repeat screening. Current OCT technology cannot be seen as replacing photographic technology for detection of other lesions of retinopathy but rather running concurrently for improved detection of DME.

What image analysis algorithms are needed for automated analysis of diabetic retinopathy? Each eye is analyzed separately. An image must be of sufficient quality, in focus, and have adequate contrast. This would need to be sampled at a number of localities across the image. One possible approach for determining contrast and focus would be to locate retinal blood vessels and determine the contrast at the vessel edges. Brightness can be manipulated to create an image of optimal parameters for analysis of a particular lesion.

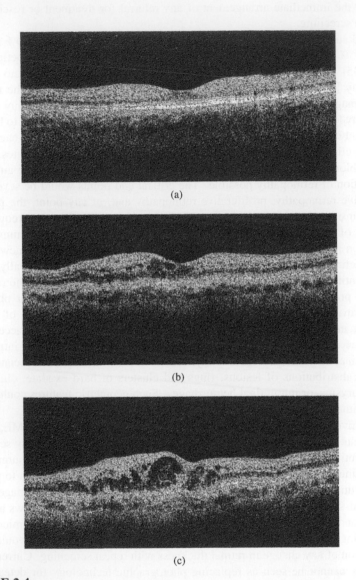

(a)

(b)

(c)

FIGURE 2.4

Optical Coherence Tomography (OCT). (a) Normal macula of a diabetic with no DR. (b) A patient with 6/6 acuity and microaneurysms close to the fovea. OCT shows intraretinal thickening and cystic spaces of intraretinal edema. Edema just involves the fovea. (c) The same patient six months later. Visual acuity has fallen to 6/12. There is increased intraretinal edema with foveal involvement. **(See color insert.)**

The minimum image field is an equivalent view to a 45° horizontal and 40° vertical image centered on the macula that includes the optic disc. More extensive coverage, that is, two or more views, provides more data and may allow for classification of retinopathy. As the optic disc is a simple landmark for the photographer to find, three 45° views with the optic disc placed at the left edge, the center, and the right edge are a simple set to obtain that cover a wide area of retina and include a view of the macula. An automated system could determine this by identifying the optic disc. It can be recognized by its approximate size, color, and the emergence of the retinal vasculature; tracking the vascular tree back to its source is an alternative. There are situations where there is difficulty in accurately identifiying the optic disc. The optic disc can be locally obscured in diabetic retinopathy either by preretinal hemorrhage, fibrovascular tissue, or retinal detachment, all advanced states of disease. Large accumulations of hard exudate could appear as an optic disc size white lesion. Uncommonly there could be other abnormalities that superficially resemble the optic disc, for example, chorioretinal scars may be white and may be associated with vessels.

Due to imperfections in centering some retinal photographs have a peripheral segment obscured while the remainder is of good quality. Poor quality areas could be enhanced or removed and analysis could also determine if there is then still sufficient area of quality image. A composite retinal image could be constructed from a set of retinal images taken widely around the retina by mapping the retinal vascular tree.

To classify retinopathy there must be an analysis of each of the four quadrants centered on the optic disc (quandants are centered on the optic disc rather than on center of the macula). To distinguish early from moderate and severe NPDR, specific lesions (intraretinal hemorrhages, venous beading, and IRMAs) must be identified and counted in each quadrant. The presence (or absence) of new vessels must be determined to identify PDR (or by their absence NPDR). Normal retinal vessels follow a particular set of parameters. They are a continuously connected tree-like structure, arising from the optic disc, have small curvatures, the vessel caliber changes gradually, and the intensity profile across a vessel is approximated by a Gaussian curve. Arterioles do not cross arterioles and veins do not cross veins. New vessels do not follow these "rules" and in particular may cross a normal vessel or themselves.

To detect DME the macula needs to be accurately identified. The macula may be identified by several strategies; for a right eye image it lies to the left of the optic disc and to the right on a left eye image, the macula is surrounded by a wreath of vasculature with branches pointing toward but not reaching the avascular center, the center has a concentration of pigment, and in a healthy eye has an optical reflex, the foveal reflex. Of these the first feature is universal, the second usually true (there are exceptions, the vascular pattern can be unreliable in a few normal eyes, and in some disease states, for example, heterotopia macula (dragged macula)), the last two features may be obscured in macular disease including diabetic retinopathy itself. With the macula identified the presence, number of, and proximity to the center of the various diabetic retinopathy lesions can be determined. This process for reading retinal images is summarized in Table 2.7.

Table 2.7: Steps in Reading a Retinal Image

1. Identify eye as right or left.
2. Identify quality view of macula as minimum image.
3. Identify lesions of retinopathy:

   microaneurysms, hemorrhages, hard exudate, (cotton wool spot,) venous beading, new vessels, fibrosis, vitreous hemorrhage.
4. Lesions' proximity to macula center as indicator for DME.
5. Grading by identification and quantification of lesions in four quadrants.

2.10.2 Frequency of screening

The optimal frequency for diabetic retinopathy screening is unknown. Without empirical data to show otherwise, annual screening is recommended [139]. Less frequent re-screening may be needed for those with no apparent retinopathy or mild NPDR with no apparent DME. For these patients, the annual incidence of progression to either PDR or DME is low and therefore a longer interval between examinations may be appropriate [140]. Based on cost effectiveness there is a clear argument for only screening those with no retinopathy every two or three years. Effectiveness is virtually unchanged for very significant screening cost savings. The need for annual screening for some type 2 diabetics has been questioned [141].

2.10.3 Cost effectiveness of screening

The cost and benefits of screening will vary depending on the perspective taken. An accepted measure of utility is the Cost per Sight Year Saved. This shows diabetic retinopathy screening to be highly effective [142; 143].

2.10.4 Access to care and screening

The size of the diabetes epidemic, socioeconomic, cultural and geographic issues, lack of patient education, limited funding with scarce health resources, incomplete communication between health care providers with broken continuity of care and incomplete patient registers all contribute to many patients missing out on adequate eye care. With effective treatment readily available, there is unnecessary loss of vision and blindness.

Access to health care is also likely to be a determinant of duration of diabetes before diagnosis, metabolic control after diagnosis, retinal screening penetration and access to early treatment. At least in Australia, there appears to be no major difference in prevalence of retinopathy between rural and urban areas although other rural-urban differences in eye disease exist [144].

As a complex, largely asymptomatic, chronic disease, there are many reasons for access to health care to be patchy. Barriers to diabetes care can be placed in five domains: psychological (i.e., behavioral), psychosocial (i.e., the way the individual and those around interact with each other such as family), internal physical (i.e., physical conditions that prevent self care), external physical (i.e., barriers relating to the health system in its widest context) and educational [145].

2.11 Conclusion

Digital photographic screening of the diabetic population is an essential health care measure for detection of early diabetic retinopathy. Automated retinal image analysis promises to provide consistently accurate and detailed screening information, an effective solution to managing the huge volume of images generated by screening the large and ever increasing diabetic population and "instant" image analysis at the time of screening.

References

[1] Fong, D.S., Aiello, L.P., and Gardner, Retinopathy in diabetes, *Diabetes Care*, 27(suppl 1), S84, 2004.

[2] Zimmet, P., Alberti, K.G., and Shaw, J., Global and societal implications of the diabetes epidemic, *Nature*, 414, 782, 2001.

[3] New Zealand Herald, World faces diabetes catastrophe, experts say, New Zealand Herald, August 26, 2003.

[4] Stumvoll, M., Goldstein, B.J., and van Haeften, T.W., Type 2 diabetes: Principles of pathogensis and therapy, *Lancet*, 365, 1333, 2005.

[5] Knowler, W.C., Barrett-Connor, E., Fowler, S.E., et al., Reduction in the incidence of type 2 diabetes with lifestyle intervention or metformin, *N Engl J Med.*, 346, 393, 2002.

[6] Tuomilehto, J., Lindstrom, J., Eriksson, J.G., et al., Prevention of type 2 diabetes mellitus by changes in lifestyle among subjects with impaired glucose tolerance, *N Engl J Med.*, 344, 1343, 2001.

[7] Ramachandran, A., Snehalatha, C., Mary, S., et al., The Indian Diabetes Prevention Programme shows that lifestyle modification and metformin prevent type 2 diabetes in Asian Indian subjects with impaired glucose tolerance (IDPP-1), *Diabetologia*, 49, 289, 2006.

[8] Daneman, D., Type 1 diabetes, *Lancet*, 367, 847, 2006.

[9] Permutt, M.A., Wasson, J., and N., C., Genetic epidemiology of diabetes, *J Clin Invest*, 115, 1431, 2005.

[10] Fagot-Campagna, A., Pettitt, D.J., Engelgau, M.M., et al., Type 2 diabetes among North American children and adolescents: An epidemiologic review and a public health perspective, *J. Pediatr.*, 136, 664, 2000.

[11] Rosenbloom, A., Joe, J.R., Young, R.S., et al., Emerging epidemic of type 2 diabetes in youth, *Diabetes Care*, 22, 345, 1999.

[12] McElduff, A., Ross, G.P., Lagström, J.A., et al., Pregestational diabetes and pregnancy: An Australian experience, *Diabetes Care*, 28, 1260, 2005.

[13] Pettitt, D.J., Bennett, P.H., Knowler, W.C., et al., Gestational diabetes mellitus and impaired glucose tolerance during pregnancy: Long terms effects on obesity and glucose tolerance in the offspring, *Diabetes*, 34(supp 2), 119, 1985.

[14] Amos, A.F., McCarty, D.J., and Zimmet, P., The rising global burden of diabetes and its complications: Estimates and projections to the year 2010, *Diab Med*, 14(supp 5), S1, 1997.

[15] International Diabetes Federation, ed., *Diabetes Atlas*, International Diabetes Federation, 2nd ed., 2003.

[16] Dorf, A. and *et al.*, Retinopathy in Pima Indians: Relationship to glucose level, duration of diabetes and age at examination in a population with a high prevalence of diabetes, *Diabetes*, 25, 554, 1976.

[17] Harris, M., Klein, R., Welborn, T., et al., Onset of NIDDM occurs at least 4–7 years before clinical diagnosis, *Diabetes Care*, 15, 815, 1992.

[18] Tapp, R.J., Shaw, J.E., Harper, C.A., et al., The prevalence of and factors associated with diabetic retinopathy in the Australian population, *Diabetes Care*, 26, 1731, 2003.

[19] Yu, T., Mitchell, P., Berry, G., et al., Retinopathy in older persons without diabetes and its relationship to hypertension, *Arch Ophthalmol*, 116, 83, 1998.

[20] Aiello, L.P., Cahill, M.T., and Wong, J.S., Systemic considerations in the management of diabetic retinopathy, *Am J Ophthalmol*, 132, 760, 2001.

[21] Klein, R., Klein, B.E., Moss, S.E., et al., The Wisconsin Epidemiologic Study of Diabetic Retinopathy. IV. Diabetic macular edema, *Ophthalmology*, 91, 1464, 1985.

[22] Williams, R., Airey, M., Baxter, H., et al., Epidemiology of diabetic retinopathy and macular oedema: A systematic review, *Eye*, 18, 963, 2004.

[23] Simmons, D., Clover, G., and Hope, C., Ethnic differences in diabetic

retinopathy, *Diabet Med*, 24, 1093, 2007.

[24] Frank, R.N., Diabetic retinopathy, *N Engl J Med*, 350, 48, 2004.

[25] Early Treatment Diabetic Retinopathy Study Research Group, Grading diabetic retinopathy from stereoscopic color fundus photographs–an extension of the modified Airlie House classification. ETDRS report number 10., *Ophthalmology*, 98, 786, 1991.

[26] Klein, R., Barriers to prevention of vision loss caused by diabetic retinopathy, *Arch Ophthalmol*, 115, 1073, 1997.

[27] American Academy of Ophthalmology, Diabetic retinopathy disease severity scale 2002, 2002, http://www.aao.org/education/library/recommendations/international_dr.cfm.

[28] Klein, R., Klein, B.E., Moss, S.E., et al., The Wisconsin Epidemiologic Study of Diabetic Retinopathy: XVII. The 14-year incidence and progression of diabetic retinopathy and associated risk factors in type 1 diabetes, *Ophthalmology*, 105, 1801, 1998.

[29] Klein, R., Klein, B.E., and Moss, S.E., How many steps of progression of diabetic retinopathy are meaningful? The Wisconsin Epidemiologic Study of Diabetic Retinopathy, *Arch Ophthalmol*, 119, 547, 2001.

[30] Klein, R., Klein, B.E., Moss, S.E., et al., The Wisconsin Epidemiologic Study of Diabetic Retinopathy. III. Prevalence and risk of diabetic retinopathy when age at diagnosis is 30 or more years, *Arch Ophthalmol*, 102, 527, 1984.

[31] Yanko, L., Goldbourt, U., Michaelson, I.C., et al., Prevalence and 15-year incidence of retinopathy and associated characteristics in middle-aged and elderly diabetic men, *Br J Ophthalmol*, 67, 759, 1984.

[32] Diabetic Retinopathy Vitrectomy Study, Early vitrectomy for severe vitreous hemorrhage in diabetic retinopathy. Four-year results of a randomized trial: Diabetic Retinopathy Vitrectomy Study Report 5, *Arch Ophthalmol*, 108, 958, 1990.

[33] The Diabetes Control and Complications Trial Research Group, The effect of intensive treatment of diabetes on the development and progression of long-term complications in insulin-dependent diabetes mellitus, *N Engl J Med*, 329, 977, 1993.

[34] Diabetes Control and Complications Trial Research Group, Progression of retinopathy with intensive versus conventional treatment in the Diabetes Control and Complications Trial, *Ophthalmology*, 102, 647, 1995.

[35] UK Prospective Diabetes Study (UKPDS) Group, Intensive blood-glucose control with sulphonylureas or insulin compared with conventional treatment and risk of complications in patients with type 2 diabetes (UKPDS 33), *Lancet*, 352, 837, 1998.

[36] Klein, R., Klein, B.E., Lee, K.E., et al., The incidence of hypertension in insulin-dependent diabetes, *Arch Intern Med*, 156, 622, 1996.

[37] Klein, R., Klein, B.E., Moss, S.E., et al., Blood pressure and hypertension in diabetes, *Am J Epidemiol*, 122, 75, 1985.

[38] UK Prospective Diabetes Study (UKPDS) Group, Tight blood pressure control and risk of macrovascular and microvascular complications in type 2 diabetes: UKPDS 38, *BMJ*, 317, 703, 1998.

[39] Park, J.Y., Kim, H.K., Chung, Y.E., et al., Incidence and determinants of microalbuminuria in Koreans with type 2 diabetes, *Diabetes Care*, 21, 530, 1998.

[40] Hasslacher, C., Bostedt-Kiesel, A., Kempe, H.P., et al., Effect of metabolic factors and blood pressure on kidney function in proteinuric type 2 (non-insulin-dependent) diabetic patients, *Diabetologia*, 36, 1051, 1993.

[41] Klein, R., Moss, S.E., and Klein, B.E., Is gross proteinuria a risk factor for the incidence of proliferative diabetic retinopathy? *Ophthalmology*, 100, 1140, 1993.

[42] Klein, R., Klein, B.E., Moss, S.E., et al., The 10-year incidence of renal insufficiency in people with type 1 diabetes, *Diabetes Care*, 22, 743, 1999.

[43] Lloyd, G., The importance of accuracy in blood pressure recording, *Br J Clin Pract*, 49, 284, 1996.

[44] UK Prospective Diabetes Study Group (UKPDS), X. Urinary albumin excretion over 3 years in diet-treated type 2, (non-insulin-dependent) diabetic patients, and association with hypertension, hyperglycaemia and hypertriglyceridaemia, *Diabetologia*, 36, 1021, 1993.

[45] Moloney, J.B. and Drury, M.I., The effect of pregnancy on the natural course of diabetic retinopathy, *Am J Ophthalmol*, 93, 745, 1982.

[46] Klein, B.E., Moss, S.E., and Klein, R., Effect of pregnancy on progression of diabetic retinopathy, *Diabetes Care*, 13, 34, 1990.

[47] Diabetes Control and Complications Trial (DCCT) Research Group, Effect of pregnancy on microvascular complications in the Diabetes Control and Complications Trial, *Diabetes Care*, 23, 1084, 2000.

[48] Sone, H., Okuda, Y., Kawakami, Y., et al., Progesterone induces vascular endothelial growth factor on retinal pigment epithelial cells in culture, *Life Sci*, 59, 21, 1996.

[49] Chen, H.C., Newsom, R.S., Patel, V., et al., Retinal blood flow changes during pregnancy in women with diabetes, *Invest Ophthalmol Vis Sci*, 35, 3199, 1994.

[50] Schocket, L.S., Grunwald, J.E., Tsang, A.F., et al., The effect of pregnancy on

retinal hemodynamics in diabetic versus nondiabetic mothers, *Am J Ophthalmol*, 128, 477, 1999.

[51] Muhlhauser, I., Cigarette smoking and diabetes: An update, *Diabet Med*, 11, 336, 1994.

[52] Sawicki, P.T., Muhlhauser, I., Bender, R., et al., Effects of smoking on blood pressure and proteinuria in patients with diabetic nephropathy, *J Intern Med*, 239, 345, 1996.

[53] Mohr, S.E. and Boswell, R.E., Genetic analysis of *Drosophila melanogaster* polytene chromosome region 44D–45F: Loci required for viability and fertility, *Genetics*, 160, 1503, 2002.

[54] Barber, A.J., Lieth, E., Khin, S.A., et al., Neural apoptosis in the retina during experimental and human diabetes. Early onset and effect of insulin, *J Clin Invest*, 102, 783, 1998.

[55] Ciulla, T.A., Harris, A., Latkany, P., et al., Ocular perfusion abnormalities in diabetes, *Acta Ophthalmol Scand*, 80, 468, 2002.

[56] Otani, T., Kishi, S., and Maruyama, Y., Patterns of diabetic macular edema with optical coherence tomography, *Am J Ophthalmol*, 127, 688, 1999.

[57] Gabbay, K.H., Hyperglycemia, polyol metabolism, and complications of diabetes mellitus, *Annu Rev Med*, 26, 521, 1975.

[58] Sato, S., Secchi, E.F., Lizak, M.J., et al., Polyol formation and NADPH-dependent reductases in dog retinal capillary pericytes and endothelial cells, *Invest Ophthalmol Vis Sci*, 40, 697, 1999.

[59] Brownlee, M., Vlassara, H., and Cerami, A., Nonenzymatic glycosylation and the pathogenesis of diabetic complications, *Ann Intern Med*, 101, 527, 1984.

[60] Friedman, E.A., Advanced glycosylated end products and hyperglycemia in the pathogenesis of diabetic complications, *Diabetes Care*, 22 Suppl 2, B65, 1999.

[61] Schmidt, A.M., Yan, S.D., Wautier, J.L., et al., Activation of receptor for advanced glycation end products: A mechanism for chronic vascular dysfunction in diabetic vasculopathy and atherosclerosis, *Circ Res*, 84, 489, 1999.

[62] Singh, R., Barden, A., Mori, T., et al., Advanced glycation end-products: A review, *Diabetologia*, 44, 129, 2001.

[63] Inoguchi, T., Battan, R., Handler, E., et al., Preferential elevation of protein kinase C isoform beta II and diacylglycerol levels in the aorta and heart of diabetic rats: Differential reversibility to glycemic control by islet cell transplantation, *Proc Natl Acad Sci USA*, 89, 11059, 1992.

[64] Xia, P., Inoguchi, T., Kern, T.S., et al., Characterization of the mechanism for the chronic activation of diacylglycerol-protein kinase C pathway in diabetes

and hypergalactosemia, *Diabetes*, 43, 1122, 1994.

[65] Nishikawa, T., Edelstein, D., and Brownlee, M., The missing link: A single unifying mechanism for diabetic complications, *Kidney Int Suppl*, 77, S26, 2001.

[66] Taher, M.M., Garcia, J.G., and Natarajan, V., Hydroperoxide-induced dia-cylglycerol formation and protein kinase C activation in vascular endothelial cells, *Arch Biochem Biophys*, 303, 260, 1993.

[67] Nagpala, P.G., Malik, A.B., Vuong, P.T., et al., Protein kinase C beta 1 overexpression augments phorbol ester-induced increase in endothelial permeability, *J Cell Physiol*, 166, 249, 1996.

[68] Xia, P., Aiello, L.P., Ishii, H., et al., Characterization of vascular endothelial growth factor's effect on the activation of protein kinase C, its isoforms, and endothelial cell growth, *J Clin Invest*, 98, 2018, 1997.

[69] Giugliano, D., Ceriello, A., and Paolisso, G., Oxidative stress and diabetic vascular complications, *Diabetes Care*, 19, 257, 1996.

[70] Sakata, K., Funatsu, H., Harino, S., et al., Relationship between macular microcirculation and progression of diabetic macular edema, *Ophthalmology*, 113, 1385, 2006.

[71] McMillan, D.E., Plasma protein changes, blood viscosity, and diabetic microangiopathy, *Diabetes*, 25, 858, 1976.

[72] McMillan, D.E., Utterback, N.G., and La Puma, J., Reduced erythrocyte deformability in diabetes, *Diabetes*, 27, 895, 1978.

[73] Schmid-Schonbein, H. and Volger, E., Red-cell aggregation and red-cell deformability in diabetes, *Diabetes*, 25, 897, 1976.

[74] Sagel, J., Colwell, J.A., Crook, L., et al., Increased platelet aggregation in early diabetus mellitus, *Ann Intern Med*, 82, 733, 1975.

[75] Miyamoto, K. and Ogura, Y., Pathogenetic potential of leukocytes in diabetic retinopathy, *Semin Ophthalmol*, 14, 233, 2000.

[76] Grant, M.B., Afzal, A., Spoerri, P., et al., The role of growth factors in the pathogenesis of diabetic retinopathy, *Expert Opin Investig Drugs*, 13, 1275, 2004.

[77] Joussen, A.M., Poulaki, V., Qin, W., et al., Retinal vascular endothelial growth factor induces intercellular adhesion molecule-1 and endothelial nitric oxide synthase expression and initiates early diabetic retinal leukocyte adhesion *in vivo*, *Am J Pathol*, 160, 501, 2002.

[78] Miller, J.W., Adamis, A.P., and Aiello, L.P., Vascular endothelial growth factor in ocular neovascularization and proliferative diabetic retinopathy, *Diabetes Metab Rev*, 13, 37, 1997.

[79] Aiello, L.P., Avery, R.L., Arrigg, P.G., et al., Vascular endothelial growth factor in ocular fluid of patients with diabetic retinopathy and other retinal disorders, *N Engl J Med*, 331, 1480, 1994.

[80] Cunha-Vaz, J., Faria de Abreu, J.R., and Campos, A.J., Early breakdown of the blood-retinal barrier in diabetes, *Br J Ophthalmol*, 59, 649, 1975.

[81] Diabetes Control and Complications Trial (DCCT), Early worsening of diabetic retinopathy in the Diabetes Control and Complications Trial, *Arch Ophthalmol*, 116, 874, 1998.

[82] Diabetic Retinopathy Study Research Group, Preliminary report on effects of photocoagulation therapy, *Am J Ophthalmol*, 81, 383, 1976.

[83] Sjolie, A.K. and Moller, F., Medical management of diabetic retinopathy, *Diabet Med*, 21, 666, 2004.

[84] Diabetic Retinopathy Study Research Group, Photocoagulation treatment of proliferative diabetic retinopathy. Clinical application of Diabetic Retinopathy Study (DRS) findings, DRS report number 8, *Ophthalmol*, 88, 583, 1981.

[85] Diabetic Retinopathy Study Research Group, Four risk factors for severe visual loss in diabetic retinopathy. the third report from the Diabetic Retinopathy Study, *Arch Ophthalmol*, 97, 654, 1979.

[86] Aiello, L.M., Perspectives on diabetic retinopathy, *Am J Ophthalmol*, 136, 122, 2003.

[87] Fong, D.S., Strauber, S.F., Aiello, L.P., et al., Comparison of the modified early treatment diabetic retinopathy study and mild macular grid laser photocoagulation strategies for diabetic macular edema, *Arch Ophthalmol*, 125, 469, 2007.

[88] Early Treatment Diabetic Retinopathy Study (ETDRS) Research Group, Photocoagulation for diabetic macular edema. Early Treatment Diabetic Retinopathy Study Report Number 1, *Arch Ophthalmol*, 103, 1796, 1985.

[89] Early Treatment Diabetic Retinopathy Study (ETDRS) Research Group, Early photocoagulation for diabetic retinopathy. ETDRS Report Number 9, *Ophthalmol*, 98(5 Suppl), 766, 1991.

[90] Luttrull, J.K., Musch, D.C., and Spink, C.A., Subthreshold diode micropulse panretinal photocoagulation for proliferative diabetic retinopathy, *Eye*, 22, 607, 2008.

[91] Luttrull, J.K., Musch, D.C., and Mainster, M.A., Subthreshold diode micropulse photocoagulation for the treatment of clinically significant diabetic macular oedema, *Br J Ophthalmol*, 89, 74, 2004.

[92] The Diabetic Retinopathy Vitrectomy Study Research Group, Early vitrectomy for severe vitreous hemorrhage in diabetic retinopathy. Two-year results

of a randomized trial. Diabetic Retinopathy Vitrectomy Study Report 2, *Arch Ophthalmol*, 103, 1644, 1985.

[93] The Diabetic Retinopathy Vitrectomy Study Research Group, Early vitrectomy for severe proliferative diabetic retinopathy in eyes with useful vision. Clinical application of results of a randomized trial—Diabetic Retinopathy Vitrectomy Study Report 4, *Ophthalmol*, 95, 1321, 1988.

[94] Smiddy, W.E. and Flynn, H.W., Vitrectomy in the management of diabetic retinopathy, *Surv Ophthalmol*, 43, 491, 1999.

[95] Sakuraba, T., Suzuki, Y., Mizutani, H., et al., Visual improvement after removal of submacular exudates in patients with diabetic maculopathy, *Ophthalmic Surg Lasers*, 31, 287, 2000.

[96] Takaya, K., Suzuki, Y., Mizutani, H., et al., Long-term results of vitrectomy for removal of submacular hard exudates in patients with diabetic maculopathy, *Retina*, 24, 23, 2004.

[97] Wada, M., Ogata, N., Minamino, K., et al., Trans-tenon's retrobulbar injection of triamcinolone acetonide for diffuse diabetic macular edema, *Jpn J Ophthalmol*, 49, 509, 2005.

[98] Bakri, S.J. and Kaiser, P.K., Posterior subtenon triamcinolone acetonide for refractory diabetic macular edema, *Am J Ophthalmol*, 139, 290, 2005.

[99] Gillies, M.C., Sutter, F.K., Simpson, J.M., et al., Intravitreal triamcinolone for refractory diabetic macular edema: Two-year results of a double-masked, placebo-controlled, randomized clinical trial, *Ophthalmology*, 113, 1533, 2006.

[100] Martidis, A., Duker, J.S., Greenberg, P.B., et al., Intravitreal triamcinolone for refractory diabetic macular edema, *Ophthalmology*, 109, 920, 2002.

[101] Massin, P., Audren, F., Haouchine, B., et al., Intravitreal triamcinolone acetonide for diabetic diffuse macular edema: Preliminary results of a prospective controlled trial, *Ophthalmology*, 111, 218, 2004.

[102] Nguyen, Q.D., Tatlipinar, S., Shah, S.M., et al., Vascular endothelial growth factor is a critical stimulus for diabetic macular edema, *Am J Ophthalmol*, 142, 961, 2006.

[103] Chun, D.W., Heier, J.S., Topping, T.M., et al., A pilot study of multiple intravitreal injections of ranibizumab in patients with center-involving clinically significant diabetic macular edema, *Ophthalmology*, 113, 1706, 2006.

[104] Adamis, A.P., Altaweel, M., Aiello, L.P., et al., A phase II randomized double-masked trial of pegaptanib, an anti-vascular endothelial growth factor aptamer, for diabetic macular edema, *Ophthalmol*, 112, 1747, 2005.

[105] Krzystolik, M.G., Filippopoulos, T., Ducharme, J.F., et al., Pegaptanib as an

adjunctive treatment for complicated neovascular diabetic retinopathy, *Arch Ophthalmol*, 124, 920, 2006.

[106] Silva Paula, J., Jorge, R., Alves Costa, R., et al., Short-term results of intravitreal bevacizumab (avastin) on anterior segment neovascularization in neovascular glaucoma, *Acta Ophthalmol Scand*, 84, 556, 2006.

[107] Comer, G.M. and Ciulla, T.A., Pharmacotherapy for diabetic retinopathy, *Curr Opin Ophthalmol*, 15, 508, 2004.

[108] Aiello, L.P., Clermont, A., Arora, V., et al., Inhibition of PKC beta by oral administration of ruboxistaurin is well tolerated and ameliorates diabetes-induced retinal hemodynamic abnormalities in patients, *Invest Ophthalmol Vis Sci*, 47, 86, 2005.

[109] Aiello, L.P., Davis, M.D., Girach, A., et al., Effect of ruboxistaurin on visual loss in patients with diabetic retinopathy, *Ophthalmology*, 113, 2221, 2006.

[110] PKC-DMES Study Group, Effect of ruboxistaurin in patients with diabetic macular edema: Thirty-month results of the randomized PKC-DMES clinical trial, *Arch Ophthalmol*, 125, 318, 2007.

[111] Kuppermann, B.D., Thomas, E.L., de Smet, M.D., et al., Pooled efficacy results from two multinational randomized controlled clinical trials of a single intravitreous injection of highly purified ovine hyaluronidase (vitrase) for the management of vitreous hemorrhage, *Am J Ophthalmol*, 140, 573, 2005.

[112] Kuppermann, B.D., Thomas, E.L., de Smet, M.D., et al., Safety results of two phase III trials of an intravitreous injection of highly purified ovine hyaluronidase (vitrase) for the management of vitreous hemorrhage, *Am J Ophthalmol*, 140, 585, 2005.

[113] Williams, J.G., Trese, M.T., Williams, G.A., et al., Autologous plasmin enzyme in the surgical management of diabetic retinopathy, *Ophthalmology*, 108, 1902, 2001.

[114] Trese, M.T., Enzymatic-assisted vitrectomy, *Eye*, 16, 365, 2002.

[115] Kristinsson, J.K., Stefansson, E., Jonasson, F., et al., Systematic screening for diabetic eye disease in insulin dependent diabetes, *Acta Ophthalmol*, 72, 72, 1994.

[116] Singer, D.E., Nathan, D.M., Fogel, H.A., et al., Screening for diabetic retinopathy, *Ann Intern Med*, 116, 660, 1992.

[117] Taylor, R. and British Diabetic Association Mobile Retinal Screening Group, Practical community screening for diabetic retinopathy using the mobile retinal camera: Report of a 12 centre study, *Diabet Med*, 13, 946, 1996.

[118] Williams, G.A., Scott, I.U., Haller, J.A., et al., Single-field fundus photography for diabetic retinopathy screening: A report by the American Academy

of Ophthalmology, *Ophthalmology*, 111, 1055, 2004.

[119] Aldington, S.J., Kohner, E.M., Meuer, S., et al., Methodology for retinal photography and assessment of diabetic retinopathy: The Eurodiab IDDM Complications Study, *Diabetologia*, 38, 437, 1995.

[120] Shiba, T., Yamamoto, T., Seki, U., et al., Screening and follow-up of diabetic retinopathy using a new mosaic 9-field fundus photography system, *Diabetes Res Clin Pract*, 55, 49, 2001.

[121] Newsom, R., Moate, B., and Casswell, T., Screening for diabetic retinopathy using digital colour photography and oral fluorescein angiography, *Eye*, 14, 579, 2000.

[122] Bursell, S.E., Cavallerano, J.D., Cavallerano, A.A., et al., Stereo nonmydriatic digital-video color retinal imaging compared with early treatment diabetic retinopathy study seven standard field 35-mm stereo color photos for determining level of diabetic retinopathy, *Ophthalmology*, 108, 572, 2001.

[123] Liesenfeld, B., Kohner, E., Piehlmeier, W., et al., A telemedical approach to the screening of diabetic retinopathy: Digital fundus photography, *Diabetes Care*, 23, 345, 2000.

[124] Pugh, J.A., Jacobson, J.M., van Heuven, W.A., et al., Screening for diabetic retinopathy. The wide-angle retinal camera, *Diabetes Care*, 16, 889, 1993.

[125] Fransen, S.R., Leonard-Martin, T.C., Feuer, W.J., et al., Clinical evaluation of patients with diabetic retinopathy: Accuracy of the inoveon diabetic retinopathy-3DT system, *Ophthalmology*, 109, 595, 2002.

[126] Scanlon, P., Screening for diabetic retinopathy in Europe: 15 years after the Saint Vincent Declaration, in *Proceedings of the Liverpool Declaration*, S.P. Harding, ed., Liverpool, UK, 2005.

[127] Bjorvig, S., Johansen, M.A., and Fossen, K., An economic analysis of screening for diabetic retinopathy, *J Telemed Telecare*, 8, 32, 2002.

[128] Cook, H.L., Heacock, G.L., Stanford, M.R., et al., Detection of retinal lesions after telemedicine transmission of digital images, *Eye*, 14 (Pt 4), 563, 2000.

[129] Gomez-Ulla, F., Fernandez, M.I., Gonzalez, F., et al., Digital retinal images and teleophthalmology for detecting and grading diabetic retinopathy, *Diabetes Care*, 25, 1384, 2002.

[130] Moss, S.E., Klein, R., Kessler, S.D., et al., Comparison between ophthalmoscopy and fundus photography in determining severity of diabetic retinopathy, *Ophthalmology*, 92, 62, 1985.

[131] Owens, D.R., Gibbins, R.L., Lewis, P.A., et al., Screening for diabetic retinopathy by general practitioners: Ophthalmoscopy or retinal photography as 35 mm colour transparencies? *Diabet Med*, 15, 170, 1998.

[132] Sussman, E.J., Tsiaras, W.G., and Soper, K.A., Diagnosis of diabetic eye disease, *JAMA*, 247, 3231, 1982.

[133] Kinyoun, J.L., Martin, D.C., Fujimoto, W.Y., et al., Ophthalmoscopy versus fundus photographs for detecting and grading diabetic retinopathy, *Invest Ophthalmol Vis Sci*, 33, 1888, 1992.

[134] Harding, S.P., Broadbent, D.M., Neoh, C., et al., Sensitivity and specificity of photography and direct ophthalmoscopy in screening for sight threatening eye disease: The Liverpool Diabetic Eye Study, *BMJ*, 311, 1131, 1995.

[135] World Health Organisation, Diabetes care and research in Europe: The St. Vincent Declaration. Diabetes mellitus in Europe: A problem for all ages in all countries. A model for prevention and self care, St. Vincent (Italy), 1989.

[136] Reda, E., Dunn, P., Straker, C., et al., Screening for diabetic retinopathy using the mobile retinal camera: The Waikato experience, *New Zealand Medical Journal*, 116(1180), 562, 2003.

[137] Jelinek, H.J., Cree, M.J., Worsley, D., et al., An automated microaneurysm detector as a tool for identification of diabetic retinopathy in rural optometric practice, *Clin Exp Optom*, 89, 299, 2006.

[138] Hipwell, J.H., Strachan, F., Olson, J.A., et al., Automated detection of microaneurysms in digital red-free photographs: A diabetic retinopathy screening tool, *Diabetic Medicine*, 17(8), 588, 2000.

[139] Fong, D.S., Aiello, L., Gardner, T.W., et al., Diabetic retinopathy, *Diabetes Care*, 26, 226, 2002.

[140] Batchelder, T.J., Fireman, B., Friedman, G.D., et al., The value of routine dilated pupil screening examination, *Arch Ophthalmol*, 115, 1179, 1997.

[141] Vijan, S., Hofer, T.P., and Hayward, R.A., Cost-utility analysis of screening intervals for diabetic retinopathy in patients with type 2 diabetes mellitus, *JAMA*, 283, 889, 2000.

[142] James, M., Turner, D.A., Broadbent, D.M., et al., Cost-effectiveness analysis of screening for sight threatening diabetic eye disease, *British Medical Journal*, 320, 1627, 2000.

[143] James, M. and Little, R., Screening for diabetic retinopathy: Report to the National Screening Committee, 2001, http://www.diabetic-retinopathy. screening.nhs.uk/decision-analysis.html.

[144] Madden, A.C., Simmons, D., McCarty, C.A., et al., Eye health in rural areas, *Clinical and Experimental Ophthalmology*, 30, 316, 2002.

[145] Simmons, D., Weblemoe, T., Voyle, J., et al., Personal barriers to diabetes care: Lessons from a multiethnic community in New Zealand, *Diabet Med*, 15, 958, 1998.

3

Detecting Retinal Pathology Automatically with Special Emphasis on Diabetic Retinopathy

Michael D. Abràmoff and Meindert Niemeijer

CONTENTS

3.1 Historical Aside 67
3.2 Approaches to Computer (Aided) Diagnosis 68
3.3 Detection of Diabetic Retinopathy Lesions................................ 70
3.4 Detection of Lesions and Segmentation of Retinal Anatomy............... 71
3.5 Detection and Staging of Diabetic Retinopathy: Pixel to Patient 71
3.6 Directions for Research 72
    References 73

3.1 Historical Aside

The idea of computer assisted and computerized detection of retinal pathology has a long history, starting in the 1970s. The earliest paper on retinal vessel segmentation of normal and abnormal vessels was published in 1973 [1]. Nevertheless, clinical application of such systems was to remain nil for an extended period of time. The reasons for this were common to most proposed systems for computer diagnosis, artificial intelligence, medical expert systems or what the fashionable term of the day might be, even outside of ophthalmology. Essentially, there was a lack of scientific evidence for disease categories and characteristics, based as they were on the implicit or explicit knowledge of one or a limited number of clinicians. At many different institutions in the world, elegant systems were designed and implemented. If a clinician from another institution came over to take a look and disagreed with the diagnosis, there would be no mechanism to decide which clinician, if any, was right. It is this fact that prevented application by anyone but the clinicians involved in the design of the system. In addition, these systems were solutions in search of a problem, not addressing diagnostic problems that were relevant to clinical practice. At that moment it was not yet appreciated that the balance of diagnostic accuracy versus system efficiency differs according to clinical need. For early detection of a disease by mass screening, high throughput at reduced accuracy is acceptable, while management of a condition, once diagnosed, requires the integration of large amounts of clinical data, and a high accuracy, with little need for high throughput. From here on, this chapter will mostly deal with early detection of eye disease.

For clinicians to appreciate the potential for these systems, several things had to change. Finally, in the 1980s and early 1990s, several positive circumstances became aligned. Most important, evidence based medicine, meaning clinical diagnoses and disease management based on scientific, well designed studies, and not on oral tradition, gained traction. Specifically in ophthalmology, the Diabetes Control and Complications Trial (DCCT, 1983–1993) [2] and the Early Treatment Diabetic Retinopathy Study (ETDRS, 1979–1989) [3–8], the largest clinical trials of their time, were monumental. As the reader may be aware, the reason we are discussing automatic screening and screening for diabetic retinopathy at all is because these trials showed that it was rational to look for early signs of retinopathy. If early diagnosis were possible, but no effective treatment had been available, there would be no rationale for screening.

Second, digital imaging of the retina became mainstream. Even though some of the most recent papers, including by our group, are still based on scanned slides because there is so much historical data available, it is clear that these systems can only work efficiently if digital images are available.

Finally, clinical data from representative patient populations, i.e., retinal photographs coupled with clinical readings, started becoming available to image analysis groups that previously had little or no access to clinicians. A pioneer was Hoover, who made available a set of 81 retinal images on the Internet to any interested researcher [9]. This contribution has allowed major strides to be made in vessel segmentation and optic disc localization [10], later enhanced by our DRIVE dataset [11]. Also, we and likely others as well have shared their expert annotated lesion image sets with other researchers on an informal basis. This sharing of clinical data is currently the most challenging issue. Though there are many advantages to sharing data, issues related to patient privacy, regulatory issues, for example, HIPAA in the United States or CBP in the Netherlands, investigational review boards requiring post hoc informed consent, fear of "losing the edge" in publishing papers, as well as patents based on supervised algorithms and therefore in part based on these datasets make this a contested area. To mitigate this, we have recently organized the first online challenge under the ROC (for Retinopathy Online Challenge) at http://roc.healthcare.uiowa.edu, and we hope to organize many of these in the future.

3.2 Approaches to Computer (Aided) Diagnosis

A system for computer aided diagnosis of the retina can either decide between disease and nondisease, i.e., diagnosis or screening, or can decide the progression of disease in the same patient between two time points, i.e., progression measurement or staging. Such a system can be built with what I term a bottom-up approach: to simulate as closely as possible the diagnosis or staging according to clinical standards as performed by human experts. For example, a system to diagnose diabetic retinopathy will detect the lesions that are known to clinicians to be related to diabetic retinopathy, such as hemorrhages and microaneurysms, and use the knowledge about the presence or absence of these lesions to estimate the probability of the presence of diabetic retinopathy. The advantages of this bottom-up approach are:

- face validity, i.e., clinicians trust the system because it mimics to some degree what they do daily, easing translation of such a system into clinical practice.

- availability of evidence showing that these classifications are valid, in other words, allow progression or outcome or need for intervention to be measured adequately. This avoids the need to evaluate the system against measures of disease or severity. Examples include the ETDRS [6] and the International Disease Severity Scale of diabetic retinopathy [12] gradings for diabetic retinopathy.

The disadvantages of the bottom-up approach are:

- a need to mimic the human visual system as closely as possible.

- a possibility of bias: the human expert may not be the optimal system for diagnosis or staging and not be fully knowledgeable or aware of all the features in the image.

- inflexibility: in the case in which imaging modalities, such as 3D Optical Coherence Tomography, are developed, human experts may not yet know what the important features are, and there is nothing to be mimicked.

Most research on computer (aided) diagnosis and staging from retinal images has used the bottom-up approach.

What we will term the top-down approach is to start with images in the one hand and diagnoses/stages or some other measurement of clinical outcome in the other, and design the system in an unbiased fashion by searching the feature detector space for the optimal characteristics of the image to predict the measurement of clinical outcome. In other words, those features of the images that are used by clinicians are simply ignored, and the system is optimized against the measurement of clinical outcome, without an intervening stage of human expert-based lesion detection.

The advantages are:

- theoretically, such a system has optimal performance that a bottom-up system cannot reach.

- if new characteristics or features are found that were not previously appreciated, these can help guide clinicians or researchers understand why these characteristics are so important.

- the system can be used on new imaging modalities, where clinicians do not (yet) know what is relevant for diagnosis or progression.

The disadvantages are:

- the system may not have face validity, making clinicians reluctant to trust it in clinical practice.

- the space of potential feature detectors may be huge, and intractable computationally.

To our knowledge, no systems based on such a top-down approach for diagnosis or staging of retinal disease from retinal images have been published. In the remainder of this chapter, we will therefore limit ourselves to a brief review of bottom-up systems.

3.3 Detection of Diabetic Retinopathy Lesions

We briefly review here the characteristic lesions that occur on the retina affected in diabetic retinopathy [8], and their approximate frequency in a typical screening population, in which 5 to 25% have some form of diabetic retinopathy [5; 8; 13–15].

- so-called "red lesions," namely microaneurysms and intraretinal hemorrhages (frequency $\sim 3.5\%$).

- so-called "bright lesions," namely exudates and cotton wool spots (most likely intraretinal infarcts) (frequency $\sim 1.6\%$).

- retinal thickening if present without bright or red lesions (frequency $\sim 1\%$).

- vascular beading (caliber changes of the vessels) (frequency $\sim 1\%$).

- intraretinal microvascular abnormalities (IRMA) (frequency $\sim 1\%$).

- new vessel growth on the optic disc (neovascularization of the disc or NVD) (frequency $< 0.1\%$).

- new vessel growth elsewhere (NVE) (frequency $< 0.1\%$).

- vitreous or subhyaloid hemorrhage (frequency $< 0.1\%$).

In previous papers, other authors as well as our group have referred to microaneurysms and intraretinal hemorrhages as "red lesions," to exudates and cotton wool spots as "bright lesions," and IRMA, NVD, and NVE as "neovascularizations." In most regions in the world, screening is performed with nonstereo digital cameras, which means that it is impossible to detect retinal thickening if no bright or red lesions are present. Neovascularizations are rare, but are important because they need urgent referral for management by an ophthalmologist. In the next section, we review the literature on how each of these objects can be detected.

3.4 Detection of Lesions and Segmentation of Retinal Anatomy

Research of methods for segmentation of retinal vessels shows that the most recent methods can segment over 99% or more of the larger vessels (arbitrarily stated here as > 2 pixels wide) [9; 11; 16–28], even in retinal images that exhibit some to severe retinopathy. The main research emphasis is on making these methods more robust in the face of more severe retinal disease, making them independent of image scale as a parameter, improving the time and memory efficiency of the algorithms, and finally detecting vessel abnormalities [29; 30].

Segmentation of red lesions (microaneurysms and hemorrhages) has also proceeded rapidly, to the point where combined sensitivity/specificity of 95%/95% are reported [16; 31–39].

Bright lesions (exudates and cotton wool spots) have received less attention, but even there, detection rates of up to 95% have been reported [40–46].

Neovascularizations have usually been grouped with red lesions, but merit a separate algorithm, because these can be subtle, which to date has not yet been published.

Many authors have successfully studied the localization of retinal landmarks, including the optic disc, large vessels, and fovea [16; 17; 42; 47–52]. In summary, as of 2007, detection of most lesions is possible with a degree of accuracy that compares favorably to human experts. We have not dealt with determination of image quality, a very important subject that is briefly discussed in Chapter 6 in regard to microaneurysm detection.

3.5 Detection and Staging of Diabetic Retinopathy: Pixel to Patient

Either implicitly or explicitly, any bottom-up system must have stages where pixels are classified into lesions or textures. Lesions or textures are detected in individual images, the presence or absence of different lesions or textures is used to determine an estimate for the presence or stage of the retinopathy for a patient. Complete systems have been published, but the authors usually have not dealt explicitly with how pixel features, lesion or texture features, and lesion location estimates are combined into this patient level estimate statement [37; 41; 44; 50; 53–55]. We have designed a supervised method for combining the output of bright-lesion and image quality algorithms and tested it on 10000 exams (40000 retinal images) from a community diabetic retinopathy screening project. Retinal images came from a variety of non-mydriatic camera types, as is typical for screening projects, and were read by only a single reader. The results of this preliminary study showed that this system could obtain an area under the ROC (receiver operating characteristic) curve of 0.84 [56]. Meanwhile we have made further improvements to the system, and at ARVO 2008 we have presented the performance of a different sample of unique patients that obtained an area under the curve of 0.88.

3.6 Directions for Research

From the above it can be concluded that there are several avenues to translate computer (aided) diagnosis of diabetic retinopathy into clinical practice. First, the value of high quality, representative, expert graded image sets cannot be overrated. High quality does not mean that the images should all be of excellent quality. High quality means that the image sets represent the type, quality, and variety of images in a real world screening setting, as well as having the same distribution of lesion types and frequency of the presence of diabetic retinopathy as true in such screening populations. In other words, the images should not come from a tertiary clinic, where diabetic retinopathy is usually much more severe and may be easier to detect than in a screening setting, where commonly only a few subtle lesions may be detectable. Also, high quality means that the images have been read by multiple, internationally respected, expert readers, so that a reference standard is available that is not subject to dispute by other experts. In the case of diabetes and diabetic retinopathy, the readings for the images of a patient, which are usually made with a nonmydriatic camera, should optimally not be obtained by having human experts read the same images, but from multiple or 7-field stereo fundus photographs read by a reading center, the gold standard for clinical trials. If such datasets can be made publicly available, evaluation and comparison of algorithms will be much easier, hopefully leading to more meaningful performance comparisons.

Second, given that the bottom-up approach, meaning detection of lesions and then estimation of diabetic retinopathy diagnosis or stage, is currently the most popular approach, it makes sense to mimic the human visual system as closely as possible, as we and other authors have either implicitly or explicitly attempted using results from visual neuroscience experiments and knowledge about the primate visual cortex [57].

Third, vessel segmentation has always been a mainstay of retinal image analysis research, even though so far it has had limited relevance for systems that screen for diabetic retinopathy. Detection of neovascularizations in diabetic retinopathy, or pigment texture changes in age-related macular degeneration, which are known to have clinical relevance, have received little or no attention in the image analysis community. If clinical needs and algorithmic development can be merged closer, this will benefit the field tremendously.

And finally, a top-down approach where images and clinical outcomes such as visual loss or need for surgery can be combined directly, so that such a system predicts the probability of outcome or of the need for treatment, has the potential to offer higher accuracy. There may well be more in retinal images than the lesions that have "met the eye" of the clinical beholder of the past. The translation of such systems into clinical practice may be problematic, unless such systems can give at least some explanation of their conclusion that is understandable by clinicians.

In summary, the field of automated detection of retinal disease, in general, and diabetic retinopathy, in particular, is currently developing rapidly. Great strides have been made already and may soon lead to the first systems tested for clinical application, and thereby to decreasing blindness and visual loss in patients with retinal diseases.

References

[1] Matsui, M., Tashiro, T., Matsumoto, K., et al., A study on automatic and quantitative diagnosis of fundus photographs. I. Detection of contour line of retinal blood vessel images on color fundus photographs, *Nippon Ganka Gakkai Zasshi*, 77(8), 907, 1973, In Japanese.

[2] DCCT Research Group, The Diabetes Control and Complications Trial (DCCT). Design and methodologic considerations for the feasibility phase, *Diabetes*, 35, 530, 1986.

[3] Early Treatment Diabetic Retinopathy Study Research Group, Photocoagulation for diabetic macular edema. Early Treatment Diabetic Retinopathy Study Report Number 1, *Arch. Ophthalmol.*, 103(12), 1796, 1985.

[4] Early Treatment Diabetic Retinopathy Study Research Group, Treatment techniques and clinical guidelines for photocoagulation of diabetic macular edema. Early Treatment Diabetic Retinopathy Study Report Number 2, *Ophthalmology*, 94(7), 761, 1987.

[5] Early Treatment Diabetic Retinopathy Study Research Group, Fundus photographic risk factors for progression of diabetic retinopathy. ETDRS Report Number 12, *Ophthalmology*, 98(5 Suppl), 823, 1991.

[6] Early Treatment Diabetic Retinopathy Study Research Group, Classification of diabetic retinopathy from fluorescein angiograms. ETDRS Report Number 11, *Ophthalmology*, 98(5 Suppl), 807, 1991.

[7] Early Treatment Diabetic Retinopathy Study Research Group, Early photocoagulation for diabetic retinopathy. ETDRS Report Number 9, *Ophthalmology*, 98(5 Suppl), 766, 1991.

[8] Early Treatment Diabetic Retinopathy Study Research Group, Focal photocoagulation treatment of diabetic macular edema. relationship of treatment effect to fluorescein angiographic and other retinal characteristics at baseline: ETDRS Report Number 19, *Arch. Ophthalmol.*, 113(9), 1144, 1995.

[9] Hoover, A., Kouznetsova, V., and Goldbaum, M., Locating blood vessels in retinal images by piecewise threshold probing of a matched filter response, *IEEE Trans. Med. Im.*, 19(3), 203, 2000.

[10] Hoover, A. and Goldbaum, M., Locating the optic nerve in a retinal image using the fuzzy convergence of the blood vessels, *IEEE Trans. Med. Im.*, 22(8), 951, 2003.

[11] Niemeijer, M., Staal, J.S., van Ginneken, B., et al., Comparative study of retinal vessel segmentation on a new publicly available database, *Proceedings of the SPIE*, 5370–5379, 2004.

[12] Wilkinson, C.P., Ferris, F. L., I., Klein, R.E., et al., Proposed international clinical diabetic retinopathy and diabetic macular edema disease severity scales, *Ophthalmology*, 110(9), 1677, 2003.

[13] Bresnick, G.H., Mukamel, D.B., Dickinson, J.C., et al., A screening approach to the surveillance of patients with diabetes for the presence of vision-threatening retinopathy, *Ophthalmology*, 107(1), 19, 2000.

[14] Lin, D.Y., Blumenkranz, M.S., Brothers, R.J., et al., The sensitivity and specificity of single-field nonmydriatic monochromatic digital fundus photography with remote image interpretation for diabetic retinopathy screening: A comparison with ophthalmoscopy and standardized mydriatic color photography, *Am. J. Ophthalmol.*, 134(2), 204, 2002.

[15] Abramoff, M.D. and Suttorp-Schulten, M.S., Web-based screening for diabetic retinopathy in a primary care population: The EyeCheck project, *Telemed. J. E. Health*, 11(6), 668, 2005.

[16] Frame, A.J., Undrill, P.E., Cree, M.J., et al., A comparison of computer based classification methods applied to the detection of microaneurysms in ophthalmic fluorescein angiograms, *Comput. Biol. Med.*, 28(3), 225, 1998.

[17] Sinthanayothin, C., Boyce, J.F., Cook, H.L., et al., Automated localisation of the optic disc, fovea, and retinal blood vessels from digital colour fundus images, *Br. J. Ophthalmol.*, 83(8), 902, 1999.

[18] Staal, J.S., Kalitzin, S.N., Abramoff, M.D., et al., Classifying convex sets for vessel detection in retinal images, in *Proceedings of the First International Symposium on Biomedical Imaging*, 2002, 269–272.

[19] Staal, J., Abramoff, M.D., Niemeijer, M., et al., Ridge-based vessel segmentation in color images of the retina, *IEEE Trans. Med. Im.*, 23(4), 501, 2004.

[20] Vermeer, K.A., Vos, F.M., Lemij, H.G., et al., A model based method for retinal blood vessel detection, *Comput. Biol. Med.*, 34(3), 209, 2004.

[21] Fang, B. and Tang, Y.Y., Elastic registration for retinal images based on reconstructed vascular trees, *IEEE Trans. Biomed. Eng.*, 53(6), 1183, 2006.

[22] Chanwimaluang, T., Fan, G., and Fransen, S.R., Hybrid retinal image registration, *IEEE Trans. Inf. Technol. Biomed.*, 10(1), 129, 2006.

[23] Huang, K. and Yan, M., A region based algorithm for vessel detection in retinal images, in *Ninth International Conference on Medical Image Computing and Computer Assisted Intervention (MICCAI'06)*, 2006, vol. 9(1), 645–653.

[24] Cai, W. and Chung, A.C., Multi-resolution vessel segmentation using normalized cuts in retinal images, in *Ninth International Conference on Medical Image Computing and Computer Assisted Intervention (MICCAI'06)*, 2006, vol. 9, Pt 2, 928–936.

[25] Soares, J.V., Leandro, J.J., Cesar Junior, R.M., et al., Retinal vessel segmentation using the 2-D Gabor wavelet and supervised classification, *IEEE Trans. Med. Im.*, 25(9), 1214, 2006.

[26] Mendonca, A.M. and Campilho, A., Segmentation of retinal blood vessels by combining the detection of centerlines and morphological reconstruction, *IEEE Trans. Med. Im.*, 25(9), 1200, 2006.

[27] Adjeroh, D.A., Kandaswamy, U., and Odom, J.V., Texton-based segmentation of retinal vessels, *J. Opt. Soc. Am. A*, 24(5), 1384, 2007.

[28] Wang, L., Bhalerao, A., and Wilson, R., Analysis of retinal vasculature using a multiresolution hermite model, *IEEE Trans. Med. Im.*, 26(2), 137, 2007.

[29] Kozousck, V., Shen, Z., Gregson, P., et al., Automated detection and quantification of venous beading using Fourier analysis, *Can. J. Ophthalmol.*, 27(6), 288, 1992.

[30] Englmeier, K.H., Schmid, K., Hildebrand, C., et al., Early detection of diabetes retinopathy by new algorithms for automatic recognition of vascular changes, *Eur. J. Med. Res.*, 9(10), 473, 2004.

[31] Baudoin, C.E., Lay, B.J., and Klein, J.C., Automatic detection of microaneurysms in diabetic fluorescein angiography, *Rev. Epidemiol. Sante Publique*, 32(3-4), 254, 1984.

[32] Spencer, T., Olson, J.A., McHardy, K.C., et al., An image-processing strategy for the segmentation and quantification of microaneurysms in fluorescein angiograms of the ocular fundus, *Comput. Biomed. Res.*, 29(4), 284, 1996.

[33] Cree, M.J., Olson, J.A., McHardy, K.C., et al., A fully automated comparative microaneurysm digital detection system, *Eye*, 11, 622, 1997.

[34] Hipwell, J.H., Strachan, F., Olson, J.A., et al., Automated detection of microaneurysms in digital red-free photographs: a diabetic retinopathy screening tool, *Diabet. Med.*, 17(8), 588, 2000.

[35] Niemeijer, M., van Ginniken, B., and Abramoff, M.D., Automatic detection and classification of microaneurysms and small hemorrhages in color fundus

photographs, in *Proceedings Computer Aided Fundus Imaging and Analysis (CAFIA)*, 2003.

[36] Larsen, M., Godt, J., Larsen, N., et al., Automated detection of fundus photographic red lesions in diabetic retinopathy, *Invest. Ophthalmol. Vis. Sci.*, 44(2), 761, 2003.

[37] Larsen, N., Godt, J., Grunkin, M., et al., Automated detection of diabetic retinopathy in a fundus photographic screening population, *Invest. Ophthalmol. Vis. Sci.*, 44(2), 767, 2003.

[38] Fleming, A.D., Philip, S., Goatman, K.A., et al., Automated microaneurysm detection using local contrast normalization and local vessel detection, *IEEE Trans. Med. Im.*, 25(9), 1223, 2006.

[39] Niemeijer, M., van Ginneken, B., Staal, J., et al., Automatic detection of red lesions in digital color fundus photographs, *IEEE Trans Med. Imaging*, 24(5), 584, 2005.

[40] Abramoff, M.D., Staal, J.S., Suttorp-van Schulten, M.S., et al., Low level screening of exudates and haemorraghes in background diabetic retinopathy, in *Proceedings Computer Assisted Fundus Imaging Workshop (CAFIA)*, Copenhagen, Denmark, 2000.

[41] Sinthanayothin, C., Boyce, J.F., Williamson, T.H., et al., Automated detection of diabetic retinopathy on digital fundus images, *Diabet. Med.*, 19(2), 105, 2002.

[42] Walter, T., Klein, J.C., Massin, P., et al., A contribution of image processing to the diagnosis of diabetic retinopathy — detection of exudates in color fundus images of the human retina, *IEEE Trans. Med. Im.*, 21(10), 1236, 2002.

[43] Osareh, A., Mirmehdi, M., Thomas, B., et al., Automated identification of diabetic retinal exudates in digital colour images, *Br. J. Ophthalmol.*, 87(10), 1220, 2003.

[44] Usher, D., Dumskyj, M., Himaga, M., et al., Automated detection of diabetic retinopathy in digital retinal images: a tool for diabetic retinopathy screening, *Diabet. Med.*, 21(1), 84, 2004.

[45] Li, H. and Chutatape, O., Automated feature extraction in color retinal images by a model based approach, *IEEE Trans. Biomed. Eng.*, 51(2), 246, 2004.

[46] Niemeijer, M., Russell, S.R., Suttorp, M.A., et al., Automated detection and differentiation of drusen, exudates, and cotton-wool spots in digital color fundus photographs for early diagnosis of diabetic retinopathy, *Invest. Ophthalmol. Vis. Sci.*, 48, 2260, 2007.

[47] Goldbaum, M.H., Katz, N.P., Nelson, M.R., et al., The discrimination of similarly colored objects in computer images of the ocular fundus, *Invest. Ophthalmol. Vis. Sci.*, 31(4), 617, 1990.

[48] Foracchia, M., Grisan, E., and Ruggeri, A., Detection of optic disc in retinal images by means of a geometrical model of vessel structure, *IEEE Trans. Med. Im.*, 23(10), 1189, 2004.

[49] Abramoff, M.D. and Niemeijer, M., Automatic detection of the optic disc location in retinal images using optic disc location regression, in *IEEE EMBC 2006*, New York, NY, 2006, 4432–4435.

[50] Singalavanija, A., Supokavej, J., Bamroongsuk, P., et al., Feasibility study on computer-aided screening for diabetic retinopathy, *Jpn. J. Ophthalmol.*, 50(4), 361, 2006.

[51] Niemeijer, M., Abramoff, M.D., and van Ginneken, B., Segmentation of the optic disc, macula and vascular arch in fundus photographs, *IEEE Trans. Med. Im.*, 26(1), 116, 2007.

[52] Tobin, K.W., Chaum, E., Priya Govindasamy, V., et al., Detection of anatomic structures in human retinal imagery, *IEEE Trans. Med. Imaging*, 26(12), 1729, 2007.

[53] Gardner, G.G., Keating, D., Williamson, T.H., et al., Automatic detection of diabetic retinopathy using an artificial neural network: a screening tool, *Br. J. Ophthalmol*, 80(11), 940, 1996.

[54] Teng, T., Lefley, M., and Claremont, D., Progress towards automated diabetic ocular screening: a review of image analysis and intelligent systems for diabetic retinopathy, *Med. Biol. Eng. Comput.*, 40(1), 2, 2002.

[55] Patton, N., Aslam, T.M., MacGillivray, T., et al., Retinal image analysis: concepts, applications and potential, *Prog. Retin. Eye Res.*, 25(1), 99, 2006.

[56] Abramoff, M.D., Niemeijer, M., Suttorp-Schulten, M.S.A., et al., Evaluation of a system for automatic detection of diabetic retinopathy from color fundus photographs in a large population of patients with diabetes, *Diabetes Care*, 31, 193, 2008.

[57] Abramoff, M.D., Alward, W.L., Greenlee, E.C., et al., Automated segmentation of the optic nerve head from stereo color photographs using physiologically plausible feature detectors, *Inv. Ophthalmol. Vis. Sci.*, 48, 1665, 2007.

4

Finding a Role for Computer-Aided Early Diagnosis of Diabetic Retinopathy

Lars B. Bäcklund

CONTENTS

4.1 Mass Examinations of Eyes in Diabetes................................... 79
4.2 Developing and Defending a Risk Reduction Program 82
4.3 Assessing Accuracy of a Diagnostic Test................................. 84
4.4 Improving Detection of Diabetic Retinopathy 90
4.5 Measuring Outcomes of Risk Reduction Programs 93
4.6 User Experiences of Computer-Aided Diagnosis 96
4.7 Planning a Study to Evaluate Accuracy 103
4.8 Conclusion.. 110
    References 110
4.A Appendix: Measures of Binary Test Performance 120

There are strong reasons why well-designed retinopathy risk reduction programs need to be implemented on a large scale. The importance of such programs, and the difficulty of achieving reliable early diagnosis of diabetic retinopathy (DR) at reasonable cost, merit considerable efforts in order to develop and evaluate computer-aided diagnosis (CAD). So why is CAD software not yet widely used in this setting? Problems and diverse application possibilities encountered by people responsible for such programs need to be considered in conjunction with the opportunities and threats facing anyone introducing computer-aided diagnosis in this field.

4.1 Mass Examinations of Eyes in Diabetes

There are many reasons why everybody who has diabetes should receive regular eye examinations. Vision loss due to diabetes is greatly feared by people with diabetes; indeed, the results of a survey conducted by the American Foundation for the Blind indicate that people with diabetes fear blindness even more than premature death [1]. Considerable income losses and costs are borne by people with diabetes and their families, by society, and by health-care providers. Ocular complications of diabetes frequently occur [2], causing major economic and social problems and impairing quality of life. Diabetic eye disease may progress to a level that is threatening sight without causing symptoms that may bring the person with diabetes to a doctor [3]. Hence, maximum uptake of screening and of timely re-screening is necessary: there is incontrovertible evidence that timely treatment prevents or delays loss of sight [4]. Large settlements have been paid to people diagnosed with sight-threatening diabetic retinopathy (STDR) — a family of conditions defined by some but not all authors as severe nonproliferative DR and/or proliferative DR and/or hard exudates within one disc diameter of the center of the fovea — too late for effective treatment. Diabetes prevalence now seems to be increasing even more rapidly than previously predicted [5].

It is thus not surprising that considerable efforts have been made to diagnose DR and STDR at early stages when timely treatment may slow or prevent worsening of DR and prevent vision loss. There are, however, important lessons to be learned regarding how to set up, carry out and monitor such a program.

4.1.1   Motive for accurate early diagnosis of retinopathy

To quote one of the maxims attributed to Publilius Syrus, who lived in the 1st century BC, "Better use medicines at the outset than at the last moment." This should be possible because accurate diagnosis of DR and its various stages can deliver feedback information to patients and other members of diabetes teams. There is clear evidence from well-designed controlled clinical trials that improved medical treatment delays or prevents the occurrence of STDR. For full effect, however, five to seven years are needed. Therefore, early diagnosis of the earliest signs of DR and accurate follow-up of progression of DR at predefined intervals will provide necessary information for diabetes management in order for prognosis to be deduced and, importantly, in time for improved treatment to be effective.

As described in a prior chapter (Section 2.9.2.1), there is clear evidence from well-designed controlled clinical trials that the right kind of timely laser photocoagulation of STDR prevents or delays worsening of visual acuity. Moreover, promising new methods for treatment of inflammation and other aspects of DR are underway, causing increased interest among diabetologists for the reliable diagnosis of DR stages preceding STDR.

From the point of view of ophthalmologists, it is important not to become overloaded with large numbers of diabetic patients not strictly needing immediate treatment by a retinal specialist. From the patient's point of view, however, securing timely treatment is of high importance. There will probably never be enough ophthalmologists to follow-up every person with diabetes by clinical examination. Thus, we need a systematic approach to delivering the right patient at the right time to the right doctor to ensure adequate and timely treatment.

4.1.2 Definition of screening

Screening may be defined as a public health intervention intended to improve the health of a precisely defined target population (in this case, people with diabetes). Within this population are individuals considered at risk of the effects of a condition (in this case, diabetic retinopathy that may threaten sight).

Screening is justified by the awareness of that condition as an important public health problem. It is the anticipated identification of those who may have a problem and who might benefit from further investigation and treatment. It therefore involves the application of a quick and simple test, usually by paramedics, to large numbers of asymptomatic persons so that those with a possible problem can be identified — and interventions can be made.

Screening does not make the final diagnosis — this is why the term *early diagnosis* is preferred by certain careful workers whose standards of image quality and reliability of grading are consistently high enough to enable a final diagnosis of DR or STDR to be made.

4.1.3 Practical importance of the concept of screening

Screening is never something that should be undertaken casually and it should always be carefully monitored and evaluated. Without strict criteria, monitoring is impossible.

"Opportunistic screening" is a concept and a term that should be avoided [6]. Unfortunately, some ophthalmologists understand "screening" to mean hurried global diagnostic impressions unworthy of adequate recording of findings. Screening, in contrast, means a systematic approach that has nothing to do with improvisation. The term "ad hoc screening" is thus a misnomer.

Screening is expensive and is an intervention that is thrust on the public rather than a response to an individual seeking help for a symptom. It must, therefore, be constantly and carefully monitored both for its processes and its effectiveness.

False negative tests are a constant source of concern, and there is often public outrage when an important condition such as STDR or cancer of the cervix has been missed. *False positive tests* cause undue anxiety and wasted resources (in the case of DR misdiagnosed as STDR, invasive tests such as fluorescein angiography may have been performed unnecessarily).

4.1.4 Coverage and timely re-examination

For the screening program to be effective, it must reach a high proportion (ideally 100%) of the population at risk. Failure to achieve this leads to the failure of the program to meet its targets. *Coverage* is defined as the proportion of the target population successfully tested in each screening activity.

Reaching out into the community is important [7]. Keep in mind that those hardest to reach in a screening program may suffer from the worst disease. In diabetes, it may be the bilateral amputee, the senior citizen who is in denial of "maybe just a touch of sugar" (and whose eyes have therefore never been examined), or the resentful/indifferent young person with diabetes who are the least likely to comply with an invitation for an eye examination — and yet they might be the most likely to be in need of treatment [6]. There is some evidence that visual handicap is associated with poor attendance at diabetes clinics [8], which underlines the importance of finding people with diabetes and making efforts to improve coverage of eye examinations.

Uptake, defined as the proportion attending of all those invited, is always higher than population coverage, because some are not invited for various reasons. Some successful programs have reached more than 75% initial screen uptake and more than 85% reattendance. Ascertainment of diabetes is difficult because early stages of the disease are asymptomatic — at best two out of three people with diabetes are diagnosed in everyday health-care settings. Coverage of DR screening is thus likely to be overestimated. Coverage and uptake affect the recorded prevalence of DR and of its various stages, thus also influencing measured sensitivity and specificity of CAD software.

Many barriers to care need to be overcome [9]. Working together with diabetes organizations, patient groups, and primary health-care staff is one way of increasing coverage [10]. Good advice on reaching out into the community is available from the Centre for Eye Research Australia [11, pp. 24–60]. Apparently, achieving timely re-screening at predefined intervals is even more difficult than optimizing coverage of first examination [12]; both are important for long-term outcomes of the program.

4.2   Developing and Defending a Risk Reduction Program

To achieve the outcome of reducing the incidence of vision loss in diabetes, early diagnosis of DR is not enough. To emphasize the objective of the program and the need to ensure timely treatment, the term *risk reduction program* is employed [12] in preference to "screening program."

4.2.1   Explaining why retinopathy is suitable for screening

To ensure its success, a risk reduction program needs to be developed in cooperation with a great number of people, institutions, companies, and organizations, and they may need convincing of the case for supporting DR screening when there are so many other screening proposals competing for interest and for resources [13]. A succinct overview of the available evidence is available from several sources, including the Scottish Intercollegiate Guidelines Network, SIGN (http://www.sign.ac.uk/guidelines/fulltext/55/section6.html#274).

4.2.2   Understanding reasons for possible criticism

A risk reduction program may meet with opposition from unexpected quarters. To try to understand why this is so, the point of view of each interested party must be taken into account. Opticians and optometrists may fear for their future income and market penetration. Ophthalmologists who cherish their clinical freedom and their power over their working day might not enjoy the feeling of being told by screeners what to do and when — even if such suggestions are being made in the nicest possible way. Economists and managers can make all sorts of objections based on the need for resources and the low probability of quick monetary return; it may be more profitable for an eye clinic to perform the extensive photocoagulation program necessary for late-stage STDR than to perform early treatment that may stop progression. Politicians are likely to show limited interest in interventions whose outcomes may not appear as good news in time for the next elections. According to folklore, vision problems are inevitable in old age and an integral part of the disease of diabetes; having read the previous chapter, however, you should be able to refute such statements. Few health economists appear to be in favor of screening programs; in the case of STDR, however, there is a good paper to cite that is based on hard evidence [14]. Be prepared to hire a health economist whose efforts could help you market your program. A good recent paper to cite comes from Scotland [15].

The word "screening" itself has a bad name in certain circles; this may be because some people think that population-oriented interventions encroach on individual freedom. Many questions of ethics have been discussed [13]. Moreover, several proposed programs such as PSA (prostate-specific antibody) screening have become the subject of considerable critical discussion, partly because their value to the individual participant is unclear. A dartboard model has been developed for use in shared decision making to show the likely consequences of one person's decision whether or not to participate in PSA screening [16]. Good DR detection programs, in contrast, are based on strong evidence and should not be lumped together with programs of unknown value.

4.2.3   Fulfilling criteria for screening tests

Some rational arguments of long standing deserve to be mentioned — at least in brief. Early enthusiasm for mass screening programs based on biochemical tests increased in the 1950s with the advent of cost-effective automated analyzers, but soon waned; for instance, if ten tests are performed, each with a reference range covering 90% or 95% of the population, the probability of at least one false positive test comes close to 50% [17].

Because such attempts at screening caused more problems than were solved, efforts were made to define why, how, and when screening for disease would be acceptable. Stringent *criteria for mass screening programs* were published [18] and several other criteria for screening tests or programs were devised later. It might seem unlikely that any disease, any screening test, or any screening program could be acceptable according to all such strict rules. Actually, DR is one of the few diseases for which screening programs exist that fulfill such criteria [19].

4.2.4   Setting quality assurance standards

There is consensus that a reliable list of patients, suitable equipment kept in good working order, trained photographers and graders, reference images, quality assurance schemes, as well as other factors ensuring good coverage and accurate diagnosis are necessary for success [20].

A particularly useful document is called *Workbook* (at the time of writing in its 4th edition, January 2007, updated March 2008) describing essential elements in developing a program [21]. You should download it and read it now.

The Scottish national standards are worth reading [22]. Furthermore, in Appendix 2 of the *Workbook* [21] there is a list of *service objectives* and *quality assurance standards*; these targets are very hard to meet but extremely important. A preliminary version of those standards was tested on 10 existing services [12] with varying results. Further information on service objectives is available on the NSC Web site (http://www.nscretinopathy.org.uk), providing links to other sites.

In 1998 the U.K. National Screening Committee, NSC, distinguished between a screening *program* and a screening *test*. A program "'consists of all those activities from the identification of the population likely to benefit through to the definitive diagnosis and treatment,' with inherent characteristics: explicit quality standards; an information system, which allows comparison of performance with these standards; managerial authority to take action to improve quality" [12].

4.2.5   Training and assessment

Training courses and competence criteria are in development in many countries. See the United Kingdom NSC Web site (http://www.nscretinopathy.org.uk) under *Training documents and advice*. The Scottish training manual [20] is highly recommended. An Australian manual [11] contains useful links. An American perspective on ophthalmic photography [23] and digital imaging for DR screening [24] is available.

4.3   Assessing Accuracy of a Diagnostic Test

Sensitivity is the proportion of disease positive individuals who are detected by the test, also known as the *true positive fraction* (TPF). An ideal test has a sensitivity of 100% (TPF = 1).

Specificity is the proportion of disease free people correctly labeled as disease free. An ideal test has a specificity of 100% meaning that the *false positive fraction* (FPF) is zero and $(1 - \text{FPF}) = 1$.

Some experts [25] desire sensitivity for detection of STDR to be at least 80% (TPF ≥ 0.8). This has reportedly been achieved by a number of studies, most of them by high-quality fundus photography through pharmacologically dilated pupils using color transparency film, trained graders, and a quality assurance system [26]. Because low sensitivity entails delayed detection of STDR and increased risk of vision loss, high sensitivity is important to the patient. Note that the less advanced is the disease, the lower the sensitivity will be [27].

Some experts [25] desire specificity for detection of STDR to be at least 95%, i.e., $(1 - FPF) \geq 0.95$, which is reportedly achievable by various methods [26] and important to the person making the final diagnosis, who might be subjected to unnecessary effort (while the patient risks unnecessary costs, travel, and workup procedures).

The "Exeter Standards" for sensitivity and specificity [25] were set in 1984 at a meeting organized by Diabetes UK (then the British Diabetic Association) and later accepted by the UK National Screening Framework. A recent review is available on the Web at http://www.nscretinopathy.org.uk/pages/nsc.asp?ModT=A&Sec=16. Most published studies have insufficient statistical power for conclusions to be made. This criticism, however, does not apply to the Gloucestershire study [28] in which one experienced ophthalmologist examined 1594 randomly selected people with diabetes who also underwent mydriatic 45° two-field imaging; sensitivity for the latter was 87.8%, specificity 86.1%. Improving on this result using new methods for imaging, quality assurance, and grading will indeed be challenging. Incidentally, this ophthalmologist did exceptionally well when compared to seven field stereo photography of 229 people with diabetes [29].

Since $(1 - TPF)$ is equal to the false negative fraction, the pair (FPF, TPF) defines the probabilities with which errors occur when using the test. A note of caution: these are proportions or probabilities — never call them "rates" in front of an epidemiologist [30]. Moreover, the pair (FPF, TPF) is just one point of the receiver operating curve and thus of limited interest; see below.

Joint confidence regions for TPF and FPF can be presented as numbers (rectangular regions derived from cross-products of confidence intervals for TPF and FPF) in order to save space. As a reader I prefer graphs showing elliptical joint confidence regions based on joint asymptotic normality. This is something to look for in published papers. Many studies of diagnostic methods are underpowered, which shows up as imprecise estimation (wide confidence regions).

4.3.1   Predictive value, estimation, power

Accuracy can be quantified by how well the test result predicts the true disease status [31]. Please note that the test should be studied in a wide variety of circumstances in which its ability to predict true clinical status may vary. *Predictive values* quantify accuracy by how well the test predicts the status. They are often presented together with sensitivity and specificity data for a test. The predictive value of a positive test, *positive predictive value* (PPV), is the probability that the subject is diseased if the test is positive. The predictive value of a negative test, *negative predictive value* (NPV), is the probability that the subject is nondiseased when the test is negative.

A perfect test will predict disease perfectly, with PPV = 1 and NPV = 1. The predictive values depend not only on the performance of the test in diseased and nondiseased subjects, but also on the prevalence of disease. A low PPV may be a result of low prevalence of disease, or an unreliable test, or both [32]. Predictive values quantify the clinical value of the test: the patient and the doctor want to know how likely it is that disease is present given the test result [33]. A screening test needs to be more accurate if it is to work well in a low-prevalence situation such as a screening program. Conversely, lower sensitivity may be acceptable in tertiary care where disease prevalence is high. A truism worth thinking about is that it is much easier to ascertain large advanced lesions (seen in a tertiary care setting) than subtle initial lesions (such as those seen in screening programs). As every grader knows, it is quite difficult for graders to agree whether minimal DR is present or absent in an image from a screening program [34]. Interestingly, the Aberdeen group has presented good results from "disease/no disease" CAD grading in Scotland [35]; their papers are recommended reading. There is a recruitment effect known from psychological research: once the first microaneurysm is identified, more of them are suddenly perceived. A good CAD algorithm could be more sensitive than humans for minimal DR but perhaps less sensitive for advanced DR with atypical manifestations. Data such as TPF, FPF, PPV, and NPV are thus context dependent.

TPF, FPF, PPV, and NPV are proportions. Authors reporting them should always provide the raw data in a contingency table. *Estimation* is preferred to hypothesis testing. Confidence intervals for proportions and for differences between proportions can be calculated and software is available in a book [36]; exact methods, which according to some statisticians may give conservative results [37], are available, e.g., in StatXact software (www.cytelsoftware.com). I repeat that you are likely to find that many studies of diagnostic tests are underpowered, yielding imprecise estimates (wide confidence intervals). This observation particularly applies when analyzing subgroups whose properties may influence the outcome of the test. Consequently, *prestudy power calculations* have been recommended [38]. For instance, when the number of patients with the target condition is 49 the two-sided 95% confidence interval of a sensitivity of 81% (40 true positives) is 68% to 91%. One of the first questions your statistician is likely to ask is whether you want to falsify a null hypothesis of *equivalence* between the index test and the reference test, or if you want to falsify a null hypothesis of *nonsuperiority*. The latter could need a larger study population, depending on design and analysis methods.

Overcalling (reporting a higher-than-warranted DR grade) needlessly causes alarm in people with diabetes and wastes ophthalmology resources. *Undercalling* (reporting a lower-than-warranted DR grade) can have serious consequences for the person with diabetes, especially when STDR is missed and laser treatment is ineffective because of delay. Slattery undertook a computer simulation of ways of sampling referral decisions during grading and criteria for initiating intensive quality assurance (QA) investigations. Assessing the effectiveness of QA systems by the ability to detect a grader (or a CAD program) making occasional errors, he found that substantial sample sizes are needed to ensure against inappropriate failure to refer (false negatives). Under certain plausible assumptions, detection of a grader who fails to refer as many as 10% of cases with referrable STDR can only be achieved with a probability of 0.58 using an annual sample size of 300, and 0.77 with 500. The same sample sizes would only have probabilities 0.33 and 0.55, respectively, of detecting a grader (or program) missing 5% of referrals [39].

Calculating statistical power, a job for your statistician, becomes more complicated when multiple tests are performed on one subject. In medical practice, the results of several different tests (or algorithms) are combined to reach a threshold value or decision rule. The diagnostic accuracy of *combinations of tests* can be assessed by applying multivariable regression analysis with receiver operating characteristic curves.

4.3.2   Receiver operating characteristic curve

The *receiver operating characteristic* (ROC) *curve* is a useful way of describing the performance of medical tests whose results are not simply positive or negative, but are measured on continuous or ordinal scales. Suitable use of ROC curves helps designers of a test choose the optimal combination of sensitivity and specificity. ROC curves, now in frequent use by developers of CAD software, were first used half a century ago. They arose in the context of signal detection theory and were first applied to radar operators, coming into use in medicine from 1960 onwards [40], particularly in radiology [41].

Assume that larger values of the test result Y are more indicative of disease. The notion of using Y to define a dichotomous decision rule is fundamental to the evaluation of medical tests. The surgeon needs a yes or no answer on the question whether to operate at once. The decision rule is based on whether or not the test result (or some transformation of it) exceeds a *threshold* value. The choice of a suitable threshold will vary with circumstances and depends on the trade-off that is acceptable between failing to detect disease and falsely identifying disease with the test. The ROC curve describes the range of trade-offs that can be achieved by the test [42].

For continuous tests (e.g., microaneurysm counts, blood vessel diameter measurements), using a threshold c, define a binary test from the continuous test result Y as positive if $Y \geq c$, negative if $Y < c$. Let the corresponding true and false positive fractions at the threshold c be $\mathrm{TPF}(c)$ and $\mathrm{FPF}(c)$, respectively. The ROC curve is the entire set of possible true and false positive fractions attainable by dichotomizing Y with different thresholds.

An *uninformative* test is one such that Y is unrelated to disease status. That is, the probability distributions for Y are the same in the diseased and the nondiseased populations, and for any threshold c we have $\mathrm{TPF}(c) = \mathrm{FPF}(c)$ and the ROC curve becomes a line with unit slope (Figure 4.1).

A *perfect* test on the other hand completely separates diseased and nondiseased subjects. That is, for some threshold c we have $\mathrm{TPF}(c) = 1$ and $\mathrm{FPF}(c) = 0$ (in other words 100% sensitivity and 100% specificity). Its ROC curve is along the left and upper borders of the positive unit quadrant (Figure 4.2).

Most tests have ROC curves that lie between those of the perfect and useless tests. Better tests have ROC curves closer to the upper left corner. The ROC curve depicts

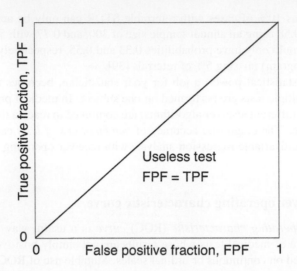

FIGURE 4.1
Receiver operating characteristic (ROC) for a useless diagnostic test shows a diagonal line. True positive fraction equals false positive fraction (TPF = FPF). Area under curve (AUC) = 0.5. (Modified from Pepe, M. S. *The Statistical Evaluation of Medical Tests for Classification and Prediction*, Oxford Statistical Science Series 28, p. 69, Oxford University Press, New York, 2003. With permission.)

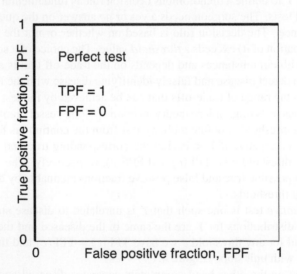

FIGURE 4.2
ROC for a perfect test. TPF = 1 and FPF = 0 (both sensitivity and specificity 100%). AUC = 1.0. (Modified from Pepe, M. S. *The Statistical Evaluation of Medical Tests for Classification and Prediction*, Oxford Statistical Science Series 28, p. 69, Oxford University Press, New York, 2003. With permission.)

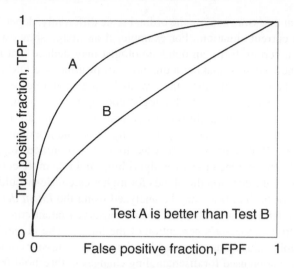

FIGURE 4.3

ROC curves for two tests, A and B, where test A is unequivocally better (ROC curve closer to upper left corner). (Modified from Pepe, M. S. *The Statistical Evaluation of Medical Tests for Classification and Prediction*, Oxford Statistical Science Series 28, p. 69, Oxford University Press, New York, 2003. With permission.)

the entire set of operating characteristics (FPF, TPF) possible with the test. Reporting of the (FPF, TPF) attained at only a single threshold conveys little useful information but this all too often occurs. That makes it difficult to compare different studies of the same test, particularly when different thresholds are employed. By reporting the entire ROC curve, information about a test can be compared and possibly combined across studies. If two diagnostic methods are applied to the same subjects, their ROC curves will be different (Figure 4.3). Confidence bands can be calculated and shown. There are several methods for comparing ROC curves for different tests [43].

4.3.3   Area under curve

The *area under the ROC curve* (AUC) is frequently reported. A perfect test has the value AUC = 1.0 and an uninformative test has AUC = 0.5, while most tests have values falling in between. The AUC is interpreted by [43] as an average TPF, averaged uniformly over the whole range of false positive fractions. Doctors sometimes rashly believe AUC to be a figure of merit for a test. This is unfortunate because surprisingly small differences in AUC can correspond to substantial differences in ROC curves. Suppose, for instance, that two ROC curves are equal over most of $(0, 1)$ but differ by 0.3 over the interval $(0.0, 0.3)$. This substantial difference in test accuracy corresponds to a difference of only 0.06 in the AUCs [43].

The ROC for *ordinal* tests is of special interest in the field of DR and STDR diagnosis. Grading scales for DR are not numeric at all but describe ordered discrete results. Different assessors can use the ordinal scale differently, depending on earlier experience and current situation. For example, if an image shows a large blotchy hemorrhage of a certain form, an ophthalmologist may deduce that it results from bleeding from new vessels, making a diagnosis of proliferative DR; a grader, however, would probably classify the same eye as having moderate or severe nonproliferative DR. In general, an ophthalmologist coming to swift judgment on an image might have a higher threshold for recognizing lesions that are not immediately sight-threatening than would a grader performing a systematic examination based on reference images. ROC curves can be used to show differences regarding thresholds between observers. One grader (or algorithm) might be more conservative than another, in which case decision thresholds for higher categories would be lower.

ROC curves for ordinal tests may be analyzed using the *latent decision variable model*. This model assumes that there is an unobserved latent continuous variable corresponding to the assessor's perception of the image. The grader has some cutpoints or threshold values that correspond to the grader's classification of the image. The ROC curve can be used for disentangling changes in threshold from changes in inherent accuracy, or to compare different imaging modalities. The ROC framework allows one to separate the discriminatory capacity of a test from the way in which the test is used to classify a positive reply, and this is particularly useful when raters use the same scale differently. A *"parametric distribution-free"* approach has been suggested for making inferences about the ROC curve from data [43]. Your statistician should be able to implement several other ways of analyzing ROC curves for ordinal tests [44]. Methods based on ROC curves have been suggested for meta-analysis of diagnostic accuracy studies [45].

4.3.4   Covariates

A covariate is a factor potentially affecting test performance. Examples could be subject's age, gender, iris color, diameter of pupil; tester's experience; qualities of test; environment, location, health-care resources; disease severity and spectrum of lesions; and manifestations of nondiabetic conditions. Your statistician should be able to help you to find several covariates and perhaps even adjust for them. Consider devising slightly different algorithms for people of different age, for instance.

4.4   Improving Detection of Diabetic Retinopathy

Standards can be set in order to evaluate *process variables* such as coverage or adherence to recommended intervals between examinations. Furthermore, *outcome variables* can be assessed. Preliminary standards were set for both kinds of variables and applied to some existing programs; these did not do well, even if one takes into account the fact that the standards had not been widely circulated and acted upon prior to the study period [12].

Judging from reports presented at a meeting in Liverpool in November 2005, it appears that far from all DR screening programs are of adequate quality, and access to ophthalmic lasers is uneven in Europe, particularly in less affluent areas. It is clear that many programs need improving. One of the methods could be the introduction of accurate CAD software.

4.4.1 Improving work environment

Keep in mind that a stressful work situation can cause decreased concentration capacity and mental fatigue that may become less easily reversible as exposure to stress is increased [46]. Thresholds for perceiving and being irritated by noise, flickering light, and so on are then lowered. Sifting input data, i.e., increasing signal-to-noise ratio, is hard work for the human brain; recall the sudden feeling of ease when subliminal noise stops, for example when an electric fan is turned off. This ability to discriminate is important for the performance of DR screening graders. To optimize their signal detection performance, it is important to protect them from unnecessary disturbances such as nagging from a computer program. Increasing signal-to-noise ratio of images by preventing artifacts and minimizing operator error also helps graders cope.

4.4.2 Going digital

Introducing digital imaging to existing risk reduction programs has not been a total success. Theoretical advantages have been described in an excellent review [47]. In practice, however, problems have occurred with many links in the chain of information gathering, transfer and assessment: fundus cameras, digital camera backs, information transfer to computers, viewing images, and the interface to existing medical records and booking systems.

4.4.3 Obtaining clear images

The main principle behind the optical design of fundus cameras produced since the 1930s has been illuminating the fundus with a hollow cone of light entering the eye at the periphery of the pupil and obtaining information through its center. The front lens system of the fundus camera is thus responsible for illumination as well as for imaging.

Should the pupil be too small, a situation that gets worse with exposure to hyperglycemia and thus with time since diagnosis of diabetes, illumination becomes uneven and shadows obscure part of the image, particularly for images of nasal and temporal fields, obtained through narrower elliptical pupil openings because the subject is asked to look aside. Photography becomes more difficult with increasing age of the subject [48], partly because the ocular lens becomes yellowed with age [49] and lets through less light.

If camera-to-eye distance is wrong, or if there is material on the front lens or in the ocular media refracting or diffracting light, both illumination and imaging suffer.

A more detailed description of the fundus camera and its use, including examples of images with optical artifacts, is recommended [23]. Keeping a fundus camera in perfect working order necessitates preventive maintenance in order to reach the goal of less than 3% technical failures [10]. Unless the front lens and other glass-air interfaces of the fundus camera are kept scrupulously clean, artifacts make diagnosis of DR difficult, tiring graders. These problems appear to be more important with digital imaging because algorithms that remove artifacts may cause loss of useful information and because existing systems have not equalled the color space, nuances, resolution, or dynamic range of film. Images from a low-resolution digital imaging screening program with 12% technical failures were analyzed by CAD software that reliably identified ungradeable images [50]. Such methods could be employed to increase reliability of diagnosis and ease of grading.

4.4.4   Avoiding loss of information

Digital cameras of today are with few exceptions one-sensor designs with Bayer color filters, necessitating interpolation and extrapolation in order for a color image to be created. Users of some digital cameras have noted that certain small lesions are suppressed while others are enlarged, apparently at random, sometimes causing dot hemorrhages/microaneurysms or small hard exudates to disappear from view when a repeat image is obtained after an interval of a few seconds.

Questions remain whether the loss of information resulting from compression of image files, conceivably impairing detection of microaneurysms and other small lesions, is acceptable [51]. Practical problems with connectors, cables, or file transfer protocols sometimes cause information to be lost.

4.4.5   Viewing images

It is still not completely known what information from images is needed for human graders to arrive at a diagnosis with optimal ease and accuracy. The reference standard remains Kodachrome color transparencies, viewed with optimum sharpness and contrast with the right color temperature of retroillumination. Today, images are usually graded using office-type LCD monitors that are not color-calibrated and whose color fidelity is dependent on angle of view. One study showed an LCD monitor to be inferior to a CRT monitor for the purpose of DR diagnosis [52]. Some information may also be lost because image files are down-sampled to screen resolution.

Many graders complain that using computer monitors for grading is more stressful and tiring than viewing slides on a lightbox using magnifiers, or by optimal-quality projection, in a darkened room. Besides, it is now being realized that certain computerized medical records and booking systems are not as safe or reliable as they ought to be. All this may combine to form a stressful environment for graders. On the other hand, one screening program manager told me, tongue in cheek, that it is usually easier to obtain funding for IT-related products and services, e.g., US$3 M for a computerized system including software and support, than to get US$0.3 M appropriated for a corresponding number of film-based fundus cameras. That said, I personally find the opportunities promised by digital image manipulation and analysis to be absolutely fascinating.

4.4.6 Ensuring accurate grading

Few DR screening programs employ double grading, whether by two independent graders with adjudication by a senior grader or grading by two persons concurrently, with STDR positive images read by a senior grader. Still fewer have fully implemented quality assurance with reference images in everyday use, systematic re-grading and external validation. As regards reference images for human graders, these images should be compatible with the magnification, field of view, and other characteristics of the program's usual screening images. A reference center for external validation of image quality and grading is the Retinopathy Grading Centre at Hammersmith Hospital, London, United Kingdom (http://www1.imperial.ac. uk/medicine/about/divisions/is/meta/diabeticretinopathy/). Data on the prowess of graders have only been published for a few community-based programs that are not part of research projects. Hence, it is far from easy to define a standard of performance that CAD software should meet or exceed.

4.4.7 Organizing for success

There are other reasons why it has been difficult to achieve on a large scale the reduction in visual loss expected to result from full implementation of findings from controlled trials of photocoagulation and diabetes treatment. Some existing programs, but not all, have up-to-date diabetes registers. Not all manage to re-screen people with diabetes at recommended intervals. Many programs, but not all, have systems in place to ensure timely photocoagulation. There is competition for scarce resources in ophthalmology; the number of people with diabetes is increasing, and so is the number of people with age-related macular degeneration now requiring or requesting costly new treatment.

4.5 Measuring Outcomes of Risk Reduction Programs

The main outcome by which success of a DR risk reduction program should be measured is *the incidence rate of blindness and visual impairment* in diabetes [53]. An important objective of diagnostic research is to evaluate the impact of one or more diagnostic strategies on therapy decisions and patient outcomes. This trend is in response to the recognition that increasing diagnostic accuracy is of little use if there is no resulting change or improvement in patient care.

In 1989 the World Health Organization European Regional Office and the European Region of the International Diabetes Federation held a joint meeting in St Vincent, Italy. Among the participants were people with diabetes, politicians, health-

care managers, doctors, and representatives of other professions. The meeting suggested many ways of improving the care of people with diabetes, setting clear aims
for reducing complications. These were published as the St. Vincent Declaration for
Diabetes Care and Research in Europe [54]. The target for ocular complications of
diabetes was to reduce new blindness due to diabetes by one-third or more within
five years.

4.5.1   Reducing new blindness and visual impairment

Meeting the St. Vincent Declaration target of reducing new blindness took longer
than hoped for. Five years after introduction of a screening system, a hospital-based
study from Lund, Sweden, showed low incidence of blindness in a group of type 1 diabetes patients [55]. Ten years after systematic fundus photography was introduced
on Iceland, covering more than 200 diabetic patients, all persons with type 1 diabetes
and a large proportion of those with type 2 diabetes, the annual number of newly
blind people with diabetes fell to 0 [56]. Reduction of a proxy measure of new blindness by more than one-third in five years was reported for Stockholm County [57].
Later, exciting data from Newcastle, United Kingdom, were published [58], confirming that a risk reduction program really can work.

Looking back, it seems that at first patients with advanced proliferative DR were
detected. In the Stockholm region, for example, this first happened on a larger scale
when greater numbers of people with diabetes were examined subsequent to a cam-
paign to increase referral rate, many of them arriving too late for effective treatment.
In that region, new blindness in diabetes peaked in 1984. Then, earlier cases of
proliferative DR were identified and treated as a result of larger-scale application of
screening tests. From 1990, when a systematic photography-based risk reduction
program took form, new blindness due to proliferative DR fell to near zero levels,
while reduction of blindness and visual impairment due to diabetic maculopathy was
achieved at a slower rate [57].

Looking forward, an additional challenge will be to identify earlier lesions so that
new drug treatments can be instituted at an early stage. Drugs now in development
are hoped to reduce inflammation or prevent capillary closure resulting from white
blood cells sticking to vessel walls and occluding capillaries. Other drugs are being
designed to reduce or prevent vascular leakage. An outcome measure for such studies
could be the proportion of subjects whose visual acuity, neither at baseline nor at
study end, falls below Snellen 20/40 or 6/12 (Monoyer 0.5). In many countries this
is a legal requirement for driving a car. That threshold represents half of the visual
acuity considered "normal" (i.e., the ability to perceive an object subtending an angle
of one minute of arc, Snellen 20/20 or 6/6, Monoyer 1.0).

4.5.2   Counting people who lost vision

There are many ways of measuring visual acuity [59]. Using an illuminated chart
(http://www.icoph.org/pdf/icovisualstandards.pdf) is regarded as good clinical practice. Several definitions of blindness exist but IRS "legal blindness" and the WHO

(ICD 10) definition are the most commonly used in the more recent literature; slight changes (http://whqlibdoc.who.int/hq/2003/WHO_PBL_03.91.pdf) are being contemplated.

The *point prevalence* of a disease is the *proportion* of a defined population at risk for the disease that is affected by it at a specified point on the time scale. Being a proportion, prevalence carries no unit, and must lie between 0 and 1 (or between 0 and 100%). The prevalence of "legal blindness" (a wide definition of blindness, coming from the U.S. Internal Revenue Service) in a population-based sample of people with diabetes can be expected to be in the region of 1 to 4% [60].

A *rate* is defined as change in number relative to change in another quantity, e.g., events per unit of time. The *incidence rate* of a disease over a specified time interval is given by the number of new cases during the interval divided by the total amount of time at risk for the disease accumulated by the entire population over the same interval. The units of a rate are thus $(time)^{-1}$.

For instance, in Stockholm County, Sweden, in the year 1984, 28 persons with diabetes were newly blind (WHO definition) in a background mid-year population of 1 556 828; incidence 1.8×10^{-5} yr^{-1} (95% confidence interval 1.2×10^{-5} yr^{-1} to 2.6×10^{-5} yr^{-1}). In 1994, 2 persons with diabetes were newly blind (WHO definition) in a background mid-year population of 1 697 366; incidence 0.12×10^{-5} yr^{-1} (95% confidence interval 0.01×10^{-5} yr^{-1} to 0.4×10^{-5} yr^{-1}) when all causes of blindness were included [57]. In the Warmia and Mazury region of Poland, recorded blindness incidence rate believed due to diabetes fell from 5.2×10^{-5} yr^{-1} to 0.8×10^{-5} yr^{-1} when the periods 1989–1994 and 2000–2004 were compared [61].

Few DR screening programs serve a large enough background population to make it possible to document reductions in new blindness during a five-year period. One may assume that scarce events, such as cases of new blindness, follow a Poisson distribution, which has the attractive property that its variance equals its mean. A table of confidence intervals for numbers of events from 1 to 40 (http://www.doh.wa.gov/Data/guidelines/ConfIntguide.htm) shows that estimation is imprecise for small numbers. Your statistician will know how to calculate exact confidence intervals and should be able to perform Poisson regression with a test for trend. Poisson regression is useful for following repeated measures such as annual numbers of newly blind.

4.5.3   Understanding the importance of visual impairment

The inclusion of visual acuity testing in a DR screening program, as in the United Kingdom, has elsewhere been questioned for reasons of cost. Visual acuity is an important process variable and a useful aid to treatment decisions. Treatable lesions such as cataracts can be discovered in time and acted upon, preserving or even increasing the patient's quality of life. Moreover, even minor loss of visual acuity greatly affects a person's social situation and activities (http://cera.unimelb.edu.au/publications/reports/Focus%20on%20LowVision.pdf). Loss of visual acuity is useful information for graders. In research settings, visual acuity is expressed as the base-10 logarithm of the minimum angle of resolution (LogMAR). These data are useful when the results of new imaging modalities showing retinal thickening are contrasted with findings from more conventional fundus images. For example, visual acuity for MAR 1 minute of arc is Snellen 20/20 and LogMAR is 0; MAR 10 minutes of arc (Snellen 20/200) corresponds to LogMAR 1. Visual acuity is a relevant outcome variable for a DR risk reduction program.

4.6   User Experiences of Computer-Aided Diagnosis

Users of DR CAD can be divided into two groups: pioneers and early adopters in one group, the other group consisting of people who have had this technology foisted on them. It is difficult to separate the performance of CAD software from the influence of patient spectrum, image quality, characteristics of users, and their workplace, including technological environment. I have listened for expressions of remaining distrust caused by inflated promises made for the primitive CAD software available 15 or even 25 years ago. Moreover, I have attempted to find out why there has been some resistance towards the adoption of this new technology.

Pioneers are often highly tolerant of program bugs and other glitches. Their screens are likely to be color-calibrated and many of them still swear by CRT monitors intended for the graphics industry. More than a few of them are proficient users of SQL database management programs under some flavor of Unix. These are inner-directed people wielding considerable power over their own working day. Pioneers tend to have experience of selected images from patients with fairly advanced DR and are likely to work in centers where standards of image quality and equipment maintenance are high; therefore, the task for CAD software is easy and its predictive value may be high as a result of high DR prevalence.

Other users, however, are more likely to be critical of factors that disturb work flow and contribute towards making the work environment more stressful. The qualities of the associated database management software and the operating system play an important part of the experiences of users not thrilled by the opportunity of matching wits with programmers, particularly if several kinds of new software begin to intrude on their work experience at the same time. Computer glitches and the qualities of the user interface are just part of the experience. Graders may not take kindly to the thought of losing their job to a machine. To add insult to injury, the machine is felt to be looking over their shoulders, usurping authority. Experienced graders with many years of reading images on film may decry the loss of information and the increase in artifacts introduced with digital cameras and grading from office-type screens with a small color space (dependent on angle of view) and poor color accuracy. Graders see images of variable quality from unselected populations for which CAD software will achieve low predictive value; this will not increase their confidence in the new technology. Moreover, a program tuned for high sensitivity will stress the grader with improbably frequently occurring indicators of putative lesions. Conversely, with software designed for high specificity, glaring errors of omission are possible, potentially giving graders and managers difficult ethical and medicolegal problems to handle. The reception of CAD software and the effects of its adoption on the work environment are suitable subjects for future research.

I have to make clear that I do not have experience of more than a few programs and about a dozen different algorithms. Most of them were in early stages of development. I do not claim to be abreast of the latest image analysis techniques and I cannot assess the quality of programming in Matlab or other environments. Neither I nor my sources from other centers felt comfortable in making judgment on the achievements of a named company, institution, or programmer. What follows is a necessarily subjective collection of partly adverse opinions.

4.6.1 Perceived accuracy of lesion detection

Accuracy of lesion detection was reported to be affected by image quality, artifacts, and operator error. There were some differences of opinion between experienced professional graders (particularly those performing systematic field-by-field, lesion-by-lesion grading) and my ophthalmologist friends (who are trained to obtain an immediate global impression of a fundus). The latter were more inclined to feel that programs (and indeed professional graders) overgrade.

Current consensus appears to be that CAD software does not yet offer potential for completely independent automated DR detection, mainly because specificity is felt to be insufficiently high. CAD is already, however, of interest for purposes such as decision support. In the near future, validated software should become useful as an integral part of well-run screening programs, safeguarding against loss of attention because of grader fatigue, monitoring image quality, and improving repeatability.

Some programs, such as those based on ContextVision technology, were more or less capable of compensating for differences in texture such as vignetting (dark edges of image); others showed poor accuracy in image areas that were underexposed because of insufficient pupil dilation, operator error (wrong distance from fundus camera to eye or camera at wrong height) or optical artifacts including effects of ocular media opacities. Depending on make and model of fundus camera (for example with Canon CR series cameras), bright reflections from the inner limiting membrane in eyes of young persons may obscure lesions inside the temporal vascular arcades within about one to three mm from fixation; the remedy is to obtain images from more nasal or temporal orientation of the eye. Indeed, imaging more than two fields and offering a stereo pair of the macula will help reduce the frequency of technical failure.

4.6.1.1 Hemorrhages and microaneurysms

Dark lesions (*dot and blot hemorrhages*): Detection was dependent on the ability of software to disregard retinal blood vessels; the RetinaLyze program was felt by some users to be particularly good in this respect, but others prefer Aberdeen software. Brown dots (*retinal pigment epithelium, RPE*) were overdiagnosed as red dots (*microaneurysms*) by several programs, particularly with monochrome images (called red-free by ophthalmologists) suffering from compression artifacts. Microaneurysm detection ability was affected by image quality including measurable resolution, subjective sharpness, number of bits (10-bit monochrome a little better than 8-bit; 16-bit color worse than 24-bit), image noise, denoising and sharpening algorithms, and compression artifacts. Indeed, most programs worked best with uncompressed files and with those only subjected to lossless compression. Another problem was repeatability; the effect of certain algorithms built into digital camera backs apparently was to give different images from the same eye obtained a few minutes apart, particularly as regards number and location of microaneurysms. Only a few cameras intended for professional photographers, such as the Canon EOS-1Ds Mk II (which is rarely used for fundus photography), allow support staff, using a special program, to turn off most image manipulation containing a memory function for earlier images and intended to deliver pleasing pictures — but possibly affecting the appearance of the retinal pigment epithelium and small details such as small hard exudates, the tips of perifoveal capillaries and small dot hemorrhages/microaneurysms, thus impairing their detection.

Microaneurysm counts are predictive of worsening of DR [62] and repeatable measurements should therefore provide useful information for members of diabetes care teams — less so for most ophthalmologists.

It should be noted that good CAD software detects more microaneurysms than do human observers who may consider this as tiresome overdiagnosis. On the other hand, I quickly stopped using some programs that were unable to identify small microaneurysms near fixation. That is a lesion widely believed to be indicative of risk for leakage and predicting possibly sight-threatening centrally located hard exudates — although this was not confirmed by one recent study [63]. Some but not all centrally located hard exudates are treatable by photocoagulation. The present consensus seems to be that centrally located microaneurysms ought not to be missed in a DR screening system.

4.6.1.2   Hard exudates

Bright lesions, also known as white lesions (for instance *hard exudates*), are reportedly accurately detected by some algorithms [64; 65] — but from what I have seen for certain earlier algorithms more easily if sufficiently large to be apparent to the trained observer. The RetinaLyze system examined "individual bright lesions without consideration of their dimension, orientation, location, pattern, chromaticity, or topographical relation to red lesion" which limited its usefulness [66]. The presence of *hard exudates within one disc diameter of the center of the fovea* is believed to be sight-threatening; this is called *macular involvement* or *diabetic maculopathy*, but confusingly sometimes referred to as "macular edema." This is an important family of conditions.

There are several possible causes of false positives. Some programs tended to confuse hard exudates with bright optical artifacts caused, for example, by dust and other material on the fundus camera's front lens or reflections from the internal limiting membrane. *Retinal pigment epithelial (RPE) defects* have existed for a long time but were not reported until a few decades ago, showing the ability of doctors to disregard information that does not fit the pattern looked for. RPE defects are highly visible as "window defects" in fluorescein angiograms. RPE defects can be distinguished from hard exudates (appearing to lie on the plane of the retina) because the defects on stereoscopic examination or in stereo images seem to lie beyond the plane of the retina. Some algorithms overdiagnose (as hard exudates) *drusen*, another retinal lesion not associated with DR. Drusen, resulting from deposition of debris from photoreceptors, are amorphous yellowish deposits beneath the sensory retina, being important as an early sign of age-related macular degeneration (AMD) and the object of current research interest [67]. Four main types of drusen can be detected in the retina. *Hard drusen* are discrete, yellow, nodular deposits, smaller than 50 microns in diameter. *Basal laminar drusen* are tiny, whitish, multiple deposits with a "starry night" appearance. *Soft drusen* are yellowish deposits with poorly defined margins, tending to coalesce, and are usually larger than 50 microns. *Crystalline drusen* are discrete, calcific, refractile deposits. Because number, size, and confluence of drusen predict development of sight-threatening AMD [68], drusen follow-up should be an important application for CAD software. New hopes for a solution to the problem of false positives caused by nondiabetic bright lesions such as drusen were recently presented [50] which is very good news for screeners.

In my opinion, overdiagnosis of hard exudates is not a problem of such dimensions as to invalidate a risk reduction program; depending on their workload, however, not all ophthalmologists might agree. Centrally located hard exudates ought not to be missed in a DR screening system. Neither should one miss hard exudates located temporal to the fovea [63].

4.6.1.3   Retinal thickening

Retinal thickening may be guessed at if parts of the macula seem structureless. Traditionally, the gold standard is examination by stereoscopic biomicroscopy or from stereo images, but there is a strong subjective element and data are very noisy. During the past decade, it has become known that human observers do not compare well with more objective methods such as the Retinal Thickness Analyzer (RTA) or time-domain optical coherence tomography (OCT). The latter [69] has been available since 1994 and yields images of sections through the retina useful for assessing morphological changes associated with retinal thickening [70]. The use of OCT, a sensitive, specific, and reproducible tool, has taught us much about the morphology and pathophysiology of macular edema [71], but one problem for the user is that the process is slow and one does not always know from what area of the retina the data are collected.

Spectral domain (SD-OCT) or frequency domain instruments (using fast-Fourier transforms; entering the market during 2007) rapidly produce images of the macula, enabling the user to place optical sections at will, through (or in the vicinity of) lesions such as vascular abnormalities, hard exudates, or foveal microaneurysms [72]. This noninvasive technology should become very useful for accurate final diagnosis of local or widespread retinal thickening in order to optimize focal and/or grid laser photocoagulation for each eye, as well as new methods of treatment. Perhaps using this method could help develop CAD for macular edema further.

4.6.1.4 Micro-infarctions

Cotton wool spots, in modern literature referred to as *micro-infarctions* (but still called soft exudates by some doctors — despite the fact that these lesions are not soft, neither do they result from exudation) are important indicators of local or widespread retinal ischemia. They tend to appear when blood glucose levels have been lowered too much too quickly, i.e., when HbA_{1c} levels are reduced by more than two percentage units in 10 to 12 months [73]. Although micro-infarctions tend to disappear with time, their presence may indicate variability in blood glucose concentration, a risk factor for painful diabetic neuropathy [74]. Micro-infarctions are part of the panorama of severe nonproliferative DR (the term "preproliferative" retinopathy was popular thirty years ago but is ill-defined and best avoided). Occasionally, photocoagulation scars or local areas of atrophy are mistaken for micro-infarctions.

Detection of micro-infarctions is easy for humans and CAD programs in case of immediately apparent lesions, but requires reasonably faithful recording of luminance data in order to identify lesions characterized by diffuse borders and minimal local increased luminance; such minimally apparent lesions seen in high-quality color images may indicate local areas of ischemia clearly confirmed on fluorescein angiography. The main reason for accurate detection of micro-infarction is that widespread ischemia is a possible indication for scatter photocoagulation.

4.6.1.5 Vascular tree abnormalities

The vascular tree can be analyzed in various ways; an excellent review is available [75]. There is considerable interest in the relationship between retinal vascular morphology and metabolic and inflammatory diseases [76]. I hope that the similarities between cerebral and retinal microcirculation will help to attract funds to the analysis of retinal vasculature by image analysis. Experimental RetinaLyze software and some published algorithms have assessed *tortuosity* of retinal blood vessels. Several researchers have measured *blood vessel diameter*, for the purposes of assessing retinal blood flow or variations of vascular diameter (*venous beading*). There have been attempts to detect *venous loops, intraretinal microvascular abnormalities* (IRMA) that predict the onset of proliferative DR, and small tufts of new blood vessels (*proliferations*) but I have not seen any algorithm in use that reliably detected such lesions. This is an area that deserves further work.

To sum up, most of the programs that I have seen in use were calibrated using images showing advanced lesions whose existence is immediately obvious to the trained observer; what I and many others would need is help finding minimal departures from normality whose presence is predictive of progression to STDR.

4.6.2 Finding and reading evaluations of software for retinopathy diagnosis

New diagnostic tests should receive thorough evaluation before being applied to medical practice; such has not always been the case in the past, and many authors including Feinstein [77] have called for reform. Published reports deserve critical reading, and methods for systematic reviews are in development, not least because methods for assessing diagnostic test accuracy differ from the well established methods for evaluating treatment methods [78]. The Cochrane Collaboration is planning a register of diagnostic test accuracy studies (http://www.cochrane.org/docs/diagnostictestreviews.htm), and a handbook for reviewers of such studies is being prepared. If you are not an experienced reader of papers published in medical journals, an introduction to EBM (evidence-based medicine) should be of interest [79].

The quality of any study can be considered in terms of internal validity, external validity, and the quality of data analysis and reporting. *Internal validity* can be defined as the degree to which estimates of diagnostic accuracy produced in a study have not been biased as a result of study design, conduct, analysis, or presentation (e.g., sample selection, problems with the reference standard and nonindependent assessment). *External validity* concerns the degree to which the results of a study can be applied to patients in practice, and is affected by factors such as spectrum of disease or nondisease, setting, other patient characteristics, how the diagnostic test was conducted, the threshold (or cut-off point) used, and the reproducibility of the test. The QUADAS checklist [80], for which a helpful manual is available on the Internet [81, Ch. 9], is a useful quality assessment tool for diagnostic accuracy studies that was recently validated and modified [82].

Reports on diabetic retinopathy CAD software are not easy to find. To search medical journals, go to PubMed Services (http://www.ncbi.nlm.nih.gov/entrez/query/static/clinical.shtml), choosing Clinical Queries, Search by Clinical Study Category, enter diabetic retinopathy and diagnosis, computer-assisted or diabetic retinopathy and image processing, computer-assisted, choose "diagnosis" and broad search. This turns up more than 140 papers of varying relevance. One hopes that a medical librarian will devise a more sensitive and specific filter to find CAD software evaluations. The situation would improve if all authors provided more useful index terms to journals and thus to the people doing the indexing for PubMed and other databases.

Several papers have described initial development and performance of the prematurely marketed (but in my opinion interesting) RetinaLyze DR CAD software [66; 83–86] whose evaluation in a well-designed multi-center trial was cut short by investors who abruptly closed down the company. Several successful ongoing projects are intended to produce CAD software useful for DR risk reduction programs. What could they have in common?

There are numerous algorithms intended for the detection of some aspect of morphology. The results of using such algorithms need to be combined into a *risk score*. This combination score can be derived from a *training dataset* of images from a DR screening system, using methods such as logistic regression, neural networks or machine learning techniques (e.g., support vector machines) and should be validated using a *test dataset* of other screening images [43]. To achieve adequate statistical power, large test sets are needed to provide a sufficient number of lesions for detection even if their prevalence is low. For example, in a Scottish study, compared to a clinical reference standard, images containing hard exudates were detected with sensitivity 95.0% and specificity 84.6% in a test set of 13 219 images of which 300 (2%) contained hard exudates [65]. Papers using this kind of approach have been appearing recently and are worthy of close study.

Algorithms now exist that can identify some, but not all, of the lesions found in the Early Treatment Diabetic Retinopathy Study (ETDRS) Standard Photographs (http: //eyephoto.ophth.wisc.edu/ResearchAreas/Diabetes/DiabStds.htm) and the publicly available images from the STARE project Web site [87]. The STARE images (http: //www.ces.clemson.edu/~ahoover/stare/) show a high proportion of advanced DR as do the ETDRS Standard Photographs. Testing CAD software on unselected populations of people with diabetes will be of greater interest but more expensive. Of course, I do not wish to discourage the creation of new CAD software, but it should be clear from the outset that the process of validating such programs entails considerable time, cost, and effort. Ideally, there should be post-marketing surveillance showing intermediate outcomes (numbers of adequate referrals vs false referrals) and final outcomes (years of sight saved) of full-scale application in DR screening programs. Until recently, we have had to make do with smaller studies on more or less selected groups of persons with diabetes.

To ensure market acceptance and approval by regulatory agencies such as the FDA (U.S. Food and Drug Administration) and from companies or government agencies paying for health-care, nowadays quite rigorous and well-documented processes of development and assessment appear to be required.

4.6.3   Opportunities and challenges for programmers

Speaking as a clinician, as a researcher, and last but not least as a senior grader with many years of experience managing a large program, I am very interested in getting help from CAD programmers. Accurate microaneurysm counts are of considerable practical importance at present because of their proven prognostic value — this work, however, is tedious; automated detection should be welcomed if reliable [88]. Methods for measuring microaneurysm turnover, for whose assessment human observers are far from ideal [89], should become an interesting research tool and are likely to become important for assessment of the earliest stages of DR [90].

Indication of image quality [91] including field definition [92] would help photographers achieve the clear sharp artifact-free images with repeatable field localization that I like to see. While detection of the optic disc and the fovea presently takes one such program 120s using a 2.4 GHz Pentium PC, near real-time speed would be most welcome. Future CAD software should help describe patterns of lesion type, location, turnover, and apparent movement, in aid of a better understanding of pathophysiology and improved prediction of STDR.

My wish list for the future, in no particular order, thus includes: Objective assessment of image quality including field definition (as feedback to photographers and for quality development), reliable early detection of changes to fundus cameras such as optical artifacts (dust on sensor, material on glass surfaces, decentered flash tube, browning of images as a result of aging flash tube), relieving graders from boredom, increasing sensitivity for early changes, help with comparisons of lesions over time, improved grading of early lesions as feedback to diabetes care teams, and maximum sensitivity for the earliest possible detection of STDR.

4.7 Planning a Study to Evaluate Accuracy

As mentioned above, the closeness of a diagnosis to the true state is termed *accuracy*. Standards for reporting of diagnostic accuracy (STARD) have been developed [93], based on available evidence [94] to improve the quality of design and reporting. A useful checklist and a clarifying flowchart are available (www.consort-statement. org/stardstatement.htm). A book describing methods for the evaluation of diagnostic tests is warmly recommended [95]. While you are looking for studies of DR CAD software, take note of how papers have been indexed (in PubMed, choose Display Citation) and list the relevant Medical Subject Headings (MeSH) index terms in your manuscript so that interested parties can find your work.

4.7.1 Getting help from a statistician

Designing studies to evaluate the accuracy of medical tests requires the expertise of a statistician with an interest in epidemiology and ideally with experience of evaluating diagnostic tests in medicine. The following treatment draws heavily on a book intended for graduates with a basic training in statistics [43]. Your statistician should read that book; useful STATA programs and help files are available (www.fhcrc.org/science/labs/pepe/book/) along with a few errata.

A commonly used design of an accuracy study compares the result of the *index* test, the test under study, with the results from applying the *reference* test, the "gold standard."

4.7.2 Choosing a measurement scale

First let us consider the *scale* for the test result. Tests for certain conditions (e.g., pregnancy, death) are expected to yield *dichotomous* results, positive if the condition is present, negative if absent; this is a *binary* scale. CAD software can be expected to help answer the question: Is any DR or STDR present or absent?

For tests that yield results on nonbinary scales, the classification rule is usually set by a threshold. Tests that yield results on a *continuous* scale (one that contains a true zero) include the measurement of fasting plasma glucose concentration, where a limit has been set for the diagnosis of diabetes from the results of repeated tests. *Categorical* data, also known as unordered discrete data, show no particular order, e.g., iris color.

Tests that involve subjective assessments are often measured on *ordinal* scales, e.g., the five main verbal categories of the 13-level ETDRS Final Scale most applicable to screening: no DR, mild-moderate-severe nonproliferative DR, proliferative DR [96; 97]. Graders of seven-field stereo images state whether a certain lesion is absent, questionably present or present in each field, referring to a Standard Photograph (SP). Stereo images are useful for the detection of retinal thickening which is however quite difficult to do reproducibly. Unless some other scale is mandated, take a look at the proposed five-level *international clinical diabetic retinopathy and diabetic macular edema disease severity scales* [98], mentioned in Chapter 2 (Section 2.5). Controversially, they do not specify distance of hard exudates from the center of the macula. The Scottish Diabetic Retinopathy Grading Scheme 2004, which does this, is now widely used in Scottish DR screening programs and in some other areas (http://www.nsd.scot.nhs.uk/services/drs/grading-scheme.pdf). Differing prevalence of diabetic macular edema has been described in mild, moderate, severe nonproliferative DR and proliferative DR, respectively [99]. Graders could use a five-point scale to express their degree of confidence in findings[100]; so could CAD programs.

There are different statistical methods for handling data from binary, continuous, and ordinal scales. A common mistake is to calculate means for numerical representations of ordinal and categorical scales, for instance 10 for no DR, 60 for proliferative DR, 99 for "cannot grade" — which of course makes no sense.

4.7.3   Optimizing design

Now consider *selection* of *study subjects*. For an *experimental study*, a fixed number of subjects with known disease and a fixed number of nondiseased subjects are selected, say, clinic attenders with diabetes with or without the kind of DR under study, and the diagnostic test is applied to both categories. This is a low-cost design, useful for early stages of development of a new test, but applicability to the entire population of, say, people with diabetes is unknown. To achieve generalizability, go on to a cohort study.

4.7.3.1   Cohort design and two-stage designs

For a *cohort study*, the diagnostic test can be applied to a set of study subjects from the population of interest, and true disease status, as measured by a *gold standard* definitive test, is also determined for all subjects [101]. The results of such a study are dependent on the accuracy of the reference test.

Suppose that the prevalence of DR is 50% and that your new test is in truth 80% sensitive and 70% specific. Consider an *imperfect reference test* (such as clinical examination by an eminent general ophthalmologist of your acquaintance) that misses disease when it is there 20% of the time but that never falsely indicates disease.

Relative to such a reference test, your new test is still 80% sensitive but only 62% specific. It will appear to be worse than it is.

On the other hand, if we also assume that both the reference test and the new test are better at detecting severe disease, the new test will appear to be better than it truly is. Finally, if the new test is perfect (100% sensitive and 100% specific) but the reference is somewhat imperfect (90% sensitive and 90% specific), the new test appears to be only 90% sensitive and only 90% specific. It is not unusual for a new test to be better than the best available standard test.

A variation on the cohort design is the two-stage design where ascertainment of true disease status depends on the result of the diagnostic test. Two-stage designs save some costs for gold-standard tests and might be ethically justified if the definitive test, i.e., fluorescein angiography, is invasive and entails some risk for the subject. In the context of a screening system, two-stage designs are fairly easy to implement. On the other hand, their statistical power is inferior to that of a true cohort study, which should be performed for a new test before two-stage designs are implemented. Special care is needed in analysis of the data, not least because results of the index test and the reference test are not independent [43].

4.7.3.2 Reference standard images and centers

The internationally recognized gold standard test for DR and STDR is seven-field stereo 30° fundus photography on color transparency film, performed by certified photographers (the original work was done using Zeiss Oberkochen FF-3 and FF-4 fundus cameras giving images with 2.5:1 magnification on Kodachrome film; certain other cameras and films are approved by the Fundus Photograph Reading Center in Madison, Wisconsin) with seven-field stereo photograph grading performed by certified graders using the set of Standard Photographs (SPs) obtainable from the *Fundus Photograph Reading Center* in Madison, Wisconsin (http://eyephoto.ophth.wisc. edu/Photography/Protocols/Mod7&FA-ver1.pdf) and special grading forms; see the ETDRS manual of operations [102].

The ETDRS Standard Photographs and data from the Wisconsin Epidemiologic Study of Diabetic Retinopathy form the basis for the proposed *international clinical diabetic retinopathy and diabetic macular edema disease severity scales* [98]. Disease severity is divided into five stages: *no apparent retinopathy* (i.e., no abnormalities), *mild nonproliferative DR* (microaneurysms only), *moderate nonproliferative DR* (more than just microaneurysms, but less than severe nonproliferative DR), *severe nonproliferative DR* follows the *4:2:1 rule* (any of the following: more than 20 intraretinal hemorrhages in each of 4 quadrants; definite venous beading in 2+ quadrants; prominent intraretinal microvascular abnormalities in 1+ quadrants — and no signs of proliferative DR), and *proliferative DR* (one or more of the following: neovascularization, vitreous/preretinal hemorrhage). The four latter categories can be combined with a separate *diabetic macular edema severity scale: diabetic macular edema apparently absent* (no apparent retinal thickening or hard exudates in posterior pole) and *diabetic macular edema apparently present* (some apparent retinal thickening or hard exudates in posterior pole). This exceptionally wide definition of macular edema is intended for general ophthalmologists and other caregivers not using stereoscopic biomicroscopy or stereo photography, being the first part of a two-tier system. The second part divides diabetic macular edema, if present, into three categories: *mild* diabetic macular edema (some retinal thickening or hard exudates in posterior pole but distant from the center of the macula), *moderate* diabetic macular edema (retinal thickening or hard exudates approaching the center of the macula but not involving the center), and *severe* diabetic macular edema (retinal thickening or hard exudates involving the center of the macula). The specific distance from the fovea is not specified. This scale was used in a recently published paper describing varying prevalence of diabetic macular edema in mild, moderate, severe nonprolifer-ative DR, and proliferative DR, respectively [99].

Another reference center is the *Retinopathy Grading Centre* at Hammersmith, London, United Kingdom (http://www1.imperial.ac.uk/medicine/about/divisions/is/meta/diabeticretinopathy/), which performs expert grading of two-field 45° images for the EURODIAB study with its useful grading scale, which was found traceable to the ETDRS scale [103], as well as different grading for other studies. Early contact with a reference center is advisable when planning a study.

You should be very wary of using the nearest ophthalmologists to perform biomi-croscopy as this kind of reference test cannot be validated. Low intra- and inter-observer agreement in assessment of retinal thickening has been described [104]. Cohort studies with adequate reference tests are necessarily expensive because a large number of subjects must be recruited and examined, but only in this way can generalizable data of practical value be obtained.

4.7.3.3   Paired or unpaired test

Diagnostic methods can be compared in two ways. When two different methods are applied to each study subject, each individual gives rise to a pair of results; this is called a *paired* design. Since an individual's results are related, the statistical method must take this into account. For paired binary data, the hypothesis test of choice is *McNemar's test*, which has the advantage of simplicity, and one may calculate *confidence intervals for the difference between paired proportions* [105]. Paired ordinal data can be analyzed using *Svensson's method* [106]; methods based on the analysis of the ROC curve are the subject of considerable current interest.

An *unpaired* design is one in which each subject receives only one of the diagnos-tic tests. Because of inter-subject variability, unpaired designs have lower statistical power and a larger study size is needed than for paired designs.

4.7.3.4   Masking

Test *integrity* is important. Knowledge of the gold standard test result (supposed to describe true disease status of the individual) must not influence the assessment of the diagnostic test, and vice versa. The persons administering and assessing the results of the diagnostic test should be *masked* to the study subject's true disease status. You should consider the ethical implications of including the diabetes patient in this group. The common term "blinded" is offensive to many ophthalmologists and to their patients [107].

One must be aware that interference can enter in some subtle ways and take precautions accordingly. For example, if there is a time delay between the experimental diagnostic test and "gold standard" assessment of disease status, altering patient management (e.g., insulin treatment) on the basis of the test might interfere with disease and lead to biased results. Knowledge of true disease status may influence the care with which the experimental diagnostic test is done [43].

4.7.3.5 Minimizing bias and variability

Bias is any systematic deviation of test results from the true state. Numerous sources of bias affect the assessment of diagnostic tests [108]. Most of them apply to previous studies comparing different imaging modalities and diagnostic methods in DR. *Verification bias* denotes nonrandom selection for definitive assessment for disease with the gold standard reference test (as in two-stage designs). *Imperfect reference test bias* means that true disease status is subject to misclassification (as when clinical examination is used instead of a validated method such as seven-field stereo photography); there is no way to compensate for this in subsequent statistical analysis. *Spectrum bias* (a form of *selection bias*) means that subjects included are not representative of the population (as when a convenience sample of diabetic patients is taken from hospital attenders). "Berkson's fallacy" denotes the choice of hospital patients to represent nondiseased subjects. *Test interpretation bias* occurs when information is available that can distort the diagnostic test (this is why persons should be masked from information from medical records and results of the reference test). *Unsatisfactory tests* are uninterpretable; they should be included among positive test results in a DR screening study because the process variable of interest usually is referral to an ophthalmologist and because media opacities and other factors causing images to be uninterpretable may be associated with presence of severe DR — but on the other hand they should not be counted in favor of the accuracy of a test in itself [109]. *Extrapolation bias* occurs when the conditions or characteristics of populations in the study are different from those in which the test will be applied (for instance, CAD software designed to detect STDR in high-quality color photographs taken through dilated pupils of young Europeans with type 1 diabetes needed extensive re-programming in order to provide acceptable accuracy when analyzing variable-quality images from undilated elderly American Indians with type 2 diabetes). Note that the implicit or explicit criterion for defining a positive versus negative test result can differ with the tester or the environment in which the test is done [110]; this is one of the reasons why published sensitivity and specificity data should be viewed with some caution. *Lead time bias,* part of screening efficacy study debates, means that earlier detection by screening may erroneously appear to indicate beneficial effects on the outcome of a progressive disease (but remember that the course of diabetic complications is modifiable when timely interventions are made). *Length bias* implies that slowly progressing disease is overrepresented in screened subjects relative to all cases of disease that arise in the population. *Overdiagnosis bias* suggests that subclinical disease may regress and never become a clinical problem in the absence of screening, but is detected by screening (this is relevant for certain mammography findings, possibly also for micro-infarctions and small hard exudates, but hardly applies to STDR). Note, however, that small microaneurysms survive for about three months, larger surviving longer, according to one classic study [111].

Variability arises from differences among studies, for example, in terms of population, setting, test protocol, or definition of the target disorder. Although variability does not lead to biased estimates of test performance, it may limit the applicability of results and thus is an important consideration when evaluating studies of diagnostic accuracy. The distinction between bias and variation is not always straightforward, and the use of different definitions in the literature further complicates this issue.

Much of the discussion of bias and variation is speculative because it is difficult to quantify their influence on the assessment of diagnostic tests. Nevertheless, evidence has been found for effects of bias and variation regarding demographic features, disease prevalence and severity, partial verification bias, clinical review bias, and observer and instrument variation [81; 112].

4.7.3.6   Choosing statistical methods

Choices made in planning each phase of a study affect choices of *methods for statistical analysis* of diagnostic tests. Formerly, papers describing new methods were widely scattered in the literature. Rating scales were discussed in psychology journals. The seminal papers warning against the use of Cohen's kappa as a measure of inter-rater agreement when true disease prevalence is close to 0 and 100%, respectively, started a debate and development work [113] that continues to this day — but were first ignored, perhaps because they were published in osteopathy or chiropractic journals. Svensson's method for analysis of paired ordinal data, discerning differences between groups from inter-individual differences, has been used in diverse fields of clinical medicine, also including ophthalmology. Radiology and clinical chemistry journals often publish excellent discussions of methods. New methods for estimation and controlling for the effects of covariates, enabling the choice of optimal tests for various categories of patients, are of increasing importance. Lately, statistics journals such as *Statistics in Medicine* have contained important advances in methodology regarding diagnostic tests. Computer-based methods such as applied multivariable regression, generalized linear models (GLM) and general estimation equations (GEE) are increasingly employed in this field [43]. Again, involve a statistician from the beginning of planning of any study!

4.7.4   Carrying out different phases of research

The process of developing a medical test begins with small exploratory studies that seek to identify how best to apply the test and whether or not it has potential for use in practice. At the end of the process there are studies that seek to determine the value of the test when applied in particular populations. Unfortunately, evaluation of most DR CAD software algorithms (or combinations thereof) never gets beyond the first phase.

Much can be learned from the procedures developed to evaluate new drugs [114] with the caveat that narrow inclusion criteria of drug trials narrow the applicability of their results to unselected populations. What now follows is an introduction adapted from Pepe [43, ch. 8].

Phase 1 is an *exploratory* investigation, intended to identify promising tests and settings for application, usually performed on subjects from a convenience sample (people with diabetes, with or without DR/STDR, attending a diabetes clinic).

Phase 2, retrospective *validation*, determines if minimally acceptable sensitivity and specificity are achieved, ideally in a population-based sample of diseased and nondiseased subjects (this is the time to reach out to primary care).

Phase 3, retrospective *refinement*, determines criteria for screen positivity and co-variates affecting ROC, comparing promising tests and developing algorithms for combining tests. Subjects are a large random sample from diseased and nondiseased subjects.

Phase 4, *prospective application*, determines positive predictive value and false referral probabilities when the test is applied in practice, using a cohort study design.

Phase 5 measures disease *impact*, determining effects of testing on cost and visual loss (and effects associated therewith) associated with DR and STDR, in a randomized prospective trial comparing the new test with an existing standard of practice.

For each phase, there are specific methodological issues that you and your statistician need to consider at the earliest possible planning stage [43].

4.7.5 An example from another field

The impact of CAD on the performance of screening mammography has recently been analyzed, with alarming results. Some background information [115] is necessary before an important recent paper is discussed. Mammography is unprofitable for radiologists in the United States. Mammograms are read by radiologists of widely varying experience. Double grading [116] — mandatory in many European countries — rarely occurs in North America. Numerous possible reasons have been suggested for the great variability of false positive fraction, and lower specificity than reported other countries, reported for North America [117]; many of those reasons also apply to DR screening programs. Screening mammography, the most common basis for lawsuits in radiology, is a particularly stressful task for radiologists, associated with a relatively high rate of burnout. CAD software developed by R2 Technologies was approved by the FDA in 1998. Medicare and many insurance companies now reimburse for its use. Within three years after FDA approval, 10% of mammography facilities in the United States had adopted it.

The association between the use of CAD and the performance of screening mammography from 1998 through 2002 at 43 facilities in three states was determined for 429 345 mammograms. Diagnostic specificity and PPV decreased after implementation, while sensitivity increased insignificantly. No more cancers were detected. Accuracy fell; area under the ROC curve, 0.871 vs 0.919 [118].

Increased frequency of recall and increased false positive fraction may have been related to increased indications of ductal carcinoma *in situ* (its hallmark, clustered microcalcifications, detected by software), a condition that develops more slowly and is less dangerous than invasive cancer. With the goal of alerting radiologists to overlooked suspicious areas on mammograms, the CAD software inserts up to four marks on the average screening mammograms. For every true positive mark (associated with underlying cancer), radiologists encounter nearly 2000 false positive marks. In other words, signal-to-noise ratio is unacceptably poor. That is a very stressful situation. One hopes that later versions of the software are more accurate.

4.8   Conclusion

There is an urgent need for reliable CAD software that will decrease the amount of stress experienced by DR graders, help increase image quality and improve quality assurance, increase accuracy of DR detection, and thus help screeners reduce the incidence of visual problems in diabetes [50]. The performance of new algorithms and of combinations thereof should be compared to the performance of the best of current practice for DR detection [119], large, well-designed multi-phase studies conducted in a variety of settings and populations. CAD programs ought to be developed in close cooperation with graders and adapted for use with electronic medical records. Proponents of CAD software will need to present high-quality evidence of a kind important to clinicians (cf. five papers by the GRADE Working Group in BMJ 2008). Forthcoming software must meet the needs of patients, programs, and staff. Evidence for CAD software needs to be of sufficient quality and relevance to form the basis of guidelines and strong recommendations according to the recently published GRADE criteria [120–124]. Such efforts should ensure market acceptance for DR CAD software.

References

[1] Lions Clubs, U.S. adults with diabetes fear blindness or vision loss more than premature death: Many respondents in international diabetes survey worried about quality of life. News release of the Lions Clubs International Foundation, 2006, http://www.lionsclubs.org/EN/content/news_news_release58.shtml (Accessed March 22, 2007).

[2] Klein, R. and Klein, B.E.K., Vision disorders in diabetes, in *Diabetes in America*, M.I. Harris, ed., National Institutes of Health, Bethesda, MD, 293–338, 2nd ed., 1995, NIH Publication No. 95-1468.

[3] Klein, R., Klein, B.E.K., Moss, S.E., et al., The validity of a survey question to study diabetic retinopathy, *Am J Epidemiol*, 124, 104, 1986.

[4] Aiello, L.P., Gardner, T.W., King, G.L., et al., Diabetic retinopathy, *Diabetes Care*, 21, 143, 1998.

[5] Lipscombe, L.L. and Hux, J.E., Trends in diabetes prevalence, incidence, and mortality in Ontario, Canada 1995–2005: A population-based study, *Lancet*, 369, 750, 2007.

[6] Wormald, R., Epidemiology in practice: Screening for eye disease, *Community Eye Health*, 12, 29, 1999, http://www.jceh.co.uk (Accessed March 22, 2007).

[7] Lee, S.J., Sicari, C., Harper, C.A., et al., Examination compliance and screening for diabetic retinopathy: A two-year study, *Clin Exp Ophthalmol*, 28, 159, 2000.

[8] Rhatigan, M.C., Leese, G.P., Ellis, J., et al., Blindness in patients with diabetes who have been screened for eye disease, *Eye*, 13 (Pt 2), 166, 1999.

[9] Moss, S.E., Klein, R., and Klein, B.E.K., Factors associated with having eye examinations in persons with diabetes, *Arch Fam Med*, 4, 529, 1995.

[10] Bäcklund, L.B., Algvere, P.V., and Rosenqvist, U., Early detection of diabetic retinopathy by a mobile retinal photography service working in partnership with primary health care teams, *Diabet Med*, 15(Suppl 3), S32, 1998.

[11] Keeffe, J., Screening for diabetic retinopathy. A planning and resource guide, 2003, http://cera.unimelb.edu.au/publications/reports/screening_for_diabetic_retinopathy.pdf.

[12] Garvican, L. and Scanlon, P.H., A pilot quality assurance scheme for diabetic retinopathy risk reduction programmes, *Diabet Med*, 21, 1066, 2004.

[13] Holland, W.W. and Stewart, S., *Screening in Disease Prevention: What works?*, Radcliffe Publishing, Abingdon, 2005.

[14] Javitt, J.C., Aiello, L.P., Chiang, Y., et al., Preventive eye care in people with diabetes is cost-saving to the federal government. implications for health-care reform, *Diabetes Care*, 17, 909, 1994.

[15] Scotland, G.S., McNamee, P., Philip, S., et al., Cost-effectiveness of implementing automated grading within the national screening programme for diabetic retinopathy in Scotland, *Br J Ophthalmol*, 91, 1518, 2007.

[16] Hoffman, J.R., Wilkes, M.S., Day, F.C., et al., The roulette wheel: An aid to informed decision making, *PLoS Med*, 3, e137, 2006.

[17] Galen, R.S. and Gambino, S.R., *Beyond Normality: The Predictive Value and Efficiency of Medical Diagnoses*, John Wiley, New York, 1975.

[18] Wilson, J.M.G. and Jungner, G., Principles and practice of screening for disease, WHO, Geneva, Switzerland, Public Health Papers No. 34, 1968.

[19] Kristinsson, J.K., Diabetic retinopathy. screening and prevention of blindness: A doctoral thesis, *Acta Ophthalmol Scand*, 223(Suppl), 1, 1997.

[20] Olson, J., ed., *Diabetic Retinopathy Screening Services in Scotland: A Training Handbook*, 2003, http://www.abdn.ac.uk/%7Eopt065/Web%20pages%20only/drh-25.htm (Accessed March 22, 2007).

[21] UK National Screening Committee, Essential elements in developing a diabetic retinopathy screening programme. Workbook 4.2, 2007, January (updated March 2008) http://www.nscretinopathy.org.uk (Accessed June 20, 2008).

[22] NHS Quality Improvement Scotland, Clinical standards for diabetic retinopathy screening, 2004, http://www.nhsqis.org.uk/nhsqis/1287.html (Accessed March 22, 2007).

[23] Saine, P.J. and Tyler, M.E., *Ophthalmic Photography: Retinal Photography, Angiography, and Electronic Imaging*, Butterworth-Heinemann, Boston, 2nd ed., 2002.

[24] Saine, P.J. and Tyler, M.E., *Practical Retinal Photography and Digital Imaging Techniques*, Butterworth-Heinemann, Boston, 2003.

[25] British Diabetic Association, *Guidelines on Screening for Diabetic Retinopathy*, British Diabetic Association, London, 1999.

[26] Hutchinson, A., McIntosh, A., Peters, J., et al., Clinical guidelines and evidence review for type 2 diabetes: Diabetic retinopathy: Early management and screening, 2001, http://guidance.nice.org.uk/page.aspx?o=28676 (Accessed March 22, 2007).

[27] Taube, A. and Tholander, B., Over- and underestimation of the sensitivity of a diagnostic malignancy test due to various selections of the study population, *Acta Oncol*, 29, 1, 1990.

[28] Scanlon, P.H., Malhotra, R., Thomas, G., et al., The effectiveness of screening for diabetic retinopathy by digital imaging photography and technician ophthalmoscopy, *Diabet Med*, 20, 467, 2003.

[29] Scanlon, P.H., Malhotra, R., Greenwood, R., et al., Comparison of two reference standards in validating two field mydriatic digital photography as a method of screening for diabetic retinopathy, *Br J Ophthalmol*, 87, 1258, 2003.

[30] Elandt-Johnson, R.C., Definition of rates: Some remarks on their use and misuse, *Am J Epidemiol*, 102, 267, 1975.

[31] Barratt, A., Irwig, L.M., Glasziou, P.P., et al., Users' guides to the medical

literature: XVII. How to use guidelines and recommendations about screening. Evidence-based medicine working group, *JAMA*, 281, 2029, 1999.

[32] Sackett, D.L., Haynes, R.B., Guyatt, G.H., et al., The selection of diagnostic tests, in *Clinical Epidemiology. A basic science for clinical medicine*, Little, Brown, London, 51–68, 2nd ed., 1991.

[33] Zweig, M.H. and Campbell, G., Receiver-operating characteristic (ROC) plots. a fundamental evaluation tool in clinical medicine, *Clin Chem*, 39, 561, 1993.

[34] von Wendt, G., Heikkila, K., and Summanen, P., Assessment of diabetic retinopathy using two-field 60 degrees fundus photography. a comparison between red-free, black-and-white prints and colour transparencies, *Acta Ophthalmol Scand*, 77, 638, 1999.

[35] Philip, S., Fleming, A.D., Goatman, K.A., et al., The efficacy of automated "disease/no disease" grading for diabetic retinopathy in a systematic screening programme, *Br J Ophthalmol*, 91, 1512, 2007.

[36] Altman, D.G., Machin, D., Bryant, T.N., et al., eds., *Statistics with Confidence*, BMJ Books, London, UK, 2nd ed., 2000.

[37] Agresti, A., Dealing with discreteness: Making "exact" confidence intervals for proportions, differences of proportions, and odds ratios more exact, *Stat Method Med Res*, 12, 3, 2003.

[38] Bachmann, L.M., Puhan, M.A., ter Riet, G., et al., Sample size of studies on diagnostic accuracy: Literature survey, *BMJ*, 332, 1127, 2006.

[39] Slattery, J., Sampling for quality assurance of grading decisions in diabetic retinopathy screening: Designing the system to detect errors, *Int J Health Care Qual Assur*, 18, 113, 2005.

[40] Metz, C.E., ROC methodology in radiologic imaging, *Invest Radiol*, 21, 720, 1986.

[41] Swets, J.A. and Pickett, R.M., *Evaluation of Diagnostic Systems: Methods from signal detection theory*, Academic Press, New York, 1982.

[42] Shapiro, D.E., The interpretation of diagnostic tests, *Stat Methods Med Res*, 8, 113, 1999.

[43] Pepe, M.S., *The Statistical Evaluation of Medical Tests for Classification and Prediction*, Oxford University Press, New York, 2003.

[44] Zhou, X.H., McClish, D.K., and Obuchowski, N.A., *Statistical Methods in Diagnostic Medicine*, Wiley, New York, 2002.

[45] Harbord, R.M., Deeks, J.J., Egger, M., et al., A unification of models for meta-analysis of diagnostic accuracy studies, *Biostatistics*, 8, 239, 2007.

[46] DeLuca, J., ed., *Fatigue as a Window to the Brain*, The MIT Press, Cambridge, London, 2005.

[47] Sharp, P.F., Olson, J., Strachan, F., et al., The value of digital imaging in diabetic retinopathy, *Health Technol Assess*, 7(30), 1, 2003.

[48] Scanlon, P.H., Foy, C., Malhotra, R., et al., The influence of age, duration of diabetes, cataract, and pupil size on image quality in digital photographic retinal screening, *Diabetes Care*, 28, 2448, 2005.

[49] Ege, B.M., Hejlesen, O.K., Larsen, O.V., et al., The relationship between age and colour content in fundus images, *Acta Ophthalmol Scand*, 80, 485, 2002.

[50] Niemeijer, M., van Ginnekan, B., Russell, S.R., et al., Automated detection and differentiation of drusen, exudates, and cotton-wool spots in digital color fundus photographs for diabetic retinopathy diagnosis, *Invest Ophthalmol Vis Sci*, 48, 2260, 2007.

[51] Basu, A., Digital image compression should be limited in diabetic retinopathy screening, *J Telemed Telecare*, 12, 163, 2006.

[52] Costen, M.T.J., Newsom, R.S.B., Parkin, B., et al., Effect of video display on the grading of diabetic retinopathy, *Eye*, 18, 169, 2004.

[53] Klein, R., Screening interval for retinopathy in type 2 diabetes, *Lancet*, 361, 190, 2003.

[54] World Health Organization Europe, European Region of International Diabetes Federation, The St. Vincent Declaration 1989, *Diabet Med*, 7, 36, 1990.

[55] Agardh, E., Agardh, C.D., and Hansson-Lundblad, C., The five-year incidence of blindness after introducing a screening programme for early detection of treatable diabetic retinopathy, *Diabet Med*, 10, 555, 1993.

[56] Kristinsson, J.K., Hauksdottir, H., Stefánsson, E., et al., Active prevention in diabetic eye disease. A 4-year follow-up, *Acta Ophthalmol Scand*, 75, 249, 1997.

[57] Bäcklund, L.B., Algvere, P.V., and Rosenqvist, U., New blindness in diabetes reduced by more than one-third in Stockholm County, *Diabet Med*, 14, 732, 1997.

[58] Arun, C.S., Ngugi, N., Lovelock, L., et al., Effectiveness of screening in preventing blindness due to diabetic retinopathy, *Diabet Med*, 20, 186, 2003.

[59] Frisén, L., *Clinical Tests of Vision*, Raven Press, New York, 1990.

[60] Olafsdottir, E., Andersson, D.K., and Stefánsson, E., Visual acuity in a population with regular screening for type 2 diabetes mellitus and eye disease, *Acta Ophthalmol Scand*, 85, 40, 2007.

[61] Bandurska-Stankiewicz, E. and Wiatr, D., Diabetic blindness significantly

reduced in the Warmia and Mazury Region of Poland: Saint Vincent Declaration targets achieved, *Eur J Ophthalmol*, 16, 722, 2006.

[62] Kohner, E.M., Stratton, I.M., Aldington, S.J., et al., Microaneurysms in the development of diabetic retinopathy (UKPDS 42), *Diabetologia*, 42, 1107, 1999.

[63] Hove, M.N., Kristensen, J.K., Lauritzen, T., et al., The relationships between risk factors and the distribution of retinopathy lesions in type 2 diabetes, *Acta Ophthalmol Scand*, 84, 619, 2006.

[64] Walter, T., Klein, J.C., Massin, P., et al., A contribution of image processing to the diagnosis of diabetic retinopathy — detection of exudates in color fundus images of the human retina, *IEEE Trans Med Imaging*, 21, 1236, 2002.

[65] Fleming, A.D., Philip, S., Goatman, K.A., et al., Automated detection of exudates for diabetic retinopathy screening, *Phys Med Biol*, 52, 7385, 2007.

[66] Larsen, M., Gondolf, T., Godt, J., et al., Assessment of automated screening for treatment-requiring diabetic retinopathy, *Curr Eye Res*, 32, 331, 2007.

[67] Gehrs, K.M., Anderson, D.H., Johnson, L.V., et al., Age-related macular degeneration — emerging pathogenetic and therapeutic concepts, *Ann Med*, 38, 450, 2006.

[68] Sarraf, D., Gin, T., Yu, F., et al., Long-term drusen study, *Retina*, 19, 513, 1999.

[69] Voo, I., Mavrofrides, E.C., and Puliafito, C.A., Clinical applications of optical coherence tomography for the diagnosis and management of macular diseases, *Ophthalmol Clin North Am*, 17, 21, 2004.

[70] Goatman, K.A., A reference standard for the measurement of macular oedema, *Br J Ophthalmol*, 90, 1197, 2006.

[71] McDonald, H.R., Williams, G.A., Scott, I.U., et al., Laser scanning imaging for macular disease: A report by the American Academy of Ophthalmology, *Ophthalmol*, 114, 1221, 2007.

[72] Srinivasan, V.J., Wojtkowski, M., Witkin, A.J., et al., High-definition and 3-dimensional imaging of macular pathologies with high-speed ultrahigh-resolution optical coherence tomography, *Ophthalmol*, 113, 2054, 2006.

[73] Funatsu, H., Yamashita, H., Ohashi, Y., et al., Effect of rapid glycemic control on progression of diabetic retinopathy, *Jpn J Ophthalmol*, 36, 356, 1992.

[74] Oyibo, S.O., Prasad, Y.D., Jackson, N.J., et al., The relationship between blood glucose excursions and painful diabetic peripheral neuropathy: A pilot study, *Diabet Med*, 19, 870, 2002.

[75] Patton, N., Aslam, T.M., MacGillivray, T., et al., Retinal image analysis. Concepts, applications and potential, *Prog Retin Eye Res*, 25, 99, 2006.

[76] Nguyen, T.T. and Wong, T.Y., Retinal vascular manifestations of metabolic disorders, *Trends Endocrinol Metab*, 17, 262, 2006.

[77] Feinstein, A.R., Misguided efforts and future challenges for research on "diagnostic tests," *J Epidemiol Community Health*, 56, 330, 2002.

[78] Deeks, J., Systematic reviews of evaluations of diagnostic and screening tests, in *Systematic Reviews in Health Care: meta-analysis in context*, M. Egger, G. Davey-Smith, and D. Altman, eds., BMJ Publ., London, 248–282, 2nd ed., 2001.

[79] Greenhalgh, T., *How to Read a Paper*, Blackwell BMJ Books, Oxford, 3rd ed., 2006.

[80] Whiting, P., Rutjes, A.W., Reitsma, J.B., et al., The development of QUADAS: A tool for the quality assessment of studies of diagnostic accuracy included in systematic reviews, *BMC Med Res Methodol*, 3, 25, 2003, http://www.biomedcentral.com/1471-2288/3/25.

[81] Whiting, P., Rutjes, A.W.S., Dinnes, J., et al., Development and validation of methods for assessing the quality of diagnostic accuracy studies, *Health Technol Assess*, 8(25), 2004, http://www.hta.nhsweb.nhs.uk/fullmono/mon825.pdf.

[82] Whiting, P.F., Weswood, M.E., Rutjes, A.W., et al., Evaluation of QUADAS, a tool for the quality assessment of diagnostic accuracy studies, *BMC Med Res Methodol*, 9, 2006, http://www.biomedcentral.com/1471-2288/6/9.

[83] Larsen, M., Godt, J., Larsen, N., et al., Automated detection of fundus photographic red lesions in diabetic retinopathy, *Invest Ophthalmol Vis Sci*, 44, 761, 2003.

[84] Larsen, N., Godt, J., Grunkin, M., et al., Automated detection of diabetic retinopathy in a fundus photographic screening population, *Invest Ophthalmol Vis Sci*, 44, 767, 2003.

[85] Hansen, A.B., Hartvig, N.V., Jensen, M.S., et al., Diabetic retinopathy screening using digital non-mydriatic fundus photography and automated image analysis, *Acta Ophthalmol Scand*, 82, 666, 2004.

[86] Bouhaimed, M., Gibbins, R., and Owens, D., Automated detection of diabetic retinopathy: results of a screening study, *Diabetes Technol Ther*, 10, 142, 2008.

[87] Hoover, A. and Goldbaum, M., Locating the optic nerve in a retinal image using the fuzzy convergence of the blood vessels, *IEEE Trans Med Imaging*, 22, 951, 2003.

[88] Fleming, A.D., Philip, S., Goatman, K., et al., Automated microaneurysm detection using local contrast normalization and local vessel detection, *IEEE Trans Med Imaging*, 25, 1223, 2006.

[89] Swensson, R.G., Unified measurement of observer performance in detecting and localizing target objects on images, *Med Phys*, 23, 1709, 1996.

[90] Goatman, K.A., Cree, M.J., Olson, J.A., et al., Automated measurement of microaneurysm turnover, *Invest Ophthalmol Vis Sci*, 44, 5335, 2003.

[91] Fleming, A.D., Philip, S., Goatman, K.A., et al., Automated assessment of diabetic retinal image quality based on clarity and field definition, *Invest Ophthalmol Vis Sci*, 47, 1120, 2006.

[92] Fleming, A.D., Goatman, K.A., Philip, S., et al., Automatic detection of retinal anatomy to assist diabetic retinopathy screening, *Phys Med Biol*, 52, 331, 2007.

[93] Bossuyt, P.M., Reitsma, J.B., Bruns, D.E., et al., Towards complete and accurate reporting of studies of diagnostic accuracy: The STARD initiative, *BMJ*, 326, 41, 2003.

[94] Bossuyt, P.M., Reitsma, J.B., Bruns, D.E., et al., The STARD statement for reporting studies of diagnostic accuracy: Explanation and elaboration, *Clin Chem*, 49, 7, 2003.

[95] Knottnerus, J.A., ed., *The Evidence Base of Clinical Diagnosis*, BMJ Books, London, 2002.

[96] Early Treatment Diabetic Retinopathy Study Research Group, Fundus photographic risk factors for progression of diabetic retinopathy. ETDRS report number 12, *Ophthalmology*, 98, 823, 1991.

[97] Early Treatment Diabetic Retinopathy Study Research Group, Grading diabetic retinopathy from stereoscopic color fundus photographs: An extension of the modified Airlie House classification. ETDRS report number 10, *Ophthalmology*, 98(suppl), 786, 1991.

[98] Wilkinson, C.P., Ferris, III, F.L., Klein, R.E., et al., Proposed international clinical diabetic retinopathy and diabetic macular edema disease severity scales, *Ophthalmology*, 110, 1677, 2003.

[99] Knudsen, L.L., Lervang, H.H., Lundbye-Christensen, S., et al., The North Jutland County Diabetic Retinopathy Study: Population characteristics, *Br J Ophthalmol*, 90, 1404, 2006.

[100] American College of Radiology, *Breast Imaging Reporting and Data System.*, American College of Radiology, Reston, Virginia, 1995.

[101] Kraemer, H.C., *Evaluating Medical Tests: Objective and Quantitative Guidelines*, Sage Publ., Newsbury Park, CA, 1992.

[102] Early Treatment Diabetic Retinopathy Study Research Group, Manual of Operations, (chapter 13), 1995, available from: National Technical Information Service, 52285 Port Royal Road, Springfield, VA 22161; Accession No. PB85

223006/AS Chapter 13, 1995.

[103] Aldington, S., Kohner, E., Meuer, S., et al., Methodology for retinal photography and assessment of diabetic retinopathy — the EURODIAB IDDM Complications Study, *Diabetologia*, 38(437-444), 1995.

[104] Knudsen, L.L. and Skriver, K., A 3-dimensional evaluation of the macular region: Comparing digitized and film-based media with a clinical evaluation, *Acta Ophthalmol Scand*, 84, 296, 2006.

[105] Swinscow, T.D.V. and Campbell, M., *Statistics at Square One*, BMJ Books, London, 10th ed., 2003.

[106] Svensson, E., Ordinal invariant measures for individual and group changes in ordered categorical data, *Stat Med*, 17, 2923, 1998.

[107] Morris, D., Fraser, S., and Wormald, R., Masking is better than blinding, *BMJ*, 334, 799, 2007.

[108] Begg, C.B., Biases in the assessment of diagnostic tests, *Stat Med*, 6, 411, 1987.

[109] Begg, C.B., Greenes, R.A., and Iglewicz, B., The influence of uninterpretability on the assessment of diagnostic tests, *J Chron Dis*, 39, 575, 1986.

[110] Irwig, L., Bossuyt, P., Glasziou, P., et al., Designing studies to ensure that estimates of test accuracy are transferable, *BMJ*, 324, 669, 2002.

[111] Kohner, E.M. and Dollery, C.T., The rate of formation and disappearance of microaneurysms in diabetic retinopathy, *Eur J Clin Invest*, 1, 167, 1970.

[112] Whiting, P., Rutjes, A.W.S., Reitsma, J.B., et al., Sources of variation and bias in studies of diagnostic accuracy. A systematic review, *Ann Intern Med*, 140, 189, 2004.

[113] Lantz, C.A. and Nebenzahl, E., Behavior and interpretation of the κ statistic: Resolution of the two paradoxes, *J Clin Epidemiol*, 49, 431, 1996.

[114] Pocock, S.J., *Clinical Trials: A Practical Approach*, John Wiley, Chichester, 1983.

[115] Hall, F.M., Breast imaging and computer-aided detection, *N Engl J Med*, 356, 1464, 2007.

[116] Thurfjell, E.L., Lernevall, K.A., and Taube, A.A., Benefit of independent double reading in a population-based mammography screening program, *Radiology*, 191, 241, 1994.

[117] Elmore, J.G., Nakano, C.Y., Koepsell, T.D., et al., International variation in screening mammography interpretations in community-based programs, *J Natl Cancer Inst*, 95, 1384, 2003.

[118] Fenton, J.J., Taplin, S.H., Carney, P.A., et al., Influence of computer-aided

detection on performance of screening mammography, *N Engl J Med*, 356, 1399, 2007.

[119] Lee, S.C., Lee, E.T., Wang, Y., et al., Computer classification of nonproliferative diabetic retinopathy, *Arch Ophthalmol*, 123, 759, 2005.

[120] Guyatt, G.H., Oxman, A.D., Kunz, R., et al., Incorporating considerations of resources use into grading recommendations, *BMJ*, 336, 1170, 2008.

[121] Schünemann, H.J., Oxman, A.D., Brozek, J., et al., Grading quality of evidence and strength of recommendations for diagnostic tests and strategies, *BMJ*, 336, 1106, 2008.

[122] Guyatt, G.H., Oxman, A.D., Kunz, R., et al., Going from evidence to recommendations, *BMJ*, 336, 1049, 2008.

[123] Guyatt, G.H., Oxman, A.D., Kunz, R., et al., What is "quality of evidence" and why is it important to clinicians? *BMJ*, 336, 995, 2008.

[124] Guyatt, G.H., Oxman, A.D., Vist, G.E., et al., GRADE: an emerging consensus on rating quality of evidence and strength of recommendations, *BMJ*, 336, 924, 2008.

4.A   Appendix: Measures of Binary Test Performance

		Disease	
		Present	Absent
Test result	pos.	a	b
	neg.	c	d

True positives Correct positive test result: $a =$ number of diseased persons with a positive test result.

True negatives Correct negative test results: $d =$ number of nondiseased persons with a negative test result.

False positives Incorrect positive test result: $b =$ number of nondiseased persons with a positive test result.

False negatives Incorrect negative test result: $c =$ number of diseased persons with a negative test result.

Sensitivity $(a/(a+c))$ proportion of people with the target disorder who have a positive test result. Known as true positive fraction (TPF).

Specificity $(d/(b+d))$ proportion of people without the target disorder who have a negative test result. False positive fraction, FPF $= (1 - \text{specificity})$.

Positive predictive value (PPV) the probability of disease among all persons with a positive test result. PPV $= a/(a+b)$.

Negative predictive value (NPV) the probability of nondisease among all persons with a negative test result. NPV $= d/(c+d)$.

5

Retinal Markers for Early Detection of Eye Disease

Alireza Osareh

CONTENTS

5.1 Abstract 121
5.2 Introduction 122
5.3 Nonproliferative Diabetic Retinopathy 123
5.4 Chapter Overview 124
5.5 Related Works on Identification of Retinal Exudates and the Optic Disc 128
5.6 Preprocessing 132
5.7 Pixel-Level Exudate Recognition 134
5.8 Application of Pixel-Level Exudate Recognition on the Whole Retinal Image 137
5.9 Locating the Optic Disc in Retinal Images 139
5.10 Conclusion 148
     References 150

5.1 Abstract

Diabetic retinopathy (DR) is a severe and widely spread eye disease that can be regarded as manifestation of diabetes on the retina. Screening to detect retinopathy disease can lead to successful treatments in preventing visual loss. Intraretinal fatty (hard) exudates are a visible sign of diabetic retinopathy and also a marker for the presence of coexistent retinal edema.

Detecting retinal exudate lesions in a large number of images generated by screening programs is very expensive in professional time and open to human error. Thus, we explore the benefits of developing an automated decision support system for the purpose of detecting and classifying exudate pathologies of diabetic retinopathy. The retinal images are automatically analyzed in terms of pixel resolution and an assessment of the level of retinopathy is derived.

Following some key preprocessing steps, color retinal image pixels are classified to exudate and nonexudate classes. *K* nearest neighbor, Gaussian quadratic, and

Gaussian mixture model classifiers are investigated within the pixel-level exudate recognition framework.

The location of the optic disc is of critical importance in retinal image analysis and is required as a prerequisite stage of exudate detection. Thus, we also address optic disc localization both to improve the overall diagnostic accuracy by masking the false positive optic disc regions from the other sought exudates and to measure its boundary precisely. We develop a method based on color mathematical morphology and active contours to accurately localize the optic disc region.

5.2 Introduction

Diabetes is an increasing health problem, both in the United Kingdom and the rest of the world. Approximately 1.4 million people in the United Kingdom are known to have diabetes [1]. One of the most feared complications of diabetes is damage to the eye. It is estimated that people with diabetes have a 25 times greater risk of going blind than the nondiabetic population. Each year around 12% of patients in the United Kingdom who are registered blind have diabetic eye disease as a cause. Diabetic retinopathy is the leading cause of blindness in the population of working age in the United Kingdom and developed nations, and is of increasing importance in developing nations [2]. Everyone who has diabetes is at risk for developing DR, but not everyone develops it. It is estimated that at any time around 10% of patients with diabetes will have DR requiring appropriate treatment [3]. The great majority of DR complications can be prevented with proper examination and treatment.

The chemical changes caused by diabetes affect retinal capillaries (the smallest blood vessels linking arteries to veins). This progressive damage is called diabetic retinopathy and occurs due to a combination of micro-vascular *leakage* and micro-vascular *occlusion*.

DR is conventionally classified according to the presence of clinical lesions indicating leakage or occlusion, and their position in the eye. The three main forms are known as nonproliferative retinopathy, maculopathy, and proliferative retinopathy.

The form of DR caused by micro-vascular leakage away from the macula is called nonproliferative diabetic retinopathy (NPDR) [4], and is shown by the presence of sacculations from the capillary walls (microaneurysms), blood (retinal hemorrhages), lipid exudates (hard exudates), and retinal edema. This stage of the disease often has no obvious warning signs and patients are unaware that they suffer from the disease until it progresses into more severe levels. Detection at this stage — one of the purposes of this work — may allow treatment to prevent future complications

When this microvascular leakage of edema, blood, and lipid occurs in the central region of the retina (the macula), it results in blurred vision, and is called diabetic maculopathy. Macular edema [4] is the most common cause of decreased vision in patients with nonproliferative DR. Less often, microvascular occlusion can also occur at the macula causing impaired vision because of an inadequate blood supply to that area (it has few clinical signs and is not usually treatable). Sometimes, there are extensive areas of microvascular occlusion throughout the retina. The retinal tissue, which depends on those vessels for its nutrition, releases a vasoproliferative factor stimulating the growth of new abnormal blood vessels where the normal capillaries have already closed. This form of DR caused by closure of capillaries and growth of new vessels is named *proliferative diabetic retinopathy*. It may result in bleeding into the cavity of the eye and scarring with loss of vision.

5.3 Nonproliferative Diabetic Retinopathy

Nonproliferative diabetic retinopathy (NPDR) is the most common type of diabetic retinopathy, accounting for approximately 80% of all patients. It can develop at any point in time after the onset of diabetes. A qualified practitioner, such as a general ophthalmologist, may detect these changes by examining the patient's retina. The physician looks for spots of bleeding, lipid exudation, or areas of retinal swelling caused by the leakage of edema, and will be more concerned if such lesions are found near the central retina (macula), when vision may become affected. Accurate assessment of retinopathy severity requires the ability to detect and record the following clinical features:

Microaneurysms: The earliest clinically recognizable characteristics of DR are microaneurysms. Retinal microaneurysms are focal dilatations of retinal capillaries. They are about 10 to 100 microns in diameter and appear as small, round, dark red dots on the retinal surface (see Figure 2.2(b) of Chapter 2) [2]. The number of microaneurysms increases as the degree of retinal involvement progresses.

Hemorrhages: As the degree of retinopathy advances retinal hemorrhages become evident. Retinal hemorrhages appear either as small red dots or blots indistinguishable from microaneurysms or as larger flame-shaped hemorrhages (Figure 2.2(c)). As the retinal vessels become more damaged and leaky, their numbers increase.

Hard Exudates: Among lesions caused by DR, exudates are one of the most commonly occurring lesions. They are associated with patches of vascular damage with leakage. The size and distribution of exudates may vary during the progress of the disease. Hard exudates represent leakage from surrounding capillaries and microaneurysms within the retina. If the lipid extends into the macula area, vision can be severely compromized. Exudates are typically manifested as random yellowish/white patches of varying sizes, shapes, and locations [2]. These are either seen as individual spots, clusters, or are found in large rings around leaking capillaries (Figures 2.2(a) and (b)). Although exudates may absorb spontaneously, they usually tend to increase in volume in an untreated retina. Occasionally, they may be confused with drusen (seen in age-related macular degeneration), which appear more regularly distributed at the macula.

The detection and quantification of exudates will significantly contribute to the mass screening and assessment of NPDR.

Cotton Wool Spots: Cotton wool spots represent a transitional stage between NPDR or maculopathy, and proliferative retinopathy. These abnormalities usually appear as little fluffy round or oval areas in the retina with a whitish color, usually adjacent to an area of hemorrhage (Figure 2.2(b)). Cotton wool spots come about due to the swelling of the surface layer of the retina, which consists of nerve fibers. This swelling occurs because the blood supply to that area has been impaired and in the absence of normal blood flow through the retinal vessels, the nerve fibers are injured in a particular location resulting in swelling and the appearance of a cotton wool spot [5].

If NPDR is not heeded and blood sugars are not controlled, the two later stages of damage to the eye may occur, i.e., diabetic maculopathy and proliferative retinopathy.

5.4   Chapter Overview

The application of digital imaging to ophthalmology has now provided the possibility of processing retinal images to assist clinical diagnosis and treatment. Retinal image analysis remarkably improves the diagnostic value of these images. In fact, with the advent of better and inexpensive ophthalmic imaging devices, along with the rapid growth of proper software for identifying those at risk of developing DR, as well as the reduction in costs and increase in computational power of computers, an advanced and cost-effective fundus image analysis system can be developed to assist ophthalmologists to make the diagnosis more efficiently. Such a system should be able to detect early signs of nonproliferative retinopathy and provide objective diagnosis based on some criteria defined by the ophthalmologists.

Intraretinal fatty exudates are a visible sign of DR and also a marker for the presence of co-existent retinal edema. If present in the macular area, edema and exudates are a major cause of visual loss in the nonproliferative forms of DR. Retinal edema and exudates in the central area are the clinical signs most closely linked with treatable visual loss.

Here, we have concentrated on detecting exudates as the prime marker because it is likely that accumulating exudates is always associated with retinal edema, and unlike edema, exudates are more visible in color retinal photographs. Detecting exudates in the retina in a large number of images generated by screening programs, which need to be repeated at least annually, is very expensive in professional time and open to human error. Thus, the main objective of the investigation described in this work is to contribute novel methods to quantitatively diagnose and classify exudate lesions in color retinal images from nonproliferative DR screening programs.

The optic disc is the entrance and exit region of blood vessels and optic nerves to the retina, and its localization and segmentation is an important task in an automated retinal image analysis system. Indeed, optic disc localization is required as a prerequisite for the subsequent stages in most algorithms applied for identification of the anatomical structures and pathologies in retinal images. Since optic disc localization is also indispensable to our exudates identification task, another objective is to develop a technique for optic disc localization and segmentation.

The overall scheme of the methods used in this work is shown in Figure 5.1. The input color retinal image is analyzed automatically and an assessment of the level of retinopathy disease is derived after analysis. The proposed method will then be able to choose diabetic patients who need further examination. In addition to the exudate detection we will also quantify the areas of exudate lesions in a pixel-based scheme. This will allow numerous measurements to be made of the deterioration in the condition over time.

In the first stage of the work, as shown at the top of Figure 5.1, we put our data through two preprocessing steps. Typically, there is a wide variation in the color of the fundus from different patients, strongly correlated to skin pigmentation and iris color. Hence, the first step is to normalize the color of the images. In the second step, the contrast between the exudates and retinal background is enhanced to facilitate later classification and segmentation. The contrast is not sufficient due to the internal attributes of exudate lesions and decreasing color saturation, especially in the peripheral retina.

Once the images have been preprocessed, exudate lesions can be identified automatically using our proposed *pixel-level exudate recognition* approach. Then, the diagnostic accuracy of this method is compared in terms of pixel resolution and image-based criteria against a provided pixel-level ground truth dataset. Here, we introduce two main criteria for assessing the diagnostic accuracy of our exudate detection techniques, i.e., lesion-based and image-based (Figure 5.2).

In lesion-based criteria each single exudate lesion is regarded as an individual connected region, where this region can be comprized of one or more pixels. Each abnormal retinal image can be segmented into a number of exudate regions. By considering a set of retinal images and applying an appropriate segmentation/classification technique, a dataset of exudate regions will be created. Then, the lesion-based accuracy can be measured in terms of lesion sensitivity and specificity by comparing the gained results against ophthalmologists' outline of the lesions.

The lesion-based accuracy can be assessed either in a pixel resolution (Figure 5.2) basis or alternatively using a bigger collection of pixels, e.g., 10×10 patches (patch resolution). Although creating an accurate pixel-based ground truth by the physician is not an easy task, a pixel resolution comparison of the results is more precise than using patch resolution, as a pixel patch may only partially cover exudate pixels. Thus, the effect of misclassification errors for individual patches (exudates/nonexudates) should be taken into consideration when the performance is not measured based on pixel resolution.

In image-based diagnostic based assessment, the objective is to provide a logical predicate of the condition of the analyzed image. In this case, each image is examined and a decision is made to illustrate whether the image has some evidence of DR, purely based on the absence or presence of exudates anywhere in the image. Hence,

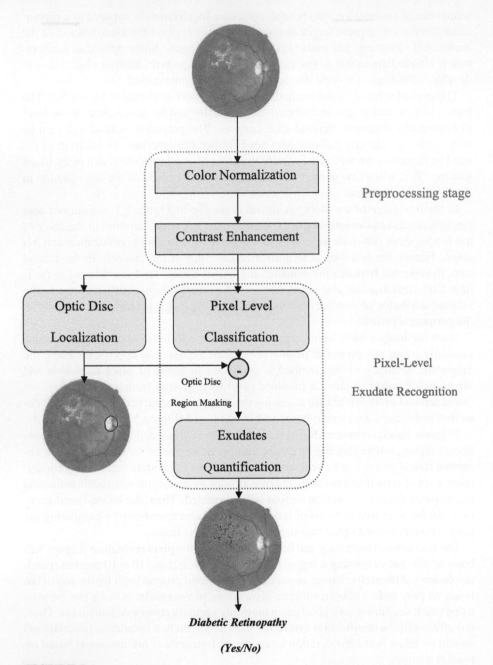

FIGURE 5.1

The outline of the proposed system for automatic identification of retinal exudates and the optic disc in color retinal images. **(See color insert following page 174.)**

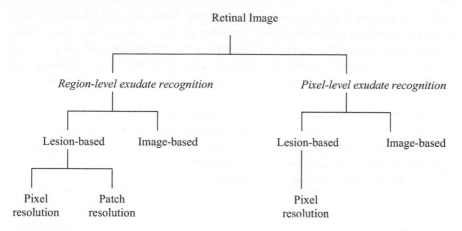

FIGURE 5.2

The stages in the scheme developed to identify the retinal exudates and different diagnostic accuracy criteria that can be used to assess the results.

the system's global image-based accuracy can be measured using a proportion of the tested normal-abnormal images to the number of images, which are correctly identified.

Three classifiers, K nearest neighbor (*KNN*), Gaussian quadratic (*GQ*), and Gaussian mixture model (*GMM*), are investigated within the *pixel-level exudate recognition* framework. Each classifier is trained and tested against four different pixel datasets of exudates and nonexudates. We consider separate *GMMs* to estimate the distribution of each class, i.e., exudates and nonexudates, and combine the models into a classifier through Bayesian theory. The *GMM* parameters are extracted by means of the expectation-maximization algorithm. To select an appropriate number of Gaussian components the minimum description length criterion is applied. The optimum *GMM* classifier is used to evaluate the effectiveness of our proposed approach by assessing the image-based accuracy of the system on a population of 67 unseen retinal images.

During our initial exudate lesion identification (*pixel-level exudate recognition*), false positive exudate candidates arise due to other pale objects including light reflection artifacts, cotton wool spots, and most significantly, the optic disc. The optic disc is detected as candidate exudate pixels/regions due to the similarity of its color to the exudates. To mask the false positive optic disc pixels/regions from the other exudate lesions, and due to the critical importance of location of the optic disc, we also address optic disc localization and segmentation problem with different levels of accuracy. Two techniques are investigated including template matching and active contours (snakes).

The first strategy provides an approximate location of the optic disc center. However, the optic disc can sometimes have an elliptical shape, and thus baseline plotting of the exact boundaries is important. Consequently, a snake-based technique is developed to generate a more accurate disc boundary. We have hand-labeled (through an expert consultant ophthalmologist) a number of optic disc regions. This allows us to develop a measure to accurately determine the performance of our proposed technique. The optic disc localization stage is shown in Figure 5.1. Its results are fed into our exudates identification scheme to mask out the optic disc regions from the computations.

Section 5.5 describes previous works on identification of retinal exudates and the optic disc. The preprocessing details are presented in Section 5.6. Sections 5.7 and 5.8 explain our proposed automatic method for identification of retinal exudates at pixel level and the application of this method on whole retinal images. Section 5.9 presents our optic disc localization techniques.

5.5 Related Works on Identification of Retinal Exudates and the Optic Disc

Currently, there is an increasing interest for setting up systems and algorithms that can screen a large number of people for sight-threatening diseases, such as DR, and then provide an automated detection of the disease. Retinal image analysis is a complicated task, particularly because of the variability of the images in terms of the color/gray-levels, the morphology of the retinal anatomical-pathological structures, and the existence of particular features in different patients, which may lead to an erroneous interpretation. Several examples of the application of digital imaging techniques in identification of DR can be found in the literature.

There have been some research investigations in the literature [6–10] to identify main components of the retina such as blood vessels, optic disc and retinal lesions including microaneurysms, hemorrhages, and exudates. Here, we review the main results, with emphasis on exudate detection and optic disc localization and segmentation.

5.5.1 Exudate identification and classification

Among lesions caused by DR, exudates are one of the most commonly occurring lesions. They are associated with patches of vascular damage with leakage. The size and distribution of exudates may vary during the progress of the disease. The detection and quantification of exudates will significantly contribute to the mass screening and assessment of NPDR.

The quantification of *diabetic maculopathy* and detection of exudates on fundus images were investigated by [11; 12]. Global and local thresholding values were used to segment exudate lesions from the red-free images. Before thresholding can be done, the digitized color photographs were preprocessed to eliminate photographic nonuniformities (shade correction), and the contrast of the exudates was then enhanced. The lesion-based sensitivity of the exudate identification technique was reported between 61% and 100% (mean 87%) [12].

In [13] an algorithm was applied to detect and measure exudates in fundus images. A fundus transparency was imaged, digitized, and then preprocessed to reduce shade variations in the image background and enhance the contrast between the background and the exudate lesions. Exudates were then separated from the background on a brightness or gray-level basis. The proposed technique required user intervention for selecting the threshold value.

In [6] a prototype was presented on automated diagnosis and understanding of retinal images. The system used images with a field of view of 10° or 60° to recognize the bright objects including exudates, cotton wool spots, drusen, and scars. Different features like color, texture, and compactness were used within the classification stage. This method achieved a lesion-based accuracy of 89% for identification of the bright objects.

Ege et al. [14] located the optic disc, fovea, and four red and yellow abnormalities (microaneurysms, hemorrhages, exudates, and cotton wool spots) in 38 color fundus images, which were previously graded by an ophthalmologist. The abnormalities were detected using a combination of template matching, region growing, and thresholding techniques. 87% of exudates were detected during the first stage while the detection rate for the cotton wool spots was up to 95% in terms of the lesion-based criterion. Following preliminary detection of the abnormalities, a Bayesian classifier was engaged to classify the yellow lesions into exudates, cotton wool spots, and noise. The classification performance for this stage was only 62% for exudates and 52% for the cotton wool spots.

Wang et al. [15] addressed the same problem by using a minimum distance discriminant classifier to categorize each pixel into yellow lesion (exudates, cotton wool spots) or nonlesion (vessels and background) class. The objective was to distinguish yellow lesions from red lesions, therefore other yellowish lesions (e.g. cotton wool spots) were incorrectly classified at the same time. The image-based diagnostic accuracy of this approach was reported as 100% sensitivity and 70% specificity.

In addition to the discussed techniques, neural networks have also been exploited to classify the retinal abnormalities in a few studies. Gardner et al. [16] broke down the retinal images into small squares and then presented them to a back propagation neural network. After median smoothing, the photographed red-free images with a field-of-view of 60° were fed directly into a large neural network (using 20×20 patches, with 400 inputs). This technique recognized the blood vessels, exudates, and hemorrhages. The neural network was trained for 5 days and the lesion-based sensitivity of the exudate detection method was 93.1%. This performance was the result of classifying the whole 20×20 pixel patches rather than a pixel resolution classification.

Walter et al. [17] identified exudates from the green channel of retinal images, according to their gray-level variation. After initial localization, the exudate contours were subsequently determined by mathematical morphology techniques. This approach had three parameters, the size of the local window, which was used for calculation of the pixel local variation, and two other threshold values. The first threshold determines the minimum variation value within each local window. The candidate exudate regions are initially found based on the first threshold value. The second threshold represents the minimum value, by which a candidate must differ from its surrounding background pixels to be classified as exudates. This technique achieved 92.8% mean sensitivity and 92.4% predictivity against a set of 15 abnormal retinal images. A set of 15 normal retinal images was also examined, of which 13 had no exudates (88.6% specificity in terms of image-based accuracy).

As is apparent from the above reviewed methods, most proposed exudate identification techniques have only been assessed in terms of *either* lesion-based *or* image-based diagnostic performance criterion and against an approximately small number of retinal images. Indeed, the reported lesion-based accuracies are often based on 10×10 or 20×20 patches (patch resolution) and pixel resolution validation has been reported in a couple of works. There are certain errors in reported patch resolution accuracies due to the small areas, which some exudates can occupy. In medical decision support systems such as ours, an accurate diagnostic accuracy assessment in terms of both pixel resolution and image-based is important.

5.5.2   Optic disc detection

Reliable and efficient optic disc localization and segmentation are significant tasks in an automatic screening system. Optic disc localization is required as a prerequisite for the subsequent stages in many algorithms applied for identification of the anatomical-pathological structures in retinal images. This is summarized in the following.

Blood vessel tracking approaches: where blood vessels positioned in the neighborhood of the optic disc are used as seeds for vessel tracking [18].

Macula localization: in this case the approximate constant distance between the optic disc and the macula can be used as *a priori* knowledge for locating the macula [19].

Diabetic retinopathy lesions identification: to improve the lesion diagnosis performance by masking or removing the false positive optic disc from the other pathologies of interest, e.g., [17] and the author's work towards exudates identification [20].

There have been relatively few works on locating the optic disc in retinal images without user intervention. In fact, most of those only locate the optic disc center and do not address the problem of optic disc boundary localization. Reliable optic disc localization is surprisingly difficult, due to its highly variable appearance in retinal images.

In [14; 21] an edge detection stage was followed by a circular Hough transform to locate the optic disc. The algorithm commenced with locating the optic disc candidate area. This was defined as a 180×180 pixels region including the highest 2% gray-level in the red color component of the retinal image. Then, the Sobel operator was used to detect the edge points of the located candidate area. The contours were then detected by means of the circular Hough transform, i.e., the gradient of the image was calculated, and the best fitting circle was then determined. These approaches are quite time consuming and rely on certain conditions regarding the shape of the optic disc that are not always met. Moreover, edge detection algorithms often fail to provide an acceptable solution due to the fuzzy boundaries, inconsistent image contrast, or missing edge features.

Li and Chutatape [19] proposed a method for locating the optic disc using a combination of pixel clustering and principal component analysis techniques. They first determined the optic disc candidate regions by clustering the brightest pixels in gray-level retinal images. This strategy can only work when there is no abnormality in the image. On the other hand, a bright pixel clustering approach will fail when there are large exudate lesions in the retinal image. This is due to the color and intensity similarities that exist between exudates and the optic disc. To cope with this difficulty principal component analysis was applied to finally locate the optic disc. They considered a small number of images as a training set and then determined the correspondent eigenvectors. Then, each new image was projected to a new space, i.e., "disc space," using its eigenvectors in a similar way to face detection. Next, the distance between the pixels belonging to the candidate regions and the provided projection was calculated and the pixel with minimum distance was finally chosen as the optic disc center. The technique was tested against 40 images and the results were reported satisfactory. However, the authors did not address the optic disc boundary localization.

Sinthanayothin [22] used an 80×80 sub-image to evaluate the intensity variance of adjacent pixels, and marking the point with the largest variance as the optic disc location. This technique has been shown to work well with 99.1% sensitivity and specificity when there are no or only few small exudate pathologies that also appear very bright and are also well contrasted. In fact, the authors made an assumption to locate the optic disc from those retinal images with no visible symptoms. This work has also mainly focused on locating the optic disc center.

Lalonde et al. [23] localized the optic disc using a combination of two procedures including a Hausdorff-based template matching technique on the edge map, guided by a pyramidal decomposition technique. *A priori* information of the image characteristics, e.g., right/left eye image and whether the input image is centered on the macula or an optic disc have to be provided. The edge maps were calculated using Canny edge detection and therefore the low and high hysteresis thresholds must be defined properly. The authors reported an average error of 7.0% in locating the disc center and 80% area overlap between their ground truth optic disc and the localized one against a database comprising 40 retinal images.

The optic disc boundary was found in Mendels et al. [24] using a twofold method. The optic disc boundary is highly influenced by the strong blood vessel edges crossing the optic disc region. Therefore, a preprocessing step was first applied based on local minima detection and morphological filtering to remove the interfering blood vessels and locate the optic disc boundary accurately. To do that, a gray-level dilation operator was applied based on a 5×5 pixel structuring element. This was followed by erosion using the same structuring element to re-establish the optic disc contour to its original place. A morphological reconstruction operator was then applied by maintaining the maximum of the dilated/eroded image and the original one. Then, the optic disc contour was located using the deformable active contours (snakes) technique. The snake was based on an external image field called Gradient Vector Flow (GVF). The technique was tested against a set of 9 retinal images and the author reported an accurate optic disc boundary localization in all the test images.

To locate the optic disc in this study, two different techniques are investigated including template matching and active contours. The first strategy provides an approximate location of the optic disc center. The optic disc can sometimes have an elliptical shape, and therefore the baseline plotting of its exact boundaries is necessary. To achieve this goal a snake technique is applied to obtain a more accurate disc boundary. We test these two approaches against an image dataset of 75 color retinal images including 25 normal and 50 abnormal images. In all cases the template image could provide a good approximate match of the optic disc center even when large, albeit scattered, areas of similarly colored exudate pathologies exist in the image.

Here, we also develop a similar approach to [25], except we introduce two novel improvements. First, we place the initial snake automatically using our earlier levels of processing. Second, we improve on the morphological step by using color morphology, which results in a more homogeneous inner disc area and aids the accuracy of the optic disc localization. We can use either of the proposed methods to automatically position an initial snake. In all our experiments this was performed successfully, however, in optic disc images a snake is significantly affected by the blood vessels present in the optic disc region.

Hence, a preparation step is necessary. To do that we devise a more basic definition of color morphology using a *reduced* ordering concept for color vectors, in which the definitions of maximum and minimum operations on color pixels reduce to the maximum and minimum of a scalar valued function in the structuring mask. Then, a closing morphological filtering is carried out in a more metric color space such as L*ab* to remove the interfering blood vessels. After the color morphological preprocessing step, the gradient image is obtained to compute the snake's external energy to drive the GVF snake towards the desired accurate optic disc boundary.

To provide a more objective assessment of the performance of our algorithm we used an effective overlap measure of the match between two regions, i.e., localized optic disc region and the optic disc region ground truth provided by an ophthalmologist. Using this measure, the GVF snake could achieve 90.32% overall accuracy against the provided image dataset when the morphological preprocessing were applied using L*ab* components respectively. We also demonstrate the improvement obtained using the proposed color morphological closing over gray-level morphology for this application. The detail of our proposed optic disc localization approaches along with a quantification of results are reported later this chapter.

5.6   Preprocessing

We used 142 color retinal images obtained from a Canon CR6-45 nonmydriatic camera with a 45° field of view. This consisted of 75 images for training and testing

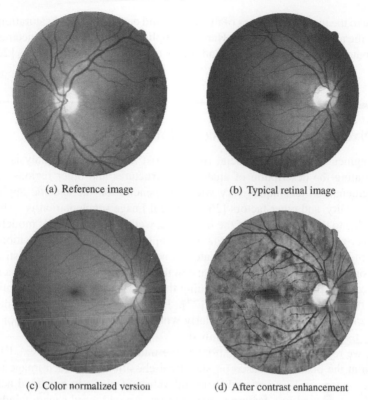

(a) Reference image   (b) Typical retinal image

(c) Color normalized version   (d) After contrast enhancement

FIGURE 5.3

Color normalization and local contrast enhancement. (**See color insert.**)

our classifiers in the pixel-level classification stage. The remaining 67 images were employed to investigate the image-based diagnostic accuracy of our system. The image resolution was 760×570 at 24-bit red-green-blue (RGB) color.

One of the main obstacles for identification of retinal exudates is the wide variability in the color of the fundus from different patients. These variations are strongly correlated to skin pigmentation and iris color. Thus, the color of exudate lesions in some region of an image may appear dimmer than the background color of other regions. As a result, the exudates can wrongly be classified as the background. In fact, without some type of color normalization the large variation in the natural retinal pigmentation across the patient dataset can hinder discrimination of the relatively small variations between the different lesion types. Thus, in the first step we selected a retinal image as a reference and applied the described histogram specification technique to modify the values of each image in the dataset such that its frequency histogram matched the reference image distribution (see Figure 5.3(c)). The color normalization process was performed using histogram specification [20].

In the second preprocessing step, the contrast between the exudates and the background is enhanced to facilitate later exudate identification. The contrast is not sufficient due to the internal attributes of the lesions and decreasing color saturation, especially in the area around the fovea. Here, we applied local contrast enhancement [22] to distribute the values of pixels around the local mean (see Figure 5.3(d)) [20].

5.7 Pixel-Level Exudate Recognition

Image segmentation plays a crucial role in most medical image analysis systems by facilitating the description of anatomical structures and other regions of interest. Segmentation techniques vary widely depending on the specific application, image modality, and other factors [26]. Medical image segmentation is a challenging task due to the complexity of the images, as well as the absence of models of the anatomical-pathological structures that fully capture the possible information.

A segmentation method ideally locates those sets that correspond to distinct anatomical or pathological regions of interest in the image. If the constraint that regions be connected is removed, then determining the sets is called pixel classification and the sets themselves are called classes [27]. Pixel classification is often a desirable objective in medical imaging, particularly when disconnected regions belonging to the same tissue class need to be identified.

Here, we report on the investigations made into the application of exudate identification at the pixel level based on statistical classifiers. For each image pixel x_0 a feature vector consisting of multi-spectral values of pixels in a defined neighborhood $N(x_0)$ was used as a feature representation. An odd-sized square window was centered on each underlying pixel x_0 in the dataset. Then the Luv color components (this color space was found the most appropriate space for our analysis) of the pixels in the window were composed into the feature vector of x_0.

The selection of a color space for image processing is application dependent. To select the most suitable space for our pixel-based classification approach, we conducted a quantitative analysis and applied a metric to evaluate the performance of various color spaces. This metric [28] estimated the class separability of our exudate and nonexudate pixel classes in different spaces and was measured using within-class and between-class scatter matrices. After within-class (S_w) and between-class (S_b) matrices are measured the following metric J can be obtained:

$$J = \mathrm{Tr}\left(\frac{S_b}{S_w}\right) \tag{5.1}$$

A higher value of J indicates that the classes are more separated while the members within each class are closer to each other. We have experimented with different color spaces and found that the Luv color space is the most appropriate space for our retinal image analysis (Table 5.1). Thus, we chose this color space to carry out our pixel-level classification task.

There might be no constraint on the neighborhood window size N in theory, but it was assumed that most contextual information was presented in a small neigh-

Table 5.1: Comparative Analysis of Different Color Spaces

Color Space	YIQ	RGB	HSL	HSI	L*ab*	L*uv*
J	2.20	2.25	2.64	2.81	3.32	**3.67**

borhood of the x_0 pixel. Here, to determine the optimal window size, we examined various pixel patch sizes, i.e., 1×1, 3×3, 5×5 and 7×7. To construct learning datasets of exudate and nonexudate (including cotton wool spots, red lesions, blood vessels, and background) pixels, a consultant ophthalmologist manually segmented 75 preprocessed images and marked the exudate lesions in these images. An almost balanced learning dataset of exudates and nonexudates was then established to eliminate any possible bias towards either of the two classes. This representative learning dataset was comprized of 62 501 exudate and 63 046 nonexudate pixels.

To model the exudate and nonexudate probability density function, we chose one very commonly used classifier for every type of probability density estimation approach, i.e., nonparametric *KNN*, parametric *GQ*, and semiparametric *GMM*. Each classifier was trained and tested against our four pixel datasets (1×1, 3×3, 5×5, and 7×7).

In *KNN* classification, the number of neighbors, i.e., K, needs to be predefined. Here, we experimented with different K values ranging from 1 to 7 (K was chosen to be odd to avoid ties), to find the optimum value with the lowest misclassification error rate. Table 5.2 summarizes the best overall performances accomplished using the *KNN* classifier. As can be seen, this classifier achieved good generalization ability, with a best overall performance of 90.26% against 5×5 pixel patch size dataset. In this case, the correct classification rate for the exudate and nonexudate classes was 88.92% and 91.60% respectively.

The Gaussian distribution is one of the most generally used density estimators. According to Bayes' theorem, the posterior probability is written as:

$$P(C_i|x) = \frac{p(x|C_i) P(C_i)}{p(x)} \tag{5.2}$$

The likelihood function $p(x|C_i)$ was defined in terms of exudates and nonexudates class mean and covariance matrix. $P(C_i)$ was the *a priori* probability denoting the probability that a pixel (exudate or nonexudate) occurs in the entire set of pixels. The posterior probability measured the probability of the pixel belonging to either the exudates (C_{Exu}) or nonexudates (C_{Non}) class once we have observed the feature vector x. Here, the class attached to each feature vector x was selected based on the maximum a posterior (MAP) rule. Table 5.2 illustrates the overall performances achieved using the *GQ* classifier. The best obtained overall classification accuracy was 88.24% for a 5×5 pixel patch size dataset, comprising 89.14% and 87.34% correct classification rates for exudates and nonexudates respectively.

A disadvantage of parametric density estimation techniques is their lack of flexibility when compared with nonparametric methods. Although single Gaussian density estimation models can be set up easily, they are restricted in their ability to

Table 5.2: The Best Overall Pixel-Level Classification Performances

Pixel Patch Size	Classifier		
	KNN	GQ	GMM
1×1	84.29% ($K = 7$)	82.25%	85.13%
3×3	86.85% ($K = 5$)	86.15%	92.35%
5×5	**90.26%** ($K = 5$)	**88.24%**	**96.49%**
7×7	89.87% ($K = 5$)	87.58%	96.32%

efficiently estimate more complex distributions [29]. *GMMs* combine much of the flexibility of nonparametric methods with certain amounts of the analytical advantages of parametric approaches.

Basically, in a mixture model distribution the data is represented as a linear combination of component densities in the form:

$$p(x_i) = \sum_{k=1}^{K} p(x_i|w_k; \Theta_k) P(w_k) \tag{5.3}$$

where K represents the number of components and each component is defined by w_k and parameterized by Θ_k (mean vector and covariance matrix). The coefficient $P(w_k)$ is called the mixing parameter. We benefited from the theory behind these models and used a separate mixture of Gaussians to estimate the class densities $p(x|C_i, \Theta)$ of exudates and nonexudates as follows:

$$p(x|C_i, \Theta) = \sum_{k=1}^{K_i} \frac{P(w_k)}{(2\pi)^{\frac{d}{2}} \det(\Sigma_k)^{\frac{1}{2}}} \exp\left\{ -\frac{1}{2} (x - \mu_k)^T \Sigma_k^{-1} (x - \mu_k) \right\} \tag{5.4}$$

where μ_k and Σ_k represent the mean and covariance of the kth component of the mixture density of class C_i. K_i denotes the numbers of components in class i and C_i refers to either the exudates or nonexudates class. Having estimated the likelihood functions of these two classes the posterior probabilities were obtained. The decision about the affiliation of each new feature vector x was then taken by applying the MAP rule. We assumed a full covariance matrix for each component, since these types of matrices have higher flexibility in estimating the underlying distributions.

To determine the parameters of a *GMM* and fit a model to the data, the expectation maximization algorithm was utilized. This algorithm started with an initial guess for the parameters of the model and then iteratively modified these parameters to decrease an error function until a minimum was reached. The parameters were initialized using a K-means clustering algorithm. The K-means algorithm partitions the feature space into K clusters. To apply the K-means algorithm, the number of clusters, i.e., K (or equivalently the number of components) needs to be known. Choosing too few components produces a model that cannot accurately model the distributions. With an increasing number of components, the probability that the model fits the dataset better will be increased, but the model also loses its capability to generalize well.

Here, the appropriate number of components was chosen by repeating the density model estimation and evaluating the minimum description length criterion [30]. We obtained the optimum mixture model of each exudate and nonexudate pixel-level dataset separately by varying the number of components within a range of 1 to 20. The optimum number of *GMM* components for exudate and nonexudate datasets were found equal to 7 and 9 (for 1×1 dataset), 10 and 11 (for 3×3 dataset), 15 and 17 (for 5×5 dataset), 19 and 23 (for 7×7 dataset) respectively. It is evident that by increasing the pixel patch size, the model complexity was also raised and necessitated a higher number of components for effective density estimation.

Table 5.2 summarizes the overall performance achieved using *GMM*. Typically, the performance of a classifier improves up to a certain point as additional features are added, and then deteriorates. This can be seen in Table 5.2, as performance continued to improve when the patch size was increased up to 5. At this point all classifiers achieved their best results. However, by increasing the pixel patch size, i.e., to 7, the accuracy decreased.

In many situations, such as our application, it is valuable to obtain a 2D or 3D projection of the original multivariate data for visual examination. Here, principal component analysis was applied to the pixel dataset that achieved the highest classification accuracy, i.e., our 5×5 dataset. The first two exudate principal modes contained 62.4% of the total variance, i.e., 49.7% + 12.7%. Similarly, the first two nonexudate principal modes represent 53.2% of the total variance (38.0% + 15.2%).

The *GMM* classifier performed better than the other two classifiers and provided the best results irrespective of the choice of pixel patch size. The best *GMM* classification demonstrated an overall performance equal to 96.49%, based on the 5×5 pixel-level dataset (Table 5.2). In this case, the correct classification rates for exudates and nonexudates were 96.15% and 96.83% respectively. Therefore, the *GMM* classifier with the 5×5 pixel level dataset was utilized to classify the pixels of a new set of images.

5.8 Application of Pixel-Level Exudate Recognition on the Whole Retinal Image

The performance of a medical diagnosis system is best described in terms of *sensitivity* and *specificity*. The *sensitivity* gives the percentage of correctly classified abnormal cases while the *specificity* defines the percentage of correctly classified normal cases. Classification of the whole retinal image pixels was required to work on an unbalanced dataset of exudate and nonexudate pixels where the number of *true negatives* (*TN*) was much higher than the *false positives* (*FPs*). The *specificity* measure was mostly near 100% and did not represent an informative measurement. Thus, we used the *predictivity* measure, which is the probability that a pixel classified as

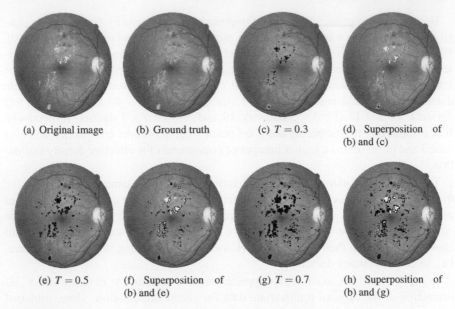

(a) Original image   (b) Ground truth   (c) $T = 0.3$ (d) Superposition of (b) and (c)

(e) $T = 0.5$ (f) Superposition of (b) and (e)   (g) $T = 0.7$ (h) Superposition of (b) and (g)

FIGURE 5.4

Pixel-level exudate recognition application on a retinal image using different ratio of exudate and nonexudate prior probabilities. The identified exudates are shown in blue and *TPs* are in white. (**See color insert.**)

exudate is really an exudate. This was defined as:

$$\text{predictivity} = \frac{TP}{TP + FP} \tag{5.5}$$

where *TP* refers to the *true positive*. In real applications, such as ours, there is no previous knowledge of actual prior probabilities of exudates and nonexudates. For example, the underlying test image can be either a normal image with no exudate, or an abnormal severe retinopathy image with a significant number of exudate pixels. Thus, to accomplish an efficient image classification process and control the balance between *sensitivity* and *predictivity*, we constructed a series of classifiers by varying the prior probability ratio of exudates to nonexudates using a decision threshold T. For instance, a threshold value equal to 0.8 sets the exudates' prior probability to 0.8 and nonexudates' prior probability equal to 0.2 (i.e., $1 - T$). Figure 5.4 shows an abnormal image that has been classified using our trained optimum *GMM* classifier. The original image and its ground truth are shown in Figure 5.4(a) and (b). The corresponding classification results for T values of 0.3, 0.5 and 0.7 are illustrated in Figure 5.4(c), (e), and (g).

By increasing the threshold value and assigning higher prior probabilities to the exudates, the number of *TPs* was increased while at the same time the *false negatives* (*FNs*) were decreased. Thus, the *sensitivity* measure was enhanced. Indeed, by increasing the threshold value another reverse trend was noticed, where the *FPs* also

Table 5.3: Pixel-Level Accuracy in Terms of
Sensitivity-Predictivity Criteria

T	Sensitivity	Predictivity
0.10	67.3	94.1
0.30	80.3	88.3
0.40	**87.2**	**83.0**
0.45	**89.2**	**81.0**
0.50	90.4	79.5
0.85	94.5	57.6

begin to intensify, which leads to a decrease in *predictivity*. The trade-off between *sensitivity* and *predictivity* measures (choice of T) needs to be appropriately balanced according to the diagnostic strategy. We considered a new set of 40 abnormal images and then each image was separately classified with different T values.

The overall pixel-level classification performance was obtained based on the average of all images' *sensitivities* and *predictivities* values. Table 5.3 summarizes some of these averaged *sensitivity-predictivity* values. As is evident, the threshold values that provided the highest average of *sensitivity* and *predictivity* values were 0.40 and 0.45. An important issue in choosing the threshold is ensuring that our classifier does not have a very high *sensitivity* for exudate detection; otherwise it can wrongly classify the normal images as abnormal. Therefore, to assess the efficiency of our proposed exudate recognition scheme in terms of image-based accuracy, we set the threshold T equal to 0.45 and classified the whole set of 67 retinal images (40 abnormal and 27 normal) using the optimum *GMM* classifier. Then a final decision was made as to whether each image had some evidence of retinopathy.

When we manually analyzed the system's decision on normal images we found that in most cases when a normal image had been wrongly identified as abnormal not many *FP* pixels had been detected. To improve the image-based *specificity* of the system without sacrificing the *sensitivity*, a threshold value was defined. Based on this threshold, each classified abnormal image with less than 50 identified exudate pixels in size was considered normal. This threshold was determined in agreement with our experiments and our consultant clinician. The *GMM* classifier could identify abnormal images with 92.5% *sensitivity* (correct identification of 37 abnormal images out of 40), while it correctly classified 81.4% (correct identification of 22 normal images out of 27) of the normal images (the *specificity*).

5.9 Locating the Optic Disc in Retinal Images

The location of the optic disc is of critical importance in retinal image analysis. Optic disc (OD) localization is necessary as a prerequisite stage in most algorithms applied for identification of the retinal anatomical structures and lesions. These can be summarized as follows:

Blood vessel detection approaches: where blood vessels positioned in the neighborhood of the optic disc provide possible seeds for vessel tracking.

Macula identification: where the approximately constant distance between the optic disc and the macula can be used as *a priori* knowledge for locating the macula.

Lesions classification: to improve the lesion diagnosis performance by masking or removing the "false positive" optic disc regions from the other required pathologies.

Optic disc localization is indispensable in our automatic exudates identification approach, since it illustrates similar attributes to the exudates in terms of color, brightness, and contrast. By detecting it we can remove it from the exudate classification process. In fact, the results reported in previous sections were all obtained *after* the removal of the optic disc using the work described in this section. Despite its importance, an accurate localization is not an easy task as some parts of the boundary are not well defined in some images and several parts are obscured by the crossing blood vessels. In these cases, the optic disc boundary is not always sharp and, more importantly, it is obscured in some places by blood vessels.

The optic disc size and shape may vary significantly. The disc diameter is about 70 to 105 pixels in our retinal images. The optic disc part located on the nasal side is usually less bright than the temporal side portion and occasionally not visible at all. Sometimes the whole optic disc is brighter than the surrounding area, thus it can be seen as a disc; in others it can appear as a hollow ring. In either case the cup appears as a smaller, brighter region within the optic disc. Whereas locating the optic disc is an apparently simple task for an expert to trace the boundary, interpolating where necessary, traditional general-purpose boundary detection algorithms have not fully succeeded in segmenting the optic disc due to fuzzy boundaries, inconsistent image contrast, variability in appearance, or missing edge features. Therefore, a reliable optic disc localization is surprisingly difficult.

To locate the optic disc in this work, two different techniques are investigated including template matching and active contours. The first strategy provides an approximate location of the optic disc center. The optic disc region can then be estimated as a circle using rough location of its center. Although template matching-based technique is enough to estimate and remove the optic disc as candidate exudate regions, but the optic disc can sometimes have an elliptical shape, and thus baseline plotting of the exact boundaries is important. Thus, a snake-based technique is also developed to generate a more accurate disc boundary.

We tested these two approaches against a dataset of 75 color retinal images including 25 normal and 50 abnormal images. In all cases the template image could provide a good approximate match of the optic disc center even when large, albeit scattered, areas of similarly colored exudate pathologies exist in the image. We also developed an active contour-based approach similar to [24], except we introduced two novel improvements. First, we placed the initial snake automatically using our earlier levels of processing. Second, we improved on the morphological step by using color morphology, which resulted in a more homogeneous inner disc area and aided the accuracy of the optic disc localization.

To provide a more objective assessment of the performance of this algorithm we used an overlap measure of the match between two regions, i.e. localized optic disc region and the optic disc ground truth provided by an ophthalmologist. According to the applied overlap measure, a gradient vector flow (GVF) based snake could achieve 90.32% overall accuracy for optic disc localization on our image dataset.

5.9.1 Template matching

Template matching is a technique used to isolate certain features in an image. This can be implemented as a correlation of the original image and a suitable template. The best match is then located based on some criterion of optimality. According to the size of the optic disc region in our retinal images, we generated a 110×110 pixels template image by averaging the optic disc region in 25 retinal images selected from our image dataset (Figure 5.5(a)). This was performed using gray levels only since the result is computationally less expensive and accurate enough. The normalized correlation coefficient is defined as follows:

$$R(i,j) = \frac{\sum_k \sum_l \left(f_{k+i,l+j} - \bar{f}_{i,j}\right)\left(t_{k,l} - \bar{t}\right)}{\sqrt{\left(\sum_k \sum_l \left(f_{k+i,l+j} - \bar{f}_{i,j}\right)^2\right)\left(\sum_k \sum_l \left(t_{k,l} - \bar{t}\right)^2\right)}} \tag{5.6}$$

where f and t represent the original image and the template respectively, $\bar{t}$ is the template pixels' mean value and similarly $\bar{f}$ denotes the image pixels' mean value in the region that is defined by the template location. We measured the normalized correlation coefficients for each retinal image to present an indication of the match between the template image and each individual pixel in the image under consideration. The highest matched point emerges as the brightest point in the correlation image. Here, we consider this point's coordinate as potential location of the optic disc center (Figure 5.5). The main weakness of template matching is that the largest correlation coefficient value does not necessarily correspond to the true optic disc center. Indeed, this technique is prone to locate the optic disc center slightly to the temporal side, due to the asymmetric nature of the optic disc (Figure 5.5).

In all 75 images the template image could provide a good approximate match of the optic disc center corresponding to the largest correlation coefficient value even when large, albeit scattered, areas of similarly colored exudate pathologies existed in the image. However, as expressed earlier, template matching only approximates the optic disc center as can be easily seen in Figure 5.5. Since our aim is a precise localization of the optic disc boundary for use in clinical analysis, we use this center approximation purely as an automatic means of initializing a snake process.

5.9.2 Color morphology preprocessing

Snake methods work on a gradient image and lock onto homogeneous regions enclosed by strong gradient information. In this application, this task is made extremely difficult since the optic disc region is invariably fragmented into multiple regions by blood vessels. Mendels et al. [24] used gray-level morphology to remove the blood

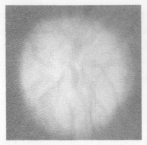 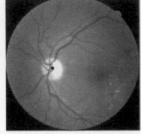 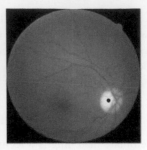

(a) Template image   (b) Localized optic disc center   (c) Localized optic disc center

FIGURE 5.5
Localization of the optic disc center. The optic disc center approximation is marked in black.

vessels to create a fairly constant region before applying a snake method. Mathematical morphology can extract important shape characteristics and also remove irrelevant information. It typically probes an image with a small shape or template known as a structuring element. Using gray-level morphology, the operation can be applied to the intensity or lightness channel. We show that better results may be obtained by using the L*ab* [31] color space using a simple definition of color morphology.

We carried out a series of experiments to determine the best method of obtaining a homogeneous optic disc region by performing gray-level morphology as in [24], gray-level morphology using the lightness channel L of the HLS (hue-lightness-saturation) color space, color morphology using the full HLS space, and two variations of color morphology using the L*ab* space. In all these cases, we performed a closing operation, i.e., a dilation to first remove the blood vessels and then an erosion to restore the boundaries to their former position. This can result in some minor inaccuracies, particularly if any boundary concavities are filled by the dilation, but in the main performs very well. We also used a symmetrical disc structuring element of size 13, since the blood vessels were determined to be not wider than 11 pixels. Standard gray-level morphology was performed after a transformation of the RGB color image into a gray-level image (see Figure 5.6(b)). The same can be performed on the L channel of the HLS color space (Figure 5.6(c)), in which the blood vessel edges are less pronounced than in a normal intensity image, so their elimination is easier.

Hanbury and Serra [32] have introduced a method for morphological preprocessing in the HLS color space using all the components. In color morphology, each pixel must be considered as a vector of color components and definitions of *maximum* and *minimum* operations on ordered vectors are necessary to perform basic operations. Hence for each arbitary point x in the color space, the definition for dilation (I_d) and erosion (I_e) by structuring element K is defined as:

$$I_d(x) = \{I(y) : I(y) = \max[I(z)], z \in K_x\} \tag{5.7}$$

$$I_e(x) = \{I(y) : I(y) = \min[I(z)], z \in K_x\} \tag{5.8}$$

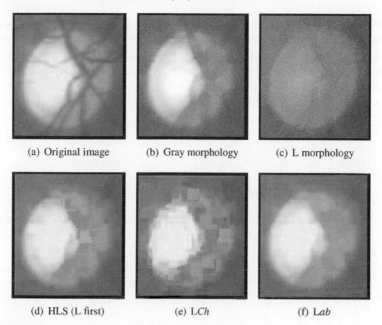

(a) Original image	(b) Gray morphology	(c) L morphology

(d) HLS (L first)	(e) L*Ch*	(f) L*ab*

FIGURE 5.6

Mathematical morphology closing in different color spaces. **(See color insert.)**

Hanbury and Serra introduced a lexicographical order to color morphology in the HLS space such that the basic morphological operations could be performed in a particular order with any one of H, L, or S in the first position. The choice was stated to be dependent on the application at hand. For example, the lexicographical order of two typical vectors x and y with saturation S in the first position was defined as:

$$x > y \quad \text{if} \quad \begin{cases} S_x > S_y \\ \text{or} \\ S_x = S_y \quad \text{and} \quad |L_x - 0.5| < |L_y - 0.5| \\ \text{or} \\ S_x = S_y \quad \text{and} \quad |L_x - 0.5| = |L_y - 0.5| \quad \text{and} \quad d(H_x, H_o) < d(H_y, H_o) \end{cases}$$
(5.9)

In this approach after choosing an origin H_o, the distance from the origin to each point H_i in the structuring element is calculated as:

$$d_i = d(H_i, H_o) = \begin{cases} |H_i - H_o| & |H_i - H_o| \leq 180° \\ 360° - |H_i - H_o| & |H_i - H_o| \geq 180° \end{cases}$$
(5.10)

Thus the point with smallest d_i is chosen as the infimum of the structuring element (erosion), and the point with the largest d_i as the supremum (dilation).

For our retinal images, operators based on the lexicographical order with L in the first position produced the best results in preserving the optic disc as the brightest object and removing the blood vessels as one of the darker objects. Figure 5.6(d) shows an example of applying a closing operation in the HLS color space with L in the first position. In a follow-up work, Hanbury and Serra [33] applied the same principles to perform color morphology in the L*Ch* color space a derivative of the L*ab* space where $C = \sqrt{(a)^2 + (b)^2}$ and $h = \arctan(b/a)$. In [33], the order of two typical vectors x and y was defined as:

$$x > y \quad \text{if} \quad \begin{cases} w_x < w_y \\ \text{or} \\ w_x = w_y \quad \text{and} \quad L_x > L_y \\ \text{or} \\ w_x = w_y \quad \text{and} \quad L_x = L_y \quad \text{and} \quad d(h_x, h_o) > d(h_y, h_o) \end{cases} \quad (5.11)$$

where w is a weighting function imposing a complete order on the L*Ch* space. It is defined so that a lower weight represents a color closer to the extremal points or a more saturated color, and a higher weight implies a color close to the luminance axis or a less saturated color. It is computed based on the image L*Ch* values and the extremal points in L and C (in the general L*Ch* space) for all values of h from 0 to 359°. Figure 5.6(e) illustrates the application of a closing operation in this L*Ch* space.

Using the perceptually uniform L*ab* color space allows us to manipulate the lightness and chromaticity of the optic disc region at the same time in a space where color differences correspond to the metric distance between them. We devised a very basic definition of color morphology in which the definition of *maxima* and *minima* operations on color pixels reduce to the maximum and minimum of the ordered set of vectors in the structuring mask.

This simple strategy works here because of the nature of the retinal image, but it may not necessarily be of use in other types of images. As expressed earlier, the optic disc region contains contrasting pixels: bright, almost saturated regions crossed by dark blood vessel regions. These color differences will reside in well separated regions of the L*ab* perceptual color space and hence our simple minima and maxima definitions work extremely well. The definitions for dilation (I_d) and erosion (I_e) in the proposed simple color morphology domain are defined by (5.7) and (5.8). The dilation is the furthest point from the origin, and the erosion is the point closest to the origin. The origin was considered at (0,0,0) for simplicity and then the maximum and minimum distances from each pixel to the reference point were obtained using the Euclidean norm within the structuring mask. An example of closing using our simple definitions of dilation and erosion in the L*ab* space is shown in Figure 5.6(f). This approach creates a more homogeneous region and preserves the optic disc edges better. As will be shown later, it also results in a more accurate localization of the optic disc.

5.9.3   Accurate localization of the optic disc-based snakes

Since the optic disc region is broken up by blood vessels, classical segmentation algorithms based exclusively on edge detection are not enough to accurately localize the optic disc as they do not incorporate the edge smoothness and continuity properties. In contrast, active contours (snakes) represent the paradigm that the presence of an edge depends not only on the gradient at a specific point but also on the spatial distribution [34]. In fact, snakes incorporate the global view of edge detection by assessing continuity and curvature, combined with the local edge strength [35]. The principal advantage of snakes is that they have the ability to interpolate missing edges of the objects while being locked on the visible parts. These properties make snakes highly suitable for our optic disc localization application.

The initial contour for a snake must be close to the desired boundary otherwise it can converge to the wrong resting place. In order to automatically position an initial snake we introduced the template-matching step in Section 5.9.1. In general, a snake is a parametric curve $X(s) = (x(s), y(s))$. The snake moves under an evolution equation that pushes it towards a configuration that minimizes internal and external energies. This energy function can be defined as:

$$E_{\text{snake}} = \int_0^1 \frac{1}{2} \left(\alpha |X'(s)|^2 + \beta |X''(s)|^2 \right) + E_{\text{ext}}(X(s)) \, ds \qquad (5.12)$$

The first two terms within the above integral stand for the internal force that is determined by the physical properties of the snake. If α and β have large values, then the snake tends to assume a smooth outline. The third term $E_{\text{ext}}(X(s))$ is the external energy, and is evaluated from the image. The external energy is the main issue discussed in active contour models. In our application this external energy is an attractor towards optic disc boundary and in the classical formulation is defined as the gradient of a low pass filtered version of the image. Considering a gray-level image $I(x, y)$ as a function of continuous variables (x, y), a typical external energy to lead the snake towards edges is defined as:

$$E_{\text{ext}}(x, y) = -|\nabla [G_\sigma(x, y) * I(x, y)]|^2 \qquad (5.13)$$

where $G_\sigma(x, y)$ is a two dimensional Gaussian function with standard deviation σ and ∇ is the gradient operator. The external energy is minimized where the image gradient is large, namely along the edges in the image. This encourages the snake to move towards the edges.

The disadvantage of this external energy field is that it may lead to many local energy minima that do not represent the desired boundary. Snakes also have difficulties progressing into boundary concavities. To overcome these problems we used the GVF field [36] that replaces the standard formulation of the external energy with a GVF field, $V(x, y) = (u(x, y), v(x, y))$, to minimize the following energy function:

$$\gamma = \iint \mu(u_x^2 + u_y^2 + v_x^2 + v_y^2) + |\nabla f|^2 |V - \nabla f|^2 \, dx \, dy \qquad (5.14)$$

Where f represents the edge gradients, μ is a regularization parameter determining a trade-off between the first and second terms of the function. GVF's larger capture range and concavity tracking abilities are attributed to the diffusion operation shown in (5.14). On the other hand, μ is a parameter that determines the trade-off between

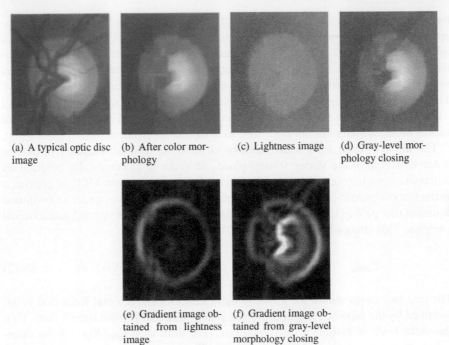

(a) A typical optic disc image   (b) After color morphology   (c) Lightness image   (d) Gray-level morphology closing

(e) Gradient image obtained from lightness image   (f) Gradient image obtained from gray-level morphology closing

FIGURE 5.7

A comparison between color morphology and gray-level morphology. **(See color insert.)**

smoothness of the vector field and how much the snake is attracted to the edge. This parameter is defined based on how much noise exists in the image, i.e., a bigger μ indicates more noise.

5.9.4   Optic disc localization results

Once the vascular structures were removed, the gradient information required for evaluating the snake's external energy to drive the snake towards the desired accurate optic disc boundary was extracted from the filtered image lightness channel. In fact, for each image pixel with RGB tristimulus, the lightness value was defined as an average between the maximum and minimum values of R, G, and B. This conversion of color images to their corresponding lightness versions provided a homogenous gray-level optic disc region as the blood vessels were less pronounced in the lightness channel. More importantly, the definition of lightness effectively suppresses the gray-level differences that naturally exist between the optic disc temporal and the nasal side and between the optic cup and its neighboring pixels.

Figure 5.7 shows an example of converting a preprocessed color optic disc region image (Figure 5.7(b)) to its corresponding lightness component (Figure 5.7(c)). As is evident, the lightness information provided a highly smoothed region with no significant difference between the temporal and nasal sides. In contrast, this difference can be clearly seen in Figure 5.7(d), which represents the gray-level morphology closing result on the gray-scale version of the original image (Figure 5.7(a)). Figure 5.7(e) and (f) show the gradient images acquired from the lightness image (Figure 5.7(c)) and the gray-level image (Figure 5.7(d)) respectively. By comparing these two gradient images, it is evident that the proposed approach provides a more accurate optic disc edge map.

Another disadvantage of the standard gray-level approach is that when applying a snake, the stronger central region gradient values in Figure 5.7(f) can force the snake to be pulled too far towards the interior part of the disc region and thus fail to locate the true optic disc boundary.

Several different values were tested for the regularization parameter of the GVF and we found $\mu = 0.27$ as the best for our images. The number of iterations during the evaluation of the GVF field was set to 40. We used $\alpha = 0.7$ and $\beta = 0.1$, which control the snake's tension and rigidity respectively. Finally, the number of iterations for the snake convergence was determined experimentally and set to 175. All these parameters were determined empirically and kept constant throughout the experiments.

The initial contour for a snake must be close to the desired boundary otherwise it can converge to the wrong resting place. Here, we initialized the snake automatically as a circle with a center at the point found through template matching and with a circular radius set to half of the width of the template. In a number of cases this initial snake intersected the real optic disc boundary, but the GVF snake has the ability to shrink or grow towards the final boundary. In Figures 5.8(a) to 5.8(d) we illustrate a typical original image, the result of L*ab* color space morphological closing, the initial snake, and the final snake. Figures 5.8(e) to 5.8(h) demonstrate a close-up of the optic disc region, L*ab* closing of optic disc region, close-up of final snake, and close-up of hand-drawn ground truth. In Figure 5.8(i) we show a combined close-up of the hand-labeled boundary and the final snake to illustrate the close match achieved.

We quantify and compare the accuracy of our active contour optic disc localization technique against the manually labeled ground truth produced by a clinician (e.g., see Figure 5.8(h)) for all the variations of optic disc morphology described earlier. These variations were closing in gray-level images, closing using L and S channels of the HLS, opening using H channel of HLS, closing in L*ab* color space and opening in L*Ch* color space. We use a simple and effective overlap measure of the match between two regions as:

$$M = \frac{n(R \cap T)}{n(R \cup T)} \tag{5.15}$$

where R and T correspond to the ground truth and the final localized optic disc region respectively and $n(.)$ is the number of pixels in a region. This measure of accuracy was used to compare a ground truth region with that inside a snake. In this case R and T notations correspond to the ground truth and the final snake localized optic disc region, respectively. Table 5.4 summarizes measure M for a selection of 10 retinal images as well as the overall average accuracy for all 75 images.

While many of the results in the 1-dimension and 3-dimension spaces are of a similar order, the best average optic disc localization performance was achieved at

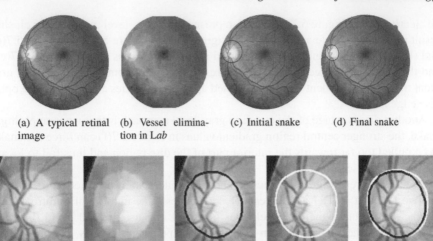

(a) A typical retinal image   (b) Vessel elimination in L*ab*   (c) Initial snake   (d) Final snake

(e) Close-up of optic disc region   (f) L*ab* closing of optic disc region   (g) Close-up of final snake   (h) Close-up of hand-drawn ground truth   (i) Overlay of (g) and (h)

FIGURE 5.8

Optic disc localization results. (**See color insert.**)

90.32% by employing a snake after our proposed L*ab* color morphological operations. The gray-level based morphological closing accomplished 89.57% accuracy, which is the best after both color morphology variations in L*ab* space. Among the HLS color morphology results, L in the first position achieved an accuracy equal to 87.12%, which is significantly better than the S (saturation) and H (hue) in the first positions. The second best performance in this color space was obtained based on S in the first position with 80.77% accuracy. However, the worst results in HLS color space were based on H in first position where we achieved an accuracy of 73.12%. The L*Ch* space-based morphological preprocessing did not achieve a high level of overall accuracy as well as being a computationally expensive method. This approach provided accuracy equal to 76.41%. Our L*ab*-based color morphological preprocessing technique was much faster than the L*Ch* where the weights had to be recomputed after each basic morphology operation in anticipation for the next operation. The L*Ch* space did not provide the same level of overall accuracy as the gray-level or HLS space when either L or S channels were assumed in the first position.

5.10   Conclusion

This chapter reported work undertaken to investigate the use of three well known statistical classifiers, i.e., *KNN*, *GQ*, and *GMM* for the *pixel-level exudate recognition*.

Table 5.4: Performance Evaluation of the Optic Disc Localization

Image	Gray	HLS (H 1st)	HLS (L 1st)	HLS (S 1st)	LCh	Lab
1	89.14	74.86	89.83	66.42	87.65	91.76
2	87.60	63.16	87.57	84.34	68.42	87.68
3	93.91	68.74	93.55	91.28	84.49	94.87
4	90.10	80.12	85.87	75.46	72.51	90.23
5	91.82	76.01	92.56	92.18	78.73	92.23
6	91.95	75.97	84.94	80.67	75.25	90.12
7	93.27	64.87	93.15	87.45	78.65	94.53
8	91.24	70.21	90.05	80.46	89.88	90.58
9	90.55	74.64	83.67	80.94	77.56	91.13
10	88.40	68.32	89.23	81.85	76.45	88.67
Average	**89.57%**	**73.12%**	**87.12%**	**80.77%**	**76.41%**	**90.32%**

The purpose was to examine parametric, nonparametric, and semiparametric probability density estimation techniques for distinguishing exudates from nonexudates and highlight areas of retinal images that contain exudate lesions. Four different datasets of exudate and nonexudate pixels were utilized to take the spatial pixels' information. A square window of pixels (1×1, 3×3, 5×5, 7×7) centered on the pixel to be classified was used to establish a feature vector for the main underlying pixel. This information was passed on to a classifier, which assigned a classification label to the pixel under consideration.

It was found that the *GMM* classifiers performed better than the other two classifiers. *KNN* classifiers could outperform the *GQs* but the latter were much quicker to develop. The effect of different pixel patch sizes was assessed for the three classifiers. There existed a distinct optimum for all the employed classifiers for a patch of 5×5 pixels.

The proposed *pixel-level exudate recognition* approach was extended to a new set of 67 retinal images, including 40 abnormal and 27 normal images. Each retinal image was then evaluated using the optimal *GMM* classifier and a final decision was made as to whether the image had some evidence of retinopathy.

An acceptable compromize between the system's sensitivity and predictivity was achieved by inspecting different ratios of exudate and nonexudate prior probabilities. The proposed scheme achieved 92.5% (correct classification of 37 abnormal images out of 40) sensitivity and 66.6% (correct classification of 18 normal images out of 27) specificity in terms of image-based classification accuracy. It also illustrated 89.2% sensitivity and 81.0% predictivity in terms of pixel resolution accuracy when the output threshold (prior probability ratio of exudates and nonexudates) was assumed to be 0.45.

Due to the importance of optic disc localization in retinal image analysis, two different approaches for locating the optic disc were investigated. Template matching could only provide an approximate location of the optic disc center. The best optic disc localization accuracy was achieved by employing a snake after morphological operations in L*ab* color space. The final localized snake and hand-labeled ground truth images were utilized to assess the performance of different employed preprocessing morphological approaches.

The purpose of locating the optic disc was twofold:

- to separate the false positive optic disc regions from the candidate segmented exudates.

- its accurate segmentation is of more use in clinical analysis, e.g., in proliferative diabetic retinopathy there may be development of new blood vessels on the optic disc and therefore baseline plotting of the exact boundaries of the disc is important.

Consequently, an active contour-based technique was developed to produce a more accurate boundary. The optic disc region is invariably fragmented into multiple regions by blood vessels. Thus, we used a color morphology preprocessing smoothing to remove the vessels and create a fairly constant region before applying a snake method. Here we implemented the concept of color morphology in different color spaces including HLS, L*Ch*, and L*ab*. As the hue component of HLS and L*Ch* color spaces is angular, the standard gray-scale morphological operations were not directly applicable to it. Thus, color morphology operations were implemented using a hue origin and lexicographical orders.

We found a highly appropriate preprocessing color morphology scheme for removing the vessels based on the L*ab* components. We also demonstrated the improvement obtained using the proposed color morphological closing over gray-level morphology for this application. The proposed method could localize the optic disc in all 75 test images. It achieved 90.32% accuracy in terms of an area overlapping between the ground truth and the identified optic disc region using a snake approach. This showed that the proposed color morphology-based preprocessing method is particularly suitable for the characteristics of our optic disc images. However, there is a degree of subjectivity in assigning the ground truth boundary in the test images and perfect correspondence would not be expected.

References

[1] Evans, J., Causes of blindness and partial sight in England and Wales 1990–1991, Technical Report 57, HMSO, London, 1995.

[2] Kanski, J., *Diabetic Retinopathy, Clinical Ophthalmology*, Butterworth-Heinmann, Oxford, UK, 1997.

[3] McLeod, B., Thompson, J., and Rosenthal, A., The prevalence of retinopathy in the insulin-requiring diabetic patients of an English country town, *Eye*, 2, 424, 1988.

[4] The Royal College of Ophthalmologists, Guidelines for diabetic retinopathy, Technical report, The Royal College of Ophthalmologists, 1997.

[5] Shah, P., Jacks, A., and Khaw, P., *Eye disease in clinical practice*, Manticore, 1999.

[6] Goldbaum, M., Moezzi, S., Taylor, A., et al., Automated diagnosis and image understanding with object extraction, object classification, and inferencing in retinal images, in *International Conference on Image Processing*, Lausanne, Switzerland, 1996, vol. 3, 695–698.

[7] Sinthanayothin, C., Boyce, J.F., Cook, H.L., et al., Automated localisation of the optic disc, fovea, and retinal blood vessels from digital colour fundus images, *British Journal of Ophthalmology*, 83(8), 902, 1999.

[8] Frame, A.J., Undrill, P.E., Cree, M.J., et al., A comparison of computer based classification methods applied to the detection of microaneurysms in ophthalmic fluorescein angiograms, *Computers in Biology and Medicine*, 28(3), 225, 1998.

[9] Lee, S.C., Wang, Y., and Lee, E.T., Computer algorithm for automated detection and quantification of microaneurysms and hemorrhages (HMAs) in color retinal images, in *Medical Imaging 1999: Image Perception and Performance*, 1999, vol. 3663 of *Proceedings of the SPIE*, 61–71.

[10] Pinz, A., Bernogger, S., Datlinger, P., et al., Mapping the human retina, *IEEE Transactions on Medical Imaging*, 17(4), 606, 1998.

[11] Phillips, R.P., Spencer, T., Ross, P.G., et al., Quantification of diabetic maculopathy by digital imaging of the fundus, *Eye*, 5(1), 130, 1991.

[12] Phillips, R., Forrester, J., and Sharp, P., Automated detection and quantification of retinal exudates, *Graefes Arch Clin Exp Ophthalmol*, 231(2), 90, 1993.

[13] Ward, N., Tomlinson, S., and Taylor, C., Image analysis of fundus photographs, *Ophthalmology*, 96, 80, 1989.

[14] Ege, B., Larsen, O.V., and Hejlesen, O.K., Detection of abnormalities in retinal images using digital image analysis, in *11th Scandinavian Conference on Image Analysis (SCIA99)*, 1999, 833–840.

[15] Wang, H., Hsu, W., Goh, K.G., et al., An effective approach to detect lesions in color retinal images, in *IEEE Conference Computer Vision and Pattern Recognition (CVPR'00)*, Hilton Head Island, SC, 2000, vol. 2, 181–186.

[16] Gardner, G.G., Keating, D., Williamson, T.H., et al., Automatic detection of diabetic retinopathy using an artificial neural network: A screening tool, *British Journal of Ophthalmology*, 80, 940, 1996.

[17] Walter, T., Klein, J.C., Massin, P., et al., A contribution of image processing to the diagnosis of diabetic retinopathy – detection of exudates in color fundus

images of the human retina, *IEEE Transactions on Medical Imaging*, 21(10), 1236, 2002.

[18] Chutatape, O., Zheng, L., and Krishman, S.M., Retinal blood vessel detection and tracking by matched Gaussian and Kalman filters, in *Proceedings of the 20th International Conference of the IEEE Engineering in Medicine and Biology Society*, 1998, vol. 6, 3144–3149.

[19] Li, H. and Chutatape, O., Automatic location of optic disk in retinal images, in *2001 International Conference on Image Processing (ICIP'01)*, 2001, vol. 2, 837–840.

[20] Osareh, A., Mirmehdi, M., Thomas, B., et al., Classification and localisation of diabetic-related eye disease, in *7th European Conference on Computer Vision (ECCV2002)*, 2002, vol. 2353 of *Lecture Notes in Computer Science*, 502–516.

[21] Liu, Z., Opas, C., and Krishnan, S.M., Automatic image analysis of fundus photograph, in *Proceedings of the 19th Annual International Conference of the IEEE Engineering in Medicine and Biology Society*, 1997, vol. 2, 524–525.

[22] Sinthanayothin, C., *Image analysis for automatic diagnosis of diabetic retinopathy*, PhD thesis, King's College of London, 1999.

[23] Lalonde, M., Beaulieu, M., and Gagnon, L., Fast and robust optic disc detection using pyramidal decomposition and Hausdorff-based template matching, *IEEE Transactions on Medical Imaging*, 20(11), 1193, 2001.

[24] Mendels, F., Heneghan, C., and Thiran, J.P., Identification of the optic disk boundary in retinal images using active contours, in *Irish Machine Vision and Image Processing Conference*, 1999, 103–115.

[25] Osareh, A., Mirmehdi, M., and Markham, R., Comparison of colour spaces for optic disc localisation in retinal images, in *16th International Conference on Pattern Recognition (ICPR'02)*, Quebec City, QC, Canada, 2002, vol. 1, 10 743–10 746.

[26] Sonka, M. and Fitzpatrick, J., *Handbook of Medical Imaging: Medical Image Processing and Analysis*, vol. 2, SPIE, 2000.

[27] Sonka, M., Hlavac, V., and Boyle, R., *Image Processing, Analysis and Machine Vision*, PWS, 1999.

[28] Fukunga, K., *Statistical Pattern Recognition*, Academic, 1990.

[29] Bishop, C., *Pattern Recognition and Machine Learning*, Springer, 2006.

[30] Rissanen, J., A universal prior for integers and estimation by minimum description length, *Annals of Statistics*, 11, 416, 1983.

[31] Lukac, R. and Plataniotis, K., eds., *Colour Image Processing: Methods and Applications*, CRC, 2006.

[32] Hanbury, A. and Serra, J., Mathematical morphology in the HLS colour spacce, in *Proceedings of the 12th British Machine Vision Conference*, 2001, 451–460.

[33] Hanbury, A. and Serra, J., Mathematical morphology in the L*ab* colour space, *Image Analysis and Stereology*, 21(3), 201, 2002.

[34] Gunn, S. and Nixon, M., A robust snake implementation; a dual active contour, *IEEE Transactions on Pattern Analysis and Machine Intelligence*, 19(1), 1, 1997.

[35] Kass, M., Witkin, A., and Terzopoulos, D., Snakes: active contour models, *International Journal of Computer Vision*, 1(4), 321, 1987.

[36] Xu, C. and Prince, J., Snakes, shapes, and gradient vector flow, *IEEE Transactions on Image Processing*, 7(3), 359, 1998.

6

Automated Microaneurysm Detection for Screening

Michael J. Cree

CONTENTS

6.1 Characteristics of Microaneurysms and Dot-Hemorrhages 155
6.2 History of Automated Microaneurysm Detection 156
6.3 Microaneurysm Detection in Color Retinal Images 165
6.4 The Waikato Automated Microaneurysm Detector 167
6.5 Issues for Microaneurysm Detection 172
6.6 Research Application of Microaneurysm Detection 177
6.7 Conclusion 178
References 178

6.1   Characteristics of Microaneurysms and Dot-Hemorrhages

Microaneurysms (MA) are small saccular bulges in the walls of the retinal capillary vessels. Although most commonly found in diabetic retinopathy, MAs may also occur in other retinopathies such as various congenital vascular abnormalities. The pathogenesis of microaneurysms is not completely understood but damage to capillary pericytes is thought to be a factor [1].

As the retinal capillaries are too small to be resolved by normal fundus photography, microaneurysms are classically described as distinct small round objects, ranging from 10 μm to 100 μm in diameter. In color fundus images they appear red and in red-free images they appear dark. With fluorescein angiography microaneurysms are hyperfluorescent, thus appear as bright dots in positive images. In practice, the appearance of microaneurysms can deviate somewhat from the classical description. They may appear in association with larger vessels or as a conglomeration of more than one MA. Microaneurysms are difficult to distinguish from dot-hemorrhages in color retinal images. Dot-hemorrhages appear as bright red dots the size of a large microaneurysm and rarely exceed 200 μm in diameter. As the clinical implications of the presence of dot-hemorrhages and MAs are sufficiently similar there is usually no need for an automated MA detector to distinguish between them.

Microaneurysms are better visualized with fluorescein angiography with more MAs visible than in color fundus images. Better discrimination between MAs and dot-hemorrhages is also achieved as dot-hemorrhages tend to block out the background choroidal fluorescence and appear hypofluorescent. Nevertheless, other features, such as retinal pigment epithelium defects and capillaries seen end on, can appear similar to MAs and some care is needed when identifying individual MAs.

Microaneurysms are often the first sign of diabetic retinopathy. A positive correlation between the number of microaneurysms and the severity and likely progression of diabetic retinopathy has been demonstrated, at least for the early stages of the disease [2–5]. Microaneurysm formation and regression is a dynamic process with over half of the MA population observed to either form or regress within a 12 month period [6]. There is evidence that the turnover of microaneurysms, in addition to absolute counts, is a predictor of retinopathy [6; 7].

As microaneurysms are reasonably easy to describe, are a well visualizable target, and their numbers have definite clinical implications, they were one of the first lesions selected for automated image analysis. Early attempts focused on the detection of MAs in fluorescein angiographic images where they are better visualized. As fluorescein angiography poses an unacceptable health risk for eye-screening and color digital camera technology has advanced sufficiently, there is now a move to perform automated MA detection on color fundus images as an adjunct to automated eye screening.

6.2   History of Automated Microaneurysm Detection

In the following an overview of the historical development of automated microaneurysm detectors is given.

6.2.1   Early morphological approaches

The first attempts at automated microaneurysm detection date back to the early 1980s, and were on fluorescein angiographic images. Laÿ et al. [8] described a morphological approach to MA detection. Image resolution and dynamic range were low (256×256 pixels with 100 gray levels), however, by using an imaging microscope to digitize film negatives, the digital image covered a small field-of-view of the macula so that MAs were well resolved. As negatives were used, the MAs appeared as dark dots, thus as localized minima in the intensity image. A tophat transform was applied to identify the local minima. Vessels were identified with the skeletonization of a further tophat transform using a linear structuring element at various orientations, and any local minima lying on vessels were eliminated as MAs. Ten angiographic images, containing a total of 177 MAs, were analyzed both by clinicians and the automated MA detector. The automated MA detector achieved 58% sensitivity with 4.2 false detections per image for detecting and locating MAs .

This process was extended by Baudoin et al. [9] with extra morphological processing to remove false detections such as objects too small to be MAs. In this study 25 retinal images centered on the macula, containing a total of 936 MAs, were analyzed both by clinicians and the automated processing. The automated MA detector achieved 70% sensitivity for detecting and locating MAs with 4.4 false detections per image.

Spencer et al. [10] used matched-filtering to detect MAs and to remove false-detections on vessels in angiographic images of the retina. Film negatives of the macula were projected onto a screen and digitized with a monochrome CCD camera at 512×512 pixel resolution. Preprocessing included radiometric correction for the illumination of the negatives, and subtractive shade-correction to remove choroidal fluorescence. MAs were identified by matched-filtering with a circularly symmetric two-dimensional Gaussian ($\sigma = 1$ pixel) and a mask of size 5×5 pixels. Vessels were identified by matched-filtering with a mask of size 5×5 pixels and $\sigma = 2$ pixels, and extra shape-analysis to identify long linear structures. Any MAs detected on the vessel network were removed. Testing was performed on six fluorescein angiographic images. Five clinicians also marked the positions of MAs, on both the digitized images and on standard photographs made from the film negatives. The automated detection performed almost as well as the clinicians working on the digitized images, however, the clinicians working on the digitized images performed poorly compared to the clinicians working on the photographs. It was concluded that the digitized image resolution was insufficient for reliable MA detection.

6.2.2 The "standard approach" to automated microaneurysm detection

In response to the limits of the morphological processing developed by Baudoin and Laÿ, and of the matched-filter approach of Spencer et al., researchers at Aberdeen University, Scotland, developed the image processing strategy for detection of MAs into what we shall call the "standard approach" of automated MA detection. This approach has since been adopted and enhanced by researchers not only at Aberdeen University, but also by a number of other groups. The standard approach [11] is described in the following and illustrated in Figure 6.1.

First, digitized retinal images are shade-corrected to even up the background illumination of the retinal image. Shade-correction is normally performed by creating an image of the background illumination often estimated by gross median or mean filtering of the retinal image. The background image is either subtracted from or divided into the retinal image. On fluorescein angiographic images subtractive shade-correction is normally performed to remove choroidal background fluorescence as the choroidal illumination is an additive process (e.g., see [11–13]; also see [14] for more description of the illumination contaminants to angiographic images). Microaneurysm detection on color retinal images is best with divisive shade-correction as

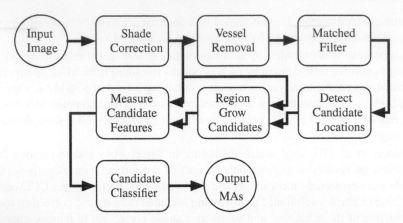

FIGURE 6.1
Flow diagram of the "standard approach" to microaneurysm detection.

intensity shading is mainly due to changing reflectances of the retina, a multiplicative process.

In the standard approach, a matched-filter with a circularly symmetric 2-D Gaussian as the kernel is used to highlight MAs, but this process tends to false-detect on vessels. Vessels are therefore first detected by the morphological opening of the shade-corrected retinal image by a long linear structuring element that is rotated to various angles to pick up all vessel segments. The length of the structuring element is chosen to be short enough to fit inside curved vessels, and long enough that it cannot fit inside MAs [11] so that it detects vessels (and other large extended features) but not MAs. The detected vessels are then subtracted from the shade-corrected retinal image to effect a tophat transform. The resultant image contains small objects such as MAs and also, in practice, small objects left over from the vessels, such as boli of fluorescein if angiographic images are used.

The tophat transformed image is thresholded to detect likely MAs, which we refer to as candidates. One could terminate the process at this stage and take all candidates as detected MAs, however it is normally found that an acceptable sensitivity leads to an unacceptable specificity. Therefore the candidate locations are used to initiate region growing on the shade-corrected retinal image to delineate the underlying morphology of the candidate. Shape and intensity features are measured on the region-grown object and a classifier is used to refine MA detection. A much better specificity can then be achieved with very little loss in sensitivity. Because the candidates are region grown this method typically cannot detect MAs attached to vessels.

This approach was first described by Spencer et al. [11], who tested the process on fluorescein angiographic film negatives digitized at a resolution of 1024×1024 pixels covering a $35°$ field of the macula. The preprocessing included illumination correction to correct for vignetting incurred in the digitization. The tophat transform used a linear structuring element 11 pixels long rotated to eight orientations. The matched filter kernel, of size 11×11 pixels, was a two-dimensional circularly symmetric Gaussian with $\sigma = 1$ pixel. Once candidate MAs were region-grown, simple shape features (area, perimeter, aspect ratio, and complexity) and intensity measures (mean intensity of object) formed the input to a rule-based classifier. Five ophthalmologists marked the positions of MAs on four high quality photographic prints of the retinal images. The automated computer detection of MAs on the four images was compared against the clinicians. The computer satisfactorily matched the response of the clinicians on a free-response receiver operating characteristic (ROC) graph.

This is the first reported use of an automated detection of MAs that compared favorably with clinicians. Note that the automated MA detector performed well compared to clinicians using photographic prints, thus the problem of poor digital resolution of their earlier study [10] was resolved. Nevertheless, the test is of limited generality as only four independent images were used and the total number of MAs present in the images used are not reported.

Further improvements to the Aberdeen automated MA detector were made by Cree et al. [12, 13]. The region-growing algorithm was made computationally efficient, and the classifier was redesigned. Extra features using intensities of candidate MAs normalized intra- and inter-image were added as was the peak response of the matched-filter that marked an object as a candidate [12]. Comparison of the manually constructed rule-based classifier with two machine learning approaches (linear discriminant analysis and a neural network), found that the manually constructed rule-based classifier provided the best result [15]. Cree et al. [12] also reported an automated method to detect the fovea based on Fourier-space correlation of a model of the gross shading of the fovea against a low-passed filtered version of the retinal image. Thus the whole process of MA detection and counting, including locating the region-of-interest centered on the fovea, was automated.

The improved Aberdeen automated MA detector for detection of MAs in fluorescein angiographic images was trained on 64 retinal images and tested against an independent test set of 20 retinal images of 1024×1024 pixel resolution of a $35°$ field-of-view of the macula [13]. The locations of MAs in the test images were established by consensus decision by a clinician and medical physicist using a computer program that enabled MAs to be highlighted on screen by mouse clicks. The test set contained 297 true MAs and the MA detector achieved a sensitivity of 82% for detecting and correctly locating MAs at 5.7 false-positives per image. MA detection performed by four independent clinicians on the same 20 test images achieved the same sensitivity at 3.2 false-positives per image. As the free-response ROC curve of the automated detector was close to that of the independent clinicians it was concluded that the computer system can reliably detect MAs. Due to the increased number of images and the various stages of retinopathy used in this study, this conclusion is more secure than that of Spencer et al. [11].

6.2.3 Extensions of the standard approach

The standard approach for automated MA detection has been embraced by a number of groups, including the University of Aberdeen, the research group established by the author at the University of Waikato, New Zealand, and by others.

Hipwell et al. [16] of Aberdeen University modified the automated MA detector of Cree et al. [13] to work on red-free images of 1024 × 1024 pixel resolution of a 50° FOV retina either centered on the macula or nasal of the optic disc. Against a testing set of 62 images, containing a total of 88 MAs that broadly reflected the level of retinopathy expected in an eye-screening population, the automated MA detector achieved 43% sensitivity with 0.11 false-positives per image for detecting and correctly locating MAs. This less sensitive operating point was chosen as being more suitable for eye-screening as only one MA per image needs to be detected to identify retinopathy. The poorer ability to detect MAs in red-free images compared to using fluorescein angiography seems to have adversely affected the overall ability of the automated MA detector in this study. In an extensive trial using 3783 directly digitized red-free images from the diabetic eye-screening program the automated MA detector achieved a sensitivity of 81% at a specificity of 93% for detecting images that contained microaneurysms, and a sensitivity of 85% at a specificity of 76% for the detection of subjects with retinopathy [16]. It was concluded that the automated MA detector would be useful in a screening context to remove half the images that contained no retinopathy, thus would reduce the load of subsequent manual screening.

The Aberdeen automated MA detector [16], in conjunction with an automated exudate detector [17], was also reported in a comparative evaluation of digital imaging, retinal photography, optometrist examination, and automated retinopathy detection [18]. The automated detection again used red-free images of 1024 × 1024 pixel resolution of a 50° field-of-view (FOV). A total of 586 participants, of which 157 had retinopathy, were included. The automated retinopathy detector achieved 83% sensitivity at a specificity of 71% for detecting any retinopathy. This compares to 83% sensitivity at 79% specificity for manual detection of retinopathy from the digital red-free images, and 89% sensitivity at 89% specificity for manual detection of retinopathy from color slides. Olson et al. [18] conclude that the automated retinopathy detection is not yet ready for sole use as the screening mechanism but could form an important adjunct to reducing the workload of manual screening.

A number of other groups have used the standard approach as a starting point for developing automated MA detectors. Mendonça et al. [19] implement the standard approach for detecting MAs in fluorescein angiographic images but only report results of testing on one image. Acha and Serrano [20] used the preprocessing of Mendonça et al. [19] and extended the classifier to include features that are based on the correlation of various shape filters with the candidates. On five angiographic images with a mean of 100 MAs per image they achieve 82% sensitivity with 3.3 false positives per image. Serrano et al. [21] further enhance the image processing strategy by using the errors of linear prediction coefficients as a means of adaptively thresholding the matched-filtered image to generate seed-points for region-growing. The classifier appears to be essentially the same as Acha and Serrano [20]. On 11 angiographic images containing a total of 711 MAs they report a sensitivity of 91% for detecting MAs at 7 false-positives per image.

Yang et al. [22] report on the detection of MAs in low-resolution color retinal images. The green-plane of the color images is used for preprocessing and detection of candidates. The removal of blood vessels in the tophat stage is improved with the use of a morphological reconstruction [23]. Notably, they dispense with the matched-filtering stage and threshold the tophat processed image to generate seed points for region growing. Basic shape features as well as the hue of the candidates as determined from the full-color information is used in classification. A preliminary test on 46 images (of healthy and diseased retinae) achieved 90% sensitivity at 80% specificity for detecting presence of MAs in the diseased retinal images. Lalonde et al. [24] use this MA detector in their RetsoftPlus retinal analysis software.

Raman et al. [25, 26] in a study on the effects of image resolution on automated diabetic retinopathy (DR) detection use an MA detector based on the standard approach. A tophat transform is used to isolate small objects in the shade-corrected image, and matched-filtering with a Gaussian model to detect vessels. Any small objects detected in the tophat that occur on vessels were removed. A genetic algorithm processes the MA detections from three 45° fields of an eye to arrive at a report on the presence of DR for the eye [26]. Color retinal images are used in the study but no mention is made of how the color information is used. On high resolution images (10 DR; 8 no diabetic retinopathy [NDR]) a sensitivity of 90% at a specificity of 88% was achieved for detecting retinopathy. The resolution of the images is not stated (other than they are digitized images of 35 mm film of 35° FOV using mydriasis), and the images were used for both training and testing. On low resolution images (640 × 480 pixels of a 45° FOV; nonmydriatic direct digitization) of 91 subjects (35 DR; 56 NDR), that form an independent test set, a sensitivity of 69% with a specificity of 66% was achieved for detecting retinopathy. This reinforces the conclusion of Spencer et al. [11] that digitization at approximately quarter megapixel resolution is insufficient for automated detection of microaneurysms.

Niemeijer et al. [27] find that the standard approach for segmenting candidates fails to segment all true MAs, thus they develop a new method to generate candidates that is based on pixel classification. After shade-correcting the image, the pixel intensities and first- and second-order Gaussian derivatives at various scales are provided to a k-nearest neighbor classifier that produces a probability map for each pixel to be a small red lesion. This is thresholded and filtered to remove vessel segments and objects that are too large, leaving the candidates. They test the standard approach and their new pixel-based approach for generating candidates and find that both methods fail to detect 14% of true microaneurysms, but when combined together into a hybrid system that figure is reduced to 10%. When coupled with the usual region-growing and final classification to detect MAs, the hybrid system achieved 100% sensitivity at 87% specificity for detecting the presence of retinopathy in the 50 training images (27 DR; 23 NDR) of 768 × 576 pixel resolution.

The standard approach suffers from other known problems. The region growing applied to delineate candidates can be unreliable if the candidate is on or near a vessel, in clusters of microaneurysms, or is in a region of unusual background texture. Most papers based on the standard approach terminate region growing when intensity increases beyond a locally determined threshold. If the resulting grown object does not accurately reflect the underlying shape, then the measured features are likely to be inaccurate, resulting in false-detections or missed microaneurysms. The other problem is local contrast variations — microaneurysms can have poor contrast in some parts of the image while background texture has higher contrast in other parts of the image. The shade-correction of the retinal image compensates for local contrast variation, nevertheless close examination of automated microaneurysm detection results suggest improvements can be made.

Fleming et al. [28] address these concerns. The region growing stopping condition is based on the mean squared gradient magnitude of the boundary of the grown object. They find that this function is maximized when region growing is terminated on the boundary of microaneurysms, and its use improves delineation of candidate shape and extent. Fleming et al. measure the background contrast in a local region about each candidate with a watershed algorithm that excludes features such as other MAs and vessels. The background local contrast is used to normalize the intensity-based features measured on the candidate. Features on the boundary of the candidate are measured as well. As a final adjunct vessels are detected in the local region about the candidate (using an efficient scheme to detect linear structures) and any candidate lying on a vessel is removed.

In an earlier study, Fleming et al. [29] showed that the use of their local contrast normalization and the detection of candidates lying on vessel improves sensitivity by about 6% and specificity by 8% for detecting retinal images containing MAs on a database of 720 good quality retinal images, of which 216 contained MAs. Fleming et al. [28] compared a number of local contrast normalization schemes and found that their proposed scheme performed best and gave a useful improvement to microaneurysm detection. The system achieved a sensitivity of 85.4% at 83.1% specificity for detecting images that contain MAs (1441 images of which 356 contain MAs).

All the above implementations of the standard approach (except [22; 27] and maybe [26]) used monochromatic images such as fluorescein angiographic images, red-free images, or the green plane only of color retinal images. Microaneurysms are well distinguished in the green plane of color retinal images, nevertheless, one wonders whether using the full color information, particularly in the final classifier, may provide an edge in sensitivity and/or specificity. This is the approach that the present author has taken, but we delay discussion to Section 6.3 as the use of color images brings in a new set of problems.

6.2.4 Other approaches

The problem that global shade-correction does not normalize the contrast of microaneurysms sufficiently has also been described by Huang and Yan [30]. They improve local contrast by first applying shade-correction coupled with a nonlinear contrast enhancing transform to local 120×120 pixel blocks of the image (that slightly overlap with one another). Candidate microaneurysms (small circular objects) are found with a tophat transform, and the area and maximum intensity of the candidates must be greater than locally determined thresholds for the candidate to be accepted as a microaneurysm. The results were determined on far too few images (12 images from six subjects) for any meaningful comparison to implementations of the standard approach. Walter et al. [31] describe a similar approach to local image contrast normalization.

Artificial neural networks have been explored for detecting microaneurysms and other lesions in retinal images [32–34]. Varying approaches, ranging from using raw pixel data to substantially processed image data as inputs to the neural network, have been tried. While Gardner et al. [32] detected lesions and features other than microaneurysms, their work is notable in that they break the image down into small windows and use the pixel data of the window (after preprocessing with median filter noise suppression) as well as the result of the Sobel edge operator as inputs to a back propagation neural network. This approach is based on the philosophy that the neural network should be able to recognize the interrelationships between pixels that enable lesions to be detected. Kamel et al. [33] take a similar approach to detect individual microaneurysms. Unfortunately the resolution and number of images used in the study are not stated, thus one cannot use the results of this study. Morganti et al. [34] seem to take a similar approach for detecting microaneurysms and other lesions, though they use a preprocessing step to locate maxima (to detect exudate) and minima (to detect microaneurysms), with the pixel data in a 5×5 pixel window about these points as input to the neural network. They also apply committee techniques to the neural networks. They use images of 512×768 pixels, which is insufficient resolution to detect microaneurysms reliably. Error rates ranging from 8.3% to 12.7% are reported for various algorithms to detect microaneurysms in small image segments. The nonstandard testing methodology makes it hard to compare to other published results.

The output of image processing operators that aid segmentation, such as matched-filters and morphological operators, can be provided as input to the neural network, thus potentially giving the neural network better information to work with. This can be taken to the extreme in which the standard approach can be used to segment candidate microaneurysms, and then use a neural network to classify the candidates as microaneurysms or spurious objects. This is the approach taken by Frame et al. [15] in which the final classification stage of the microaneurysm detector of Cree et al. [13] was tested with various classifiers including a neural network. The manually constructed rule-based classifier, as used by Cree et al. [13], was found to be best.

A variety of general purpose operators, other than those typified by the standard approach, can be used to segment microaneurysms in retinal images. Huang et al. [35], after shade-correcting the retinal image, generate an edge map of the retinal image with the Canny edge detector. The idea is to detect the closed circular edge that surrounds a microaneurysm. Edges that are too long or too short to be a microaneurysm, as well as edges weak in intensity, are removed from the edge map. Edges that resemble small circles are identified and, with reference to the green plane of the retinal image, those that enclose a low-intensity region inside the circle are retained as candidate microaneurysms. This still contains some false-detections, so intensity and shape features are measured on the candidates and used in a classifier to improve specificity. An advantage of this method is that the segmentation algorithm naturally provides the underlying boundary of the microaneurysm without resorting to region growing.

Walter et al. [31] note that the tophat transform of the standard approach tends to detect tortuous vessels as round small objects. This is because the linear structuring element fails to fit inside such vessels at any orientation. They overcome this problem by using a morphological "bounding box" [36] or "diameter" [31] closing (similar to the "area closing" described by Vincent [37]) to segment microaneurysms. Intensity and shape features are extracted for the candidates and classified with the Bayes classifier with kernel density estimation. The system achieved 89% sensitivity at 2.13 false-positives per images for detecting microaneurysms in 94 images (640×480 pixel resolution; 68 DR, 26 NDR) containing a total of 373 microaneurysms [31]. This result compared favorably with the three human graders reported. One may question the low resolution of the images, however, it is to be noted they do use a 3 CCD color camera that produces better quality images than the equivalent resolution (and typically used) 1 CCD camera with Bayer mask.

Quellec et al. [38] use a wavelet approach to detect microaneurysms. Out of three wavelets tested they find the Haar wavelet performed best with 88% sensitivity at 96% specificity for detecting microaneurysms in retinal images. Their database included 995 images (1280×1008 pixel resolution) including both angiographic images and photographs. It is not clear how many images were used for training and how many were used for testing. It is hard to believe that all 995 images were manually segmented by graders, as that is a very time-intensive task!

6.2.5　General red lesion detection

All the studies described above aim to detect microaneurysms and dot-hemorrhages, i.e., small red lesions, only. For diabetic eye screening, detecting more extensive hemorrhage in addition to microaneurysms and dot-hemorrhages would be beneficial. Some research groups have aimed at developing general automated red lesion detection.

Lee et al. [39] present a system for the detection of a number of retinal features including flame and blot hemorrhages as well as dot-hemorrhages and microaneurysms. They use two separate processing pathways, one to detect the large hemorrhages and the other to detect the dot-hemorrhages and MAs. Unfortunately their paper (and an earlier one [40]) provide little detail on the algorithms. In a later paper [41] they report on comparison of their automated computer system against retinal specialists though no details on the algorithms are given and their earlier papers are not cited. On a test set of 428 color fundus images (resolution not stated; 129 contain MAs; 275 without MAs; 24 images excluded due to questionable lesions) the computer system has a sensitivity of 87% at a specificity of 98% for detecting images with microaneurysms. They also report results for automated detection of exudate and cotton wool spots.

Larsen et al. [42, 43] report on testing of the RetinaLyze fundus analysis system. This system can detect a variety of retinal lesions, including hemorrhages and microaneurysms, but no detail is given of the algorithm. On a test set of 400 images of 100 patients digitized from slide film at 1448×1296 pixel resolution (30 patients

DR; 70 NDR) the computerized system detected patients with diabetic retinopathy with 97% sensitivity at 71% specificity [43].

Sinthanayothin et al. [44] described a system for the detection of retinopathy. They detect hemorrhages, microaneurysms (HMAs), and other lesions with use of the "moat operator" (the subtraction of a high pass filtered version of the image from the image) to create a trough around lesions in the image. The lesions are segmented by region growing that is terminated at the troughs. A neural network is used to classify segmented objects into HMAs and non-HMAs. On 30 images (570×550 pixel resolution; 14 contain hemorrhages and/or microaneurysms) the system achieved a sensitivity of 78% and specificity of 89% for detection of hemorrhage/microaneurysms.

6.3 Microaneurysm Detection in Color Retinal Images

Most publications on automated microaneurysm detection use monochromatic data, even if full color information is available. The green part of the spectrum contains the most useful information for discriminating microaneurysms and vascular structure, but whether there is any useful extra information in the red and blue parts of the spectrum is an open question. It is interesting to note that Olson et al. [18] reported improved sensitivity and specificity for manual screening for DR with color slides compared to manual screening with red-free images, though that may be linked to factors other than the presence of color. Monochromatic automated microaneurysm detection has achieved reasonable results and any possible further improvements are likely to be small. Nevertheless, if using color enables a small improvement in specificity for no loss in sensitivity, then this may be important for automated eye screening.

It is normally said that in retinal images, the green plane contains the best detail; the red plane, while brighter and sometimes saturated, has poorer contrast; and the blue plane is dark and typically not much better than noise. Explanations of the color content of fundus images based on radiation transport models [45; 46] tell us that the violet and blue light entering the eye is mostly absorbed by the lens, is further absorbed by melanin and hemoglobin, and is the most scattered light, thus does not contain much contrast. Hemoglobin has an absorption peak in the green part of the spectrum, thus features containing hemoglobin (e.g., microaneurysms) absorb more green light than surrounding tissues, and appear dark and well contrasted in the green part of the spectrum. The red light penetrates deeper into the layers of the inner eye and is primarily reflected in the choroid, explaining the reddish appearance of fundus images. Because red light has a lower absorption coefficient in the tissues of the eye than green, the red part of the spectrum is less contrasted. It also depends on the melanin concentration in the choroid.

The author has observed retinal images of Polynesian subjects to have a much increased blue component. This observation agrees with the results of Preece and Claridge [46], who show that for a non-Caucasian subject the reflectance of the eye in the red and green parts of the spectrum is much reduced when compared to Caucasian subjects, whereas the blue reflectance remains similar. Assuming that the photographer adjusts the fundus camera shutter exposure to increase the brightness for non-Caucasian subjects to better expose the captured image, this will appear in captured retinal images as an increase in the blue component.

The upshot is that the appearance of color retinal images can vary between subjects considerably due to changing shifts in balance between red and green, and between red-green and blue. If microaneurysm detection is to use all color information then some form of color normalization is needed, particularly for mixed populations.

Histogram specification to force color retinal images to a reference histogram has been investigated by a couple of groups [47; 48]. A comparison between gray world normalization, color histogram equalization and color histogram specification to a standard image was undertaken by Goatman et al. [48]. Interestingly they found histogram specification performed best in the sense that the class separateness between exudates, cotton wool spots, hemorrhage, and blot hemorrhages in the chromaticity components was best with this method. This result is a little surprising as certain lesions (such as exudate) are often evident in the shape of the histogram and reshaping of the histogram to a reference that does not necessarily contain the lesion is likely to mask the lesion.

This criticism of histogram specification lead Erin Gamble, a former master student of the author, to use a straightforward and general purpose scheme for color normalization of retinal images [49] in order to modify the automated microaneurysm detector of Cree et al. [13] to work on color retinal images. Each color plane of the red-green-blue (RGB) color retinal image is processed independently of the others. First, divisive shade-correction to correct for illumination variation intra-image is applied, then contrast normalization to a specified mean and standard deviation is applied to correct for illumination variation inter-image. This process retains the overall shape of the color image histogram, but shifts the hue (which is often dominated by the ratio of green to red in retinal images) to be consistent between images.

In the top line of Figure 6.2 is shown two color retinal images, one of a Caucasian and one of a Polynesian. The corresponding color normalized images, using the procedure of Cree et al. [49] are shown in the bottom line of Figure 6.2. The color normalized images may not appear familiar to an ophthalmologist, nevertheless the color between the images is much more consistent than in the original retinal images.

This scheme for color normalization is straightforward, and now can be implemented very efficiently with the discovery of a median filter algorithm whose speed is (almost) independent of the kernel size [50]. It can be criticized for processing the color planes independently (with the potential for unwanted chromaticity shifts) and not being based on a more robust model of illumination of retinal images. With high resolution color retinal imaging becoming widely available, further research into better color normalization of retinal images, particularly to normalize images of different ethnic groups, is required.

Of the few papers on automated MA detection that use color information [22; 27; 31], we leave discussion of their findings on the importance of the color features for MA detection to after discussion of the Waikato Automated Microaneurysm Detector in the next section.

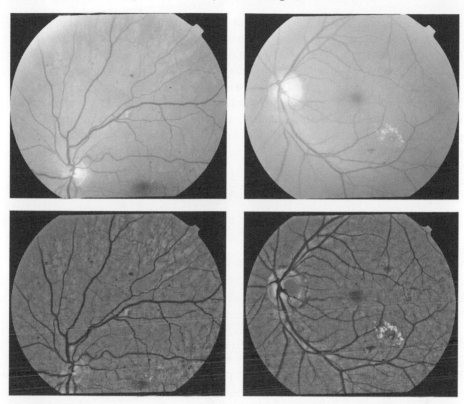

FIGURE 6.2
Color normalization of retinal images. Top: color retinal images of a Caucasian and a Polynesian. Bottom: color normalized version of the image directly above. (**See color insert following page 174.**)

6.4 The Waikato Automated Microaneurysm Detector

The automated microaneurysm detector, developed by the authors and co-workers at the University of Waikato [49; 51], is a modification of the standard approach to work on color retinal images. The processing of the images for microaneurysms is as follows: The green plane only of the retinal image is used to segment candidate microaneurysms. It is divisive shade-corrected and then lightly median filtered for noise-suppression. The tophat transform is followed by a morphological reconstruction [23] to improve the removal of vessels from the image. A circularly symmetric 2-D Gaussian is used as the template for matched-filtering to highlight microaneurysms. An adaptive threshold then isolates candidates from the match-filtered image, and region-growing on the shade-corrected green plane at the positions of candidates is used to isolate the morphology of the underlying candidate.

The full color information is only used in the classification stage. The retinal image is color normalized by the process described above. In the training stage 52 features involving color, intensity, and shape were analyzed, but it was found that microaneurysm detection was almost optimal using only seven of the features. Taking r, g, and b to be the red components of the original retinal image, $\hat{r}$, $\hat{g}$, and $\hat{b}$ to be the color normalized retinal image, m to be the result of the matched-filter, Ω to be the set of pixels of a candidate microaneurysm, $A = \sum_\Omega 1$ to be the area identical to the number of pixels in the candidate, and μ_{ij}^x to be the 2D central moment of order i, j of the candidate calculated over image x (where x can be any of r, g, etc.) then,

Red Mean $$\bar{R} = \frac{1}{A} \sum_{i \in \Omega} r_i \tag{6.1}$$

Norm Red Mean $$\bar{\hat{R}} = \frac{1}{A} \sum_{i \in \Omega} \hat{r}_i \tag{6.2}$$

Green Std. Dev. $$\sigma_g = \sqrt{\frac{1}{A} \left(\sum_{i \in \Omega} (g_i^2) - \left(\sum_{i \in \Omega} g_i \right)^2 / A \right)} \tag{6.3}$$

Norm Blue Std. Dev. $$\sigma_{\hat{b}} = \sqrt{\frac{1}{A} \left(\sum_{i \in \Omega} (\hat{b}_i^2) - \left(\sum_{i \in \Omega} \hat{b}_i \right)^2 / A \right)} \tag{6.4}$$

Matched Filter Mean $$\bar{M} = \frac{1}{A} \sum_{i \in \Omega} m_i \tag{6.5}$$

Norm Green Rot. Inert. $$I_{\hat{G}} = \frac{1}{A} \left(\mu_{20}^{\hat{g}} + \mu_{02}^{\hat{g}} \right) \tag{6.6}$$

Minor Axis Length $$l_- \tag{6.7}$$

The minor axis length l_- is the length of the minor axis of the ellipse that has the same normalized second moments as the candidate.

The feature "norm green rot. inert.," is the rotational inertia about the centroid of a flat plate of the same shape as the candidate and with density given by the color normalized green component, and scaled by the area. It depends usefully on both the shape and intensity distribution (in the color normalized green plane) of the microaneurysm. In the green plane microaneurysms are darker than the surrounding tissue, hence the normalized green rotational inertia feature is typically small for microaneurysms. The further the candidate deviates from being a perfectly round disc, the greater this feature, and if the boundary of the candidate does not approach the background retinal intensity in the normal way this feature is likely to be increased. This feature proves to be the most powerful of the list above for discriminating microaneurysms from spurious objects.

The microaneurysm detector was trained on 80 retinal images (60 DR; 20 NDR), captured at 50° field-of-view with a Topcon fundus camera and a Nikon D1X 6 megapixel digital camera. The images contained JPEG quantization tables identical to those produced by the Independent JPEG Group's opensource code* when set to 95% quality. A later closer examination of the images revealed an unusual distribution in the raw JPEG stream suggestive that these images have been JPEG compressed at least twice, putting into question the 95% quality claim. It also raises questions about quality control of retinal images, of which we have more to say in Section 6.5.2 below.

The microaneurysm detector was run on the images to the stage of segmenting the candidates. Each candidate was labeled as a microaneurysm or a spurious object by an expert in the field. The features listed above (plus others) were measured over each candidate. There were 3053 candidates detected on the sixty, images of which 401 were marked as microaneurysms by the expert, leaving the other 2652 as spurious objects. The expert identified another 14 microaneurysms in the images that were not segmented as candidates by the automated software, for a total of 415 microaneurysms.

The retinal images used in this study were obtained from a mobile eye-screening program, and the Nikon digital camera had to be removed from the fundus camera to fit it in the vehicle for transport from one eye center to another. Unfortunately dust got into the camera optics, and the dust marks in the image bear a striking similarity to microaneurysms. Indeed the trained expert originally identified 465 "microaneurysms" in the training images before it was realized some were dust and removed to leave the 415 microaneurysms in the gold standard. Because at least four retinal images were captured per patient at a visit on the same day, it was straight-forward to analyze all images of a patient with the automated microaneurysm detector and remove detections of candidates that occur at the same position in a majority of the patient's images. Presence of dust as a confounding issue for detecting microaneurysms, even using direct digital retinal photography, has been noted elsewhere [52].

A number of different classifiers were tested for their ability to distinguish microaneurysms [49], and the naïve Bayes classifier [53] was finally chosen for implementation. Despite the potentially flimsy assumption it is based upon (statistical independence of the features) it is known to perform surprisingly well in some domains, and is very fast to run [54]. In our tests more sophisticated (and slower) classifiers only gave marginal improvements.

The receiver operating characteristic (ROC) curve for classifying the 3053 candidates correctly as microaneurysms or spurious objects is shown in Figure 6.3. The nonparametric curve does not quite approach 100% (except at 0% specificity) as there are 14 microaneurysms that are not detected by the candidate generation algorithm. The parametric curve is a fitting of the bi-normal ROC model [55] by a nonlinear least squares fit to the nonparametric curve.

The detection of microaneurysms in an image can be used to predict the presence of diabetic retinopathy. We use the number of detected microaneurysms in an image as the predictor for the presence of diabetic retinopathy. The resultant ROC curve is

---

*libjpeg version 6b, downloadable from www.ijg.org.

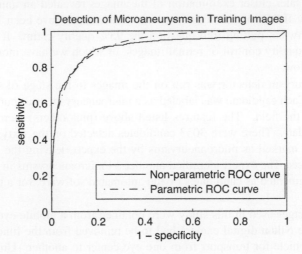

FIGURE 6.3
Result of classification of candidates as microaneurysms by the naïve Bayes classifier.

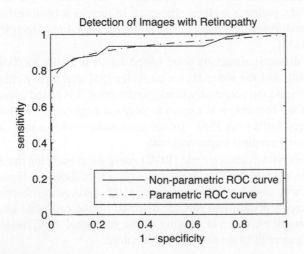

FIGURE 6.4
ROC graph for determining presence of diabetic retinopathy by the number of detected microaneurysms in the training images.

shown in Figure 6.4. This result is after a few false detections of microaneurysms that were in fact dust marks were automatically removed, however, dust detection only gave a marginal improvement, indicating that the microaneurysm detector is distinguishing microaneurysms from dust reasonably reliably.

The Waikato Automated Microaneurysm Detector has been tested on images from a completely different source that was not affected by dust [56]. These images were acquired at 2.8 megapixel resolution and were approximately 1560×1360 pixels after cropping the black regions of the images away. As this is a lower resolution than the microaneurysm detector was trained on, the parameters (such as the tophat linear structure size, and the matched filter template diameter) were adjusted proportionally to match. No changes were made to the naïve Bayes classifier. The automated detector was run on 745 color retinal images (145 DR; 600 NDR). There were 34 images with extensive white reflections (sometimes seen in retinal images of young people), and the microaneurysm detector false-detected extensively as the white reflections broke up the vessels into small segments. Such images were not present in the database the automated microaneurysm detector was trained on, and are unlikely to be seen in any numbers in an eye-screening program so were removed from this study. The automated microaneurysm detector achieved 85% sensitivity and 90% specificity for detecting diabetic retinopathy on the remaining 711 images [56].

6.4.1 Further comments on the use of color

We return to further consider whether the use of full color information in color retinal images provides a useful benefit over use of the green plane alone. In the Waikato Automated Microaneurysm Detector two red features and one blue feature (Equations 6.1 through 6.7) were found to be beneficial. It is interesting that the standard deviation of the normalized blue component over the candidate provided a small but useful improvement in microaneurysm detection. Since only eighty images are used in training, there remains a possibility that this improvement may be due to the particular training set used, and would not be replicated with a much larger testing database. But there is another possibility: it is possible that the blue field enabled the classifier to better distinguish microaneurysms from the dust marks, and would not be replicated in a study with clean retinal images.

This reliance on color-based features for classification of microaneurysms was not replicated by Walter et al. [31]. They explored the use of various color features, but found that only the Euclidean color difference measured in Lab color space provided extra discriminatory power. Yang et al. [22] find the hue of the candidate useful for discrimination but do not indicate whether they explored other color features. Niemeijer et al. [27] include a variety of color features (the contrast in red, green, blue, and hue) in their k-nearest neighbor classifier. They ran feature selection tests and report that no subset of their original set of 68 features improved classification, but do not report whether the removal of any features (such as the color features) impacts negatively on classification.

These experiences of using color to aid MA detection seem a little contradictory, and it remains an open question as to whether the use of color features, when color retinal images are being analyzed, provides a useful improvement to automated MA detection.

6.5   Issues for Microaneurysm Detection

There are a number of issues for successful use of automated microaneurysm detection in diabetic eye screening. We can split these into two classes: the actual issues that impact negatively on reliable microaneurysm detection, and the means of verifying that an automated microaneurysm detection system is reliable enough for its intended use. In this section we first discuss things that impact negatively on reliable microaneurysm detection, namely poor image quality, the use of lossy image compression, and the causes of false detections of microaneurysms. We then turn to the issue of verifying automated microaneurysm detectors in a meaningful way that allows cross-comparisons.

6.5.1   Image quality assessment

Largely ignored in the literature is the effect of image quality on automated microaneurysm detection (notable exceptions are [57; 58]). In eye screening studies a not insignificant proportion of images are of poor contrast or blurred due to factors such as lens cataract and teary eyes. In such situations automated microaneurysm detection is impaired at best and may completely fail at worst. If automated microaneurysm detection is to be used as a means of determining the presence of diabetic retinopathy, then retinal image quality assessment needs to be automated, so that poor quality images can be reported. This is an area that needs further investigation.

Also not often realized is that the single lens reflex (SLR) digital cameras now typically used with fundus cameras do not record full color at each pixel. A Bayer mask is placed over the light sensor so that only one of the primary colors (in some cases secondary colors) of light is measured at each pixel. Software interpolation (within the camera) is used to estimate full color information at each pixel from lower resolution measurements of different colors in its neighborhood. In contrast a 3-CCD camera has three CCD sensors, one CCD for each primary color, so that full color is acquired at full resolution. A 3-CCD camera normally performs substantially better than a camera with a Bayer mask rated at the same resolution.

There is a criticism that high resolution digital cameras (greater than say 1 megapixel) are unnecessary for imaging the retina as their resolution exceeds the limit of resolvable detail imageable through the eye. But considering the loss in detail due to the typically used Bayer mask it is prudent to use a camera of higher specified resolution to ensure that the observeable detail is actually captured.

6.5.2 Image compression implications

The use of JPEG (Joint Photographic Experts Group) compression[†] at source in digital retinal image acquisition is ubiquitous. JPEG compression is a lossy compression. Not only is it impossible to recover the original image data as provided by the camera sensor, there is also a loss of general image quality due to smoothing of image data and introduced blockiness and ringing artifacts.

It is almost unavoidable to work with anything but JPEG compressed images in retinal imaging. The author is aware of one research center that purchased a fundus camera and retinal imaging suite, and were assured by the distributor that the system could capture and store the original uncompressed image data, but later found that the images saved in uncompressed TIFF format by the system contained the blatant signatures of JPEG compression in the image data. It is likely the digital camera JPEG compressed the image data before sending it to the client computer, despite the client software's claim it was handling and saving uncompressed image data. We have already noted above how the training images for the Waikato Automated Microaneurysm Detector contain evidence of being saved at least twice with JPEG compression. Each compression with JPEG degrades image data, and retinal imaging systems do not provide audit trials of degraded image data.

A number of studies on the ability of ophthalmologists to detect and grade the presence of clinically significant disease in JPEG degraded retinal images have supported the not uncommon assumption that a certain amount of JPEG compression can safely be tolerated in retinal images. All of these studies have focused on the ability of expert graders and ophthalmologists to grade retinal images. There appear to be only two studies that consider the effect of JPEG compression on automated detection of retinal lesions, both focusing on microaneurysm detection.

First it is worth summarizing the results of studies that consider the effect of JPEG compression on manual grading of retinal images. Studies using questionable resolution (about 800×600 pixels) find that specialists overly misgrade retinal images with compression ratios (raw image data size to JPEG compressed image size) as low as 30:1 [59–61], whereas those that use a more suitable higher original image resolution find that higher compression ratios can be sustained [62; 63]. For example, Baker et al. [64], who used image resolution of 3040×2008 pixels[‡] (6 megapixel) found no problems with image compression ratios as large as 113:1. This result is not unexpected: the better the original image resolution and quality, the larger the compression ratios that can be withstood.

It is typical, as in the above reported studies, to report JPEG compression ratios as a measure of how much the images are compressed. Typically the larger the compression ratio, the lower the quality of the image and the more noticeable the introduced artifacts. Nevertheless compression ratios do not fully characterize the resultant image quality and may not be directly comparable between studies. There

---

[†]http://www.jpeg.org. The JPEG standard is available as ISO/IEC IS 10918-1.

[‡]Baker et al. reported resolution as 2008×3040 pixels, however, it is likely they have reported rows by columns rather than the more commonly reported width by height.

are two reasons for this. First, JPEG compression involves a number of steps and quite a few parameters that are not directly accessible to the user. The mapping of the user-specified *quality factor* to the internal parameters (particularly the quantization tables used for JPEG compression) is software package dependent, thus the quality factor of one package need not produce the same compression and image quality as that of another package. The second reason arises from the final step in JPEG compression, namely lossless Huffman encoding, which is used to further compress the image bitstream. The amount of compression achieved by Huffman encoding is dependent on the nature of the original image. For example, areas of entirely black pixels can be compressed very efficiently, so retinal images with large surrounding black areas (which sometimes happens with digital camera backends that have a 3:2 aspect ratio) achieve larger compression ratios, for the same image quality, than retinal images where the fundus camera aperture is much more tightly cropped.

JPEG compression has three major effects: it smoothes image data, it introduces ringing about sharp edges (a similar effect to the Gibbs phenomenon of the Fourier transform) and it introduces blockiness artifacts on an 8×8 pixel basis. Many implementations of JPEG compression also halve the resolution (at least in the vertical direction) of the chroma components of color images. The smoothing of image data, provided that compression ratios are not too high, can actually be a benefit as it acts as a noise-suppression technique. In contrast, the blockiness artifacts, since they can be of similar scale to microaneurysms, are particularly likely to be detrimental to microaneurysm detection. The ringing about sharp edges is likely to be detrimental to measuring fine vessel characteristics and the detection of finely detailed lesions such as neovascularization.

Of importance here is Hänsgen et al. [65] in which automated microaneurysm detection on JPEG and wavelet compressed fluorescein angiographic images was tested with the microaneurysm detector of Cree et al. [13]. Using a test-bed of 20 retinal images of 35° field-of-view (FOV) at 1024×1024 resolution, they found that a loss of sensitivity and an increasing false-positive detection rate of microaneurysms was noticeable at a JPEG compression ratio of 10:1 and started to become severe at about 20:1 compression ratio. The wavelet compression proved to be less disastrous for microaneurysm detection.

That wavelet compression is a better compression method than the discrete cosine transform (DCT) used in standard JPEG compression has been recognized by JPEG. The newer 2000 standard replaces the DCT with a wavelet compression and potentially provides better image quality for the same compression ratio. Unfortunately adoption of this standard has been slow.

The most recent study on the effect of JPEG compression on automated microaneurysm detection [66] was performed by the current author. The eighty training images for the Waikato Automated Microaneurysm Detector were further compressed with the Independent JPEG Group's software to 70%, 50%, 30%, and 10% quality (recall the original images appeared to be 95% quality). The result of using the automated microaneurysm detection to detect retinopathy based on the presence of microaneurysms is shown in Figure 6.5. Note the drop-off in sensitivity for the 50% and 30% quality curves compared to the 75% and 95% quality curves. Assuming the drop in sensitivity for the 50% quality can be replicated with testing on a

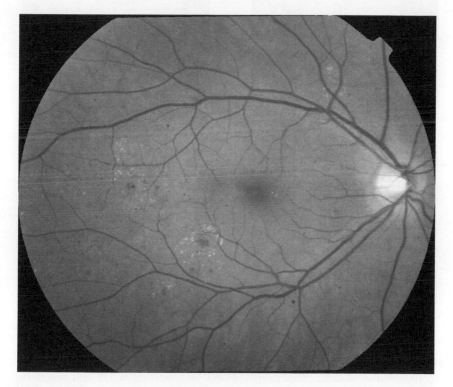

FIGURE 2.1
Moderate nonproliferative diabetic retinopathy with moderate diabetic macular edema.

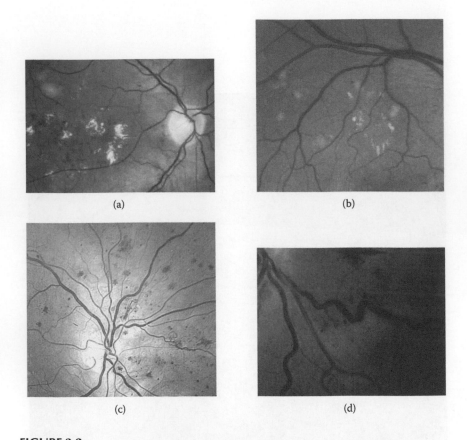

FIGURE 2.2
Nonproliferative diabetic retinopathy (NPDR). (a) Moderate NPDR and severe diabetic macular edema; hard exudates involve the center of the macula. (b) Moderate NPDR; microaneurysms/dot hemorrhages, hard exudate (ring) and cotton wool spots. (c) Severe NPDR; > 20 intraretinal hemorrhages in four quadrants (three shown here) and IRMA (possibly NVE). Biomicroscopy showed the latter lesion to be intraretinal, hence it is IRMA. (d) Venous beading.

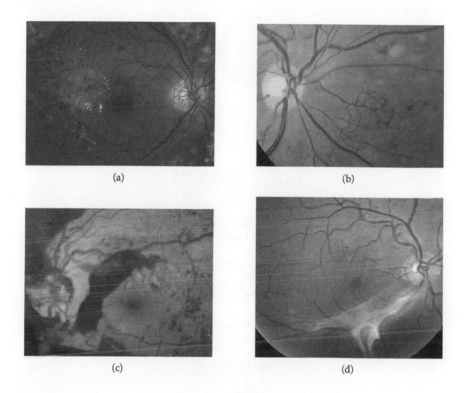

(a)

(b)

(c)

(d)

FIGURE 2.3

Proliferative diabetic retinopathy (PDR) (a) PDR with moderate diabetic macular edema. There are new vessels disc, new vessels elsewhere, IRMA, blotchy hemorrhages, microaneurysms/dot hemorrhages, and hard exudates. Hard exudate approach the center of the macula. Pan retinal photocoagulation scars are seen in the top left and top and bottom far right. (b) New vessels elsewhere. (c) PDR with preretinal hemorrhage. Hemorrhage is contained within the space between the retina and the posterior vitreous face. The hemorrhage obscures the retinal new vessels. (d) Fibrous proliferation with traction macular detachment. PDR has regressed. Regressed fibro-vascular tissue along the inferior temporal vascular arcade has contracted causing traction macular detachment. Traction lines can be seen extending into the central macula.

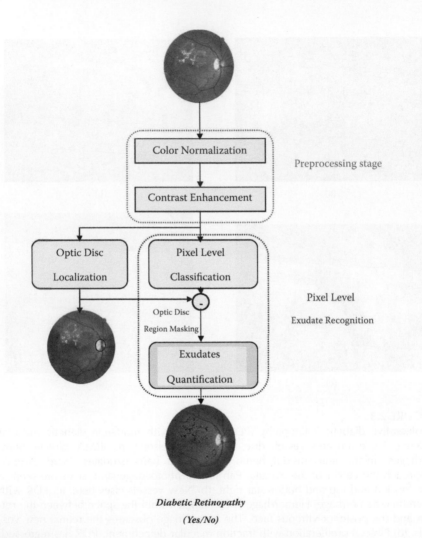

Diabetic Retinopathy

(Yes/No)

FIGURE 5.1

The outline of the proposed system for automatic identification of retinal exudates and the optic disc in color retinal images.

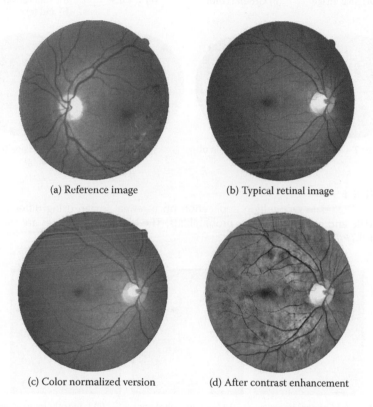

(a) Reference image   (b) Typical retinal image

(c) Color normalized version   (d) After contrast enhancement

FIGURE 5.3
Color normalization and local contrast enhancement.

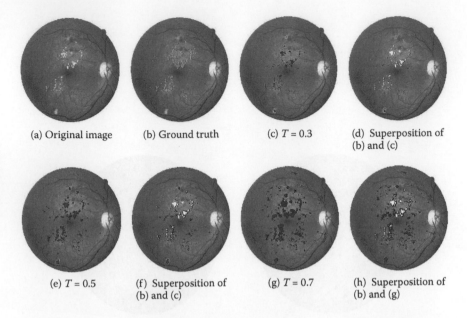

(a) Original image   (b) Ground truth   (c) $T = 0.3$ (d) Superposition of (b) and (c)

(e) $T = 0.5$ (f) Superposition of (b) and (c)   (g) $T = 0.7$ (h) Superposition of (b) and (g)

FIGURE 5.4
Pixel-level exudate recognition application on a retinal image using different ratio of exudate and nonexudate prior probabilities. The identified exudates are shown in blue and *TPs* are in white.

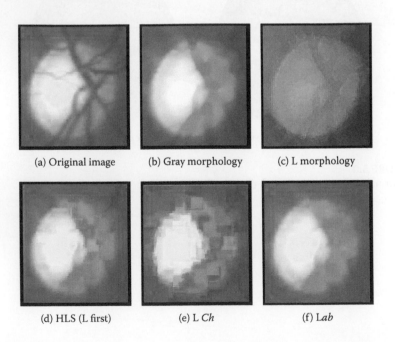

(a) Original image   (b) Gray morphology   (c) L morphology

(d) HLS (L first)   (e) L *Ch*   (f) L*ab*

FIGURE 5.6
Mathematical morphology closing in different color spaces.

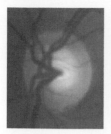 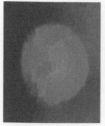 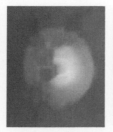 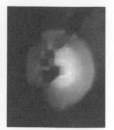

(a) A typical optic disc image   (b) After color morphology   (c) Lightness image   (d) Gray-level morphology closing

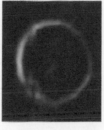 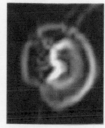

(e) Gradient image obtained from lightness image   (f) Gradient image obtained from gray-level morphology closing.

FIGURE 5.7

A comparison between color morphology and gray-level morphology.

(a) A typical retinal image   (b) Vessel elimination in *Lab*   (c) Initial snake   (d) Final snake

(e) Close-up of optic disc region   (f) *Lab* closing of optic disc region   (g) Close-up of final snake   (h) Close-up of hand-drawn ground truth   (i) Overlay of (g) and (h)

FIGURE 5.8

Optic disc localization results.

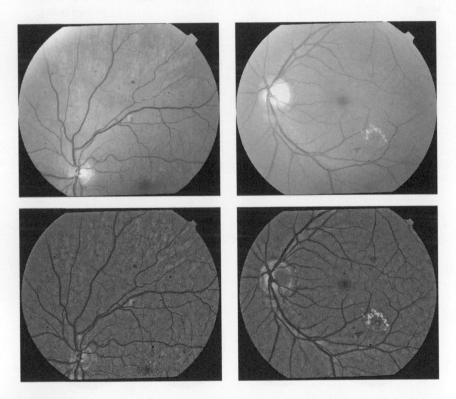

FIGURE 6.2
Color normalization of retinal images. Top: color retinal images of a Caucasian and a Polynesian. Bottom: color normalized version of the image directly above.

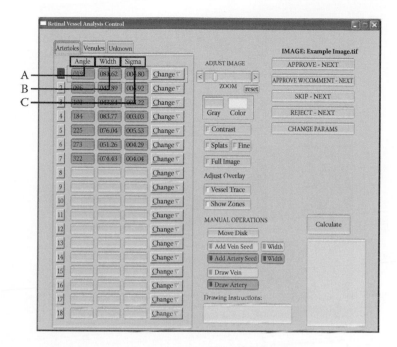

FIGURE 7.A.2

Secondary monitor — control panel (in arteriole view). The labels are: (A) angle of vessel in degrees, (B) mean width, and (C) standard deviation (sigma).

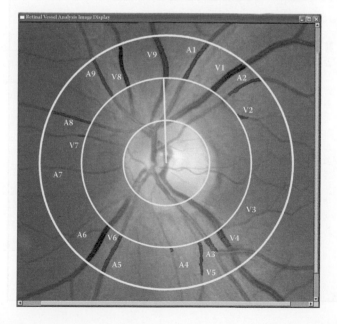

FIGURE 7.A.3

Automated display before grader interaction.

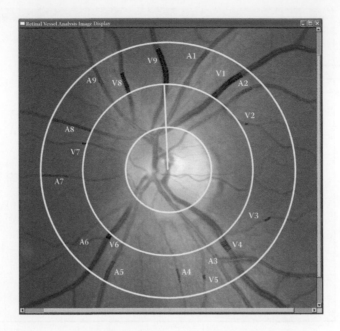

FIGURE 7.A.4
Completed grading with grader interaction.

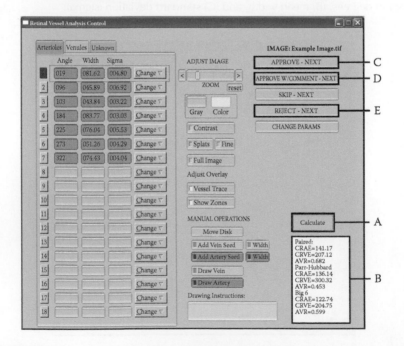

FIGURE 7.A.5
Control panel view after calculation. The labels are: (A) Calculate button, (B) Results panel, (C) APPROVE, (D) APPROVE W/COMMENT, and (E) REJECT.

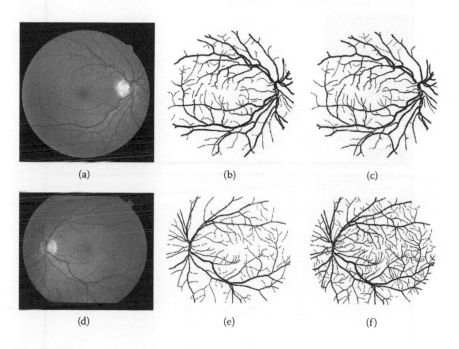

FIGURE 8.6

Images from the DRIVE and STARE databases and their respective manual segmentations: (a) normal image from the test set of the DRIVE database; (b) manual segmentation from set A; (c) manual segmentation from set B; (d) normal image from the STARE database; (e) manual segmentation by the first observer; and (f) manual segmentation by the second observer.

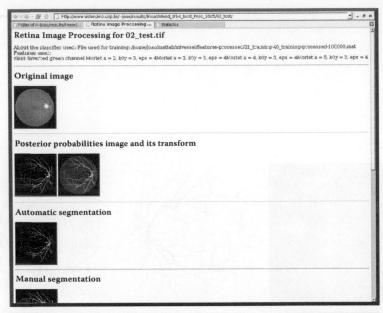

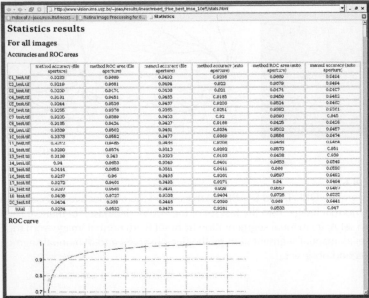

FIGURE 8.8
Examples of HTML outputs produced using the mlvessel package. Top: segmentation results for an image from the DRIVE database. Bottom: statistics and ROC graphs for results on the DRIVE database.

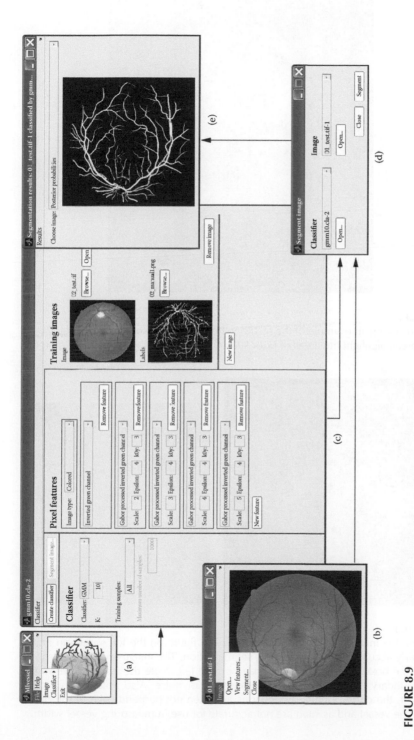

FIGURE 8.9

Windows and dialogues from the GUI illustrating the supervised image segmentation process: (a) main window; (b) image window; (c) classifier window; (d) image segmentation dialogue; and (e) segmentation result window.

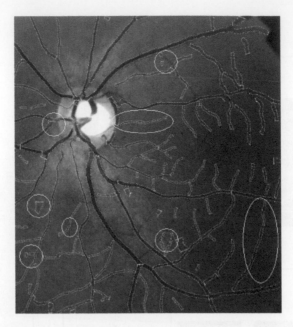

FIGURE 9.2
Figure illustrating an example of the results generated by the vessel-tracing algorithm.
Circled areas highlight the areas of poor smoothness or erroneous vessel detection.

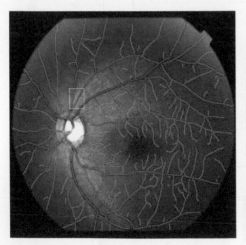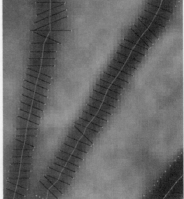

FIGURE 9.3
Illustrating the inaccuracy in the boundaries. The figure on the left shows an image
with a fairly accurate vessel (centerline) segmentation. The image on the right, shows
in detail the boxed region from the image on the left. Note the inaccuracies in the
vessel boundary points caused by poor contrast or noise. Also note how for each
trace point, the corresponding boundaries are often not perpendicular to the orientation of the vessel and as such are not accurate for use in measuring vessel width.

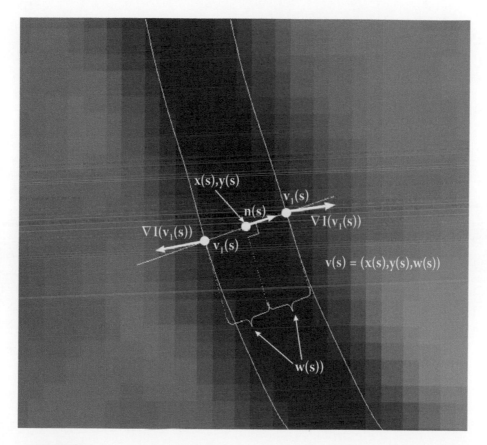

FIGURE 9.7
Illustration showing the parameters of a ribbon snake. Note the projection of the gradient on the unit norm (n(s)) used to further improve the boundary extraction.

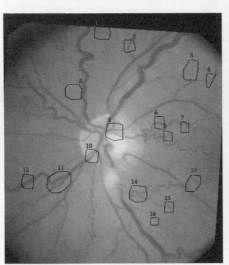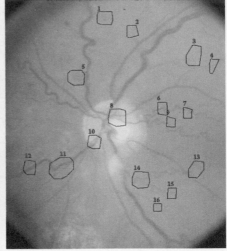

FIGURE 9.9

Illustrating the results of change detection. Boxes are drawn around vessels with suspected width change. The image on the left has been transformed into the samecoordinate system as the image on the right.

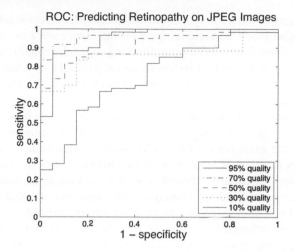

FIGURE 6.5

Predicting retinopathy based on the presence of microaneurysms on images that have been degraded by JPEG compression. (From Cree, M. J. and Jelinek, H. F. *The Effect of JPEG Compression on Automated Detection of Microaneurysms in Retinal Images*, Proc. SPIE, 6813, p. 68130M-6, 2008. With permission.)

larger independent dataset, then the loss of sensitivity might mean the difference in meeting required reliability targets for microaneurysm detection in an eye-screening program.

Ideally the test should be performed on a larger independent set of retinal images that are acquired without any JPEG compression so that a baseline can be set to compare minimal JPEG compression against original image data. Cree and Jelinek [66] do present results using an independent test set, but it is only 20 images (12 DR; 8 NDR) and the results are somewhat inconclusive due to too few images. Further research into the effects of JPEG image compression on automated retinal pathology detection is required.

6.5.3 Optic disc detection

False detections of microaneurysms can occur on the optic disc. An effective automated microaneurysm detector must detect the optic disc so that it can remove any detections of microaneurysms in the vicinity of the optic disc. There are a number of proposals for optic disc detection, however, many of them fail to detect abnormal optic discs reliably or false detect in the presence of extensive yellow lesions.

6.5.4 Meaningful comparisons of implementations

In the review above results of testing of automated microaneurysm detectors have been reported whenever the studies have included results in their publications. It would be a dangerous thing to say that one automated MA detector is better or more suited than another based on these reported results. There are a number of reasons why this is so, ranging from a failure to sufficiently report the conditions under which the study has been performed, to testing on an image database, whether by number or type of images included, that is not reflective of the anticipated application for the automated MA detector.

A common failure is to test on image databases of far too few images. Some studies hide this fact by breaking images down into small image segments, thus inflating the numbers of test cases but not their independence. Admittedly researchers often have access only to a limited number of images that have suitable annotations of the presence of lesions by experts. Nevertheless, if results are to be meaningful, automated MA detectors (indeed any computer-aided detection of retinal lesions) must be tested on a large number of images that embody the breadth in quality, of appearance, levels of retinopathy, and of confounding lesions that occur in practice. For example, to compare two systems, one with a true area under the curve (AUC) of 0.85 and the other with a true AUC of 0.9, one should plan on 350 healthy images and 350 diseased images to achieve statistical significance at the 80% level to establish the difference between the two systems [67].

Studies vary in the level of retinopathy present in their image databases, which may bias results from study to study. Microaneurysm detection on images with lots of microaneurysms is likely to produce high false-positive rates because of the presence of doubtful microaneurysms. Even expert human observers have a certain level of disagreement not only with others but also with themselves on such images. It is important to report the level of retinopathy and the number of microaneurysms in the test database.

Some studies have used images of low resolution in which microaneurysms are too poorly resolved to be reliably detected. It is the opinion of this author that resolutions below 1000×1000 pixels are suboptimal for microaneurysm detection. If a color digital camera is used then even higher resolution is preferable to counteract the degradation in image quality at capture due to the camera Bayer mask and subsequent image degradation due to JPEG compression.

Researchers are also developing automated lesion detection for various reasons. If the aim is a research tool that grades retinopathy by microaneurysm counts then it is important to test the system for the ability to both detect and accurately locate microaneurysms in retinal images. On the other hand, if the aim is to develop a system for the detection of diabetic retinopathy, say for use in eye screening, then accurate microaneurysm counts are not necessary. As long as one microaneurysm is detected per image that contains microaneurysms then the system may be quite successful.

Thus meaningful comparisons between published studies are often hard to draw due to variation in testing methodologies and test image banks. There is a need for a publicly accessible and generally approved database of images with marked microaneurysms for testing automated microaneurysm detectors. The STARE [68] and DRIVE [69] databases of images with accompanying gold standards for vessel detection, and the acceptance of testing new vessel detection algorithms against these databases, are shining examples of what can be achieved. The recently announced Retinopathy Online Challenge§ is an interesting development in this area, and we await the results of the competition.

6.6   Research Application of Microaneurysm Detection

While much work on automated microaneurysm detection is motivated by the need to reduce costs in diabetic eye screening, some work is aimed at enabling otherwise labor-intensive research studies. That the number of microaneurysms reflect the severity of diabetic retinopathy and its likely progression was established by labor-intensive research studies conducted over many years and involving a large number of patients [3–5]. A computer system that could automatically grade retinal images would make collecting and analyzing data for such large studies more manageable.

The work of Goatman et al. [6] using automated microaneurysm detection to study the life cycle of microaneurysms is a noteable move in this direction. In this study two fluorescein angiographic images of 35 patients with diabetic retinopathy were taken (nominally) a year apart. The images of 10 patients (image set 1) were analyzed by manual grading and by automated detection of microaneurysms, and the images of the remaining 25 patients (image set 2) by automated detection of microaneurysms only. The small increase in the number of microaneurysms between baseline and 1-year follow-up did not reach statistical significance.

The ability of the microaneurysm detector to detect *new* microaneurysms (that is, MAs seen at 1-year follow-up but not at baseline), *static* microaneurysms (MAs seen at baseline and 1-year follow-up), and *regressed* microaneurysms (MAs seen at baseline and have disappeared at 1-year follow-up) was verified to be comparable to the manual graders. The determination of the total number of microaneurysms is somewhat resistant to operator error as errors of omissions tend to balance out errors in inclusion. In contrast, detection of microaneurysm turnover (new and regressed MAs) is degraded by such errors.

Manual annotation of microaneurysms is subject to intra-observer variation. Expert graders' decisions can vary from one session to another, with a reproducibility (the ratio of the number of MAs that matched in both sessions to the number of unique MAs found in both sessions) of 78%, the best reported [6; 70–72]. An automated system is not subject to this error and has a 100% reproducibility. Even though the automated system is not quite as sensitive as the manual observers, that it is exactly consistent may be more important for determining microaneurysm turnover.

Goatman et al. [6] found that 57% of microaneurysms at baseline of image set 1, (respectively 53% of image set 2) were present a year later (static MAs), the balance being regressed microaneurysms. The small increase in the number of microaneurysms between baseline and follow-up did not reflect the high level of turnover

---

§http://roc.healthcare.uiowa.edu/.

of microaneurysms measured. They suggest that turnover data may be more sensitive than counts of microaneurysms at predicting progression of diabetic retinopathy. Further larger studies are needed to test this claim, and are an area where automated analysis can have a role to play.

6.7   Conclusion

Because microaneurysms are normally the first lesion seen in early diabetic retinopathy and microaneurysm counts have an established relationship to severity of diabetic retinopathy, there is some impetus to develop CAD software for the automated detection of microaneurysms in retinal images. Early attempts focused on detection in fluorescein angiographic images where MAs are better visualized, whereas there is now a drive to develop software for use on color retinal images for the automated detection of diabetic retinopathy in eye-screening programs.

A range of image processing strategies have been proposed for automated MA with a number of systems achieving over 80% sensitivity and 80% specificity for the detection of images containing microaneurysms. Still better is required for an eye-screening program. Some systems have claimed sensitivities or specificities near 90%, however, the variation in testing methodologies and substantial weaknesses and differences in test image sets make it difficult to compare systems or to assess whether they would be suitable for their intended purpose. There is a need to establish testing methodologies that enable useful comparison of automated MA detection systems.

In addition to the problems in testing methodologies, we have highlighted issues in using color images, and the need for image quality assessment and optic disc detection for an effective automated MA detector. In addition, being able to determine the retinal field and which eye is being viewed would be useful. Automated microaneurysm detection may be useful to reduce the workload of manual screening, however, for a fully automated eye screening system it will be necessary to be able to detect less commonly occurring lesions. Systems to meet such needs include exudate and hemorrhage detection, however, for a robust system, being able to detect vessel lesions, such as venous beading and new vessel growth, will be essential.

References

[1] Crick, R.P. and Khaw, P.T., *A textbook of clinical ophthalmology*, World Scientific, New Jersey, 3rd ed., 2003.

[2] Kohner, E.M., Sleightholm, M., and KROC Collaborative Study Group, Does microaneurysm count reflect severity of early diabetic retinopathy? *Ophthalmology*, 93, 586, 1986.

[3] Kohner, E.M., Stratton, I.M., Aldington, S.J., et al., Microaneurysms in the development of diabetic retinopathy (UKPDS 42), *Diabetologia*, 42(9), 1107, 1999.

[4] Klein, R., Meuer, S.M., Moss, S.E., et al., The relationship of retinal micro-aneurysm counts to the 4-year progresssion of diabetic retinopathy, *Archives of Ophthalmology*, 107, 1780, 1989.

[5] Klein, R., Meuer, S.M., Moss, S.E., et al., Retinal microaneurysm counts and 10-year progression of diabetic retinopathy, *Archives of Ophthalmology*, 113(11), 1386, 1995.

[6] Goatman, K.A., Cree, M.J., Olson, J.A., et al., Automated measurement of microaneurysm turnover, *Investigative Ophthalmology & Visual Science*, 44(12), 5335, 2003.

[7] Kohner, E.M. and Dollery, C.T., The rate of formation and disapearance of microaneurysms in diabetic retinopathy, *Eur J Clin Invest*, 1(3), 167, 1970.

[8] Lay, B., Baudoin, C., and Klein, J.C., Automatic detection of microaneurysms in retinopathy fluoro-angiogram, *Proceedings of the SPIE*, 432, 165, 1983.

[9] Baudoin, C.E., Lay, B.J., and Klein, J.C., Automatic detection of microa-neurysms in diabetic fluorescein angiography, *Rev. Epidém. et. Santé Publ.*, 32, 254, 1984.

[10] Spencer, T., Phillips, R.P., Sharp, P.F., et al., Automated detection and quan-tification of microaneurysms in fluorescein angiograms, *Graefes Arch Clin Exp Ophthalmol*, 230(1), 36, 1992.

[11] Spencer, T., Olson, J.A., McHardy, K.C., et al., An image-processing strategy for the segmentation and quantification of microaneurysms in fluorescein an-giograms of the ocular fundus, *Computers and Biomedical Research*, 29, 284, 1996.

[12] Cree, M.J., Olson, J.A., McHardy, K.C., et al., Automated microaneurysm de-tection, in *International Conference on Image Processing*, Lausanne, Switzer-land, 1996, vol. 3, 699–702.

[13] Cree, M.J., Olson, J.A., McHardy, K.C., et al., A fully automated comparative microaneurysm digital detection system, *Eye*, 11, 622, 1997.

[14] Cree, M.J., Olson, J.A., McHardy, K.C., et al., The preprocessing of retinal im-ages for the detection of fluorescein leakage, *Physics in Medicine and Biology*, 44(1), 293, 1999.

[15] Frame, A.J., Undrill, P.E., Cree, M.J., et al., A comparison of computer based

classification methods applied to the detection of microaneurysms in ophthalmic fluorescein angiograms, *Computers in Biology and Medicine*, 28(3), 225, 1998.

[16] Hipwell, J.H., Strachan, F., Olson, J.A., et al., Automated detection of microaneurysms in digital red-free photographs: A diabetic retinopathy screening tool, *Diabetic Medicine*, 17(8), 588, 2000.

[17] Phillips, R., Forrester, J., and Sharp, P., Automated detection and quantification of retinal exudates, *Graefes Arch Clin Exp Ophthalmol*, 231(2), 90, 1993.

[18] Olson, J.A., Strachan, F.M., Hipwell, J.H., et al., A comparative evaluation of digital imaging, retinal photography and optometrist examination in screening for diabetic retinopathy, *Diabetic Medicine*, 20(7), 528, 2003.

[19] Mendonça, A.M., Campilho, A.J., and Nunes, J.M., Automatic segmentation of microaneurysms in retinal angiograms of diabetic patients, in *10th International Conference on Image Analysis and Processing*, 1999, 728–733.

[20] Acha, B. and Serrano, C., Automatic detection of microaneurysms in retinal angiograms, *International Congress Series*, 1256, 1328, 2003.

[21] Serrano, C., Acha, B., and Revuelto, S., 2D adaptive filtering and region growing algorithm for the detection of microaneurysms in retinal angiograms, in *Medical Imaging 2004*, San Diego, CA, 2004, vol. 5370 of *Proceedings of the SPIE*, 1924–1931.

[22] Yang, G., Gagnon, L., Wang, S., et al., Algorithm for detecting microaneurysms in low-resolution color retinal images, in *Proceedings of Vision Interface 2001*, Ottawa, Canada, 2001, 265–271.

[23] Vincent, L., Morphological grayscale reconstruction in image analysis: Applications and efficient algorithms, *IEEE Transactions on Image Processing*, 2, 176, 1993.

[24] Lalonde, M., Laliberté, F., and Gagnon, L., Retsoftplus: A tool for retinal image analysis, in *17th IEEE Symposium on Computer-Based Medical Systems (CBMS'04)*, Bethesda, MD, 2004, 542–547.

[25] Raman, B., Wilson, M., Benche, I., et al., A JAVA-based system for segmentation and analysis of retinal images, in *16th IEEE Symposium on Computer-Based Medical Systems (CBMS'03)*, 2003, 336–339.

[26] Raman, B., Bursell, E.S., Wilson, M., et al., The effects of spatial resolution on an automated diabetic retinopathy screening system's performance in detecting microaneurysms for diabetic retinopathy, in *17th IEEE Symposium on Computer-Based Medical Systems (CBMS'04)*, 2004, 128.

[27] Niemeijer, M., van Ginneken, B., Staal, J., et al., Automatic detection of red lesions in digital color fundus photographs, *IEEE Transactions on Medical Imaging*, 24(5), 584, 2005.

[28] Fleming, A.D., Philip, S., Goatman, K.A., et al., Automated microaneurysm detection using local contrast normalization and local vessel detection, *IEEE Transactions on Medical Imaging*, 25(9), 1223, 2006.

[29] Fleming, A.D., Goatman, K.A., Philip, S., et al., Local environment analysis to aid microaneurysm detection, in *Medical Image Understanding and Analysis (MIUA2005)*, Bristol, UK, 2005, 15–18.

[30] Huang, K. and Yan, M., A local adaptive algorithm for microaneurysms detection in digital fundus images, in *Computer Vision for Biomedical Image Applications*, 2005, vol. 3765 of *Lecture Notes in Computer Science*, 103–113.

[31] Walter, T., Massin, P., Erginay, A., et al., Automatic detection of microaneurysms in color fundus images, *Medical Image Analysis*, 11, 555, 2007.

[32] Gardner, G.G., Keating, D., Williamson, T.H., et al., Automatic detection of diabetic retinopathy using an artificial neural network: A screening tool, *British Journal of Ophthalmology*, 80, 940, 1996.

[33] Kamel, M., Belkassim, S., Mendonça, A.M., et al., A neural network approach for the automatic detection of microaneurysms in retinal angiograms, in *International Joint Conference on Neural Networks (IJCNN'01)*, Washington, DC, 2001, vol. 4, 2695–2699.

[34] Morganti, M., Sperduti, A., and Starita, A., A multiple classifier system for the automatic localization of anomalies in retinas of diabetic patients, in *3rd International Conference on Neural Networks and Expert Systems in Medicine and Healthcare*, Pisa, Italy, 1998, 101–108.

[35] Huang, K., Yan, M., and Aviyente, S., Edge directed inference for microaneurysms detection in digital fundus images, in *Medical Imaging 2007: Image Processing*, 2007, vol. 6512 of *Proceedings of the SPIE*, 51237.

[36] Walter, T. and Klein, J.C., Automatic detection of microaneurysms in color fundus images of the human retina by means of the bounding box closing, in *Medical Data Analysis, Proceedings*, 2002, vol. 2526 of *Lecture Notes in Computer Science*, 210–220.

[37] Vincent, L., Morphological area openings and closings for greyscale images, in *NATO Shape in Picture Workshop*, Driebergen, The Netherlands, 1992, 197–208.

[38] Quellec, G., Lamard, M., Josselin, P.M., et al., Detection of lesions in retina photographs based on the wavelet transform, in *28th IEEE EMBS Annual International Conference*, New York City, 2006, 2618–2621.

[39] Lee, S.C., Wang, Y., and Lee, E.T., Computer algorithm for automated detection and quantification of microaneurysms and hemorrhages (HMAs) in color retinal images, in *Medical Imaging 1999: Image Perception and Performance*, 1999, vol. 3663 of *Proceedings of the SPIE*, 61–71.

[40] Lee, S.C. and Wang, Y., A general algorithm for recognizing small, vague, and imager-alike objects in a nonuniformly illuminated medical diagnostic image, in *32nd Asilomar Conference on Signals, Systems and Computers*, Pacific Grove, CA, 1998, vol. 2, 941–943.

[41] Lee, S.C., Wang, Y., and Tan, W., Automated detection of venous beading in retinal images, *Proceedings of the SPIE*, 4322, 1365, 2001.

[42] Larsen, N., Godt, J., Grunkin, M., et al., Automated detection of diabetic retinopathy in a fundus photographic screening population, *Investigative Ophthalmology & Visual Science*, 44(2), 767, 2003.

[43] Larsen, M., Godt, J., Larsen, N., et al., Automated detection of fundus photographic red lesions in diabetic retinopathy, *Invest Ophthalmol Vis Sci*, 44(2), 761, 2003.

[44] Sinthanayothin, C., Boyce, J.F., Williamson, T.H., et al., Automated detection of diabetic retinopathy on digital fundus images, *Diabet Med*, 19(2), 105, 2002.

[45] Delori, F.C. and Pflibsen, K.P., Spectral reflectance of the human ocular fundus, *Applied Optics*, 28(6), 1061, 1989.

[46] Preece, S.J. and Claridge, E., Monte Carlo modelling of the spectral reflectance of the human eye, *Physics in Medicine and Biology*, 47, 2863, 2002.

[47] Osareh, A., Mirmehdi, M., Thomas, B., et al., Classification and localisation of diabetic-related eye disease, in *7th European Conference on Computer Vision (ECCV2002)*, 2002, vol. 2353 of *Lecture Notes in Computer Science*, 502–516.

[48] Goatman, K.A., Whitwam, A.D., Manivannan, A., et al., Colour normalisation of retinal images, in *Proceedings of Medical Image Understanding and Analysis*, Sheffield, UK, 2003, 49–52.

[49] Cree, M.J., Gamble, E., and Cornforth, D.J., Colour normalisation to reduce inter-patient and intra-patient variability in microaneurysm detection in colour retinal images, in *APRS Workshop on Digital Image Computing (WDIC2005)*, Brisbane, Australia, 2005, 163–168.

[50] Perreault, S. and Hébert, P., Median filtering in constant time, *IEEE Transactions on Image Processing*, 16, 2389, 2007.

[51] Streeter, L. and Cree, M.J., Microaneurysm detection in colour fundus images, in *Proceedings of the Image and Vision Computing New Zealand Conference (IVCNZ'03)*, Palmerston North, New Zealand, 2003, 280–285.

[52] Sharp, P.F., Olson, J., Strachan, F., et al., The value of digital imaging in diabetic retinopathy, *Health Technology Assessment*, 7(30), 1, 2003.

[53] Bayes, T., An essay towards solving a problem in the doctrine of chances, *Philosophical Transactions of the Royal Society of London*, 53, 370, 1763.

[54] Han, J. and Kamber, M., *Data Mining Concepts and Techniques*, Morgan Kaufman, 2001.

[55] Metz, C.E., ROC methodology in radiologic imaging, *Investigative Radiology*, 21, 720, 1986.

[56] Jelinek, H.F., Cree, M.J., Worsley, D., et al., An automated microaneurysm detector as a tool for identification of diabetic retinopathy in rural optometric practice, *Clinical and Experimental Optometry*, 89(5), 299, 2006.

[57] Lee, S.C. and Wang, Y., Automatic retinal image quality assessment and enhancement, in *Medical Imaging 1999: Image Processing*, 1999, vol. 3661 of *Proceedings of the SPIE*, 1581–1590.

[58] Fleming, A., Philip, S., Goatman, K., et al., Automated assessment of retinal image field of view, in *Medical Image Understanding and Analysis (MIUA 2004)*, London, UK, 2004, 129–132.

[59] Newsom, R.S.B., Clover, A., Costen, M.T.J., et al., Effect of digital image compression on screening for diabetic retinopathy, *British Journal of Ophthalmology*, 85(7), 799, 2001.

[60] Basu, A., Kamal, A.D., Illahi, W., et al., Is digital image compression acceptable within diabetic retinopathy screening? *Diabetic Medicine*, 20(9), 766, 2003.

[61] Stellingwerf, C., Hardus, P.L.L.J., and Hooymans, J.M.M., Assessing diabetic retinopathy using two-field digital photography and the influence of JPEG-compression, *Documenta Ophthalmologica*, 108(3), 203, 2004.

[62] Anagnoste, S.R., Orlock, D., Spaide, R., et al., Digital compression of ophthalmic images: Maximum JPEG compression undetectable by retina specialists, *Investigative Ophthalmology & Visual Science*, 39, S922, 1998.

[63] Lee, M.S., Shin, D.S., and Berger, J.W., Grading, image analysis, and stereopsis of digitally compressed fundus images, *Retina*, 20(3), 275, 2000.

[64] Baker, C.F., Rudnisky, C.J., Tennant, M.T.S., et al., JPEG compression of stereoscopic digital images for the diagnosis of diabetic retinopathy via teleophthalmology, *Canadian Journal of Ophthalmology*, 39(7), 746, 2004.

[65] Hänsgen, P., Undrill, P.E., and Cree, M.J., The application of wavelets to retinal image compression and its effect on automatic microaneurysm analysis, *Computer Methods and Programs in Biomedicine*, 56(1), 1, 1998.

[66] Cree, M.J. and Jelinek, H.F., The effect of JPEG compression on automated detection of microaneurysms in retinal images, in *Electronic Imaging Symposium: Image Processing: Machine Vision Applications*, San Jose, CA, 2008, vol. 6813 of *Proceedings of the SPIE*, 68 130M–1.

[67] Hanley, J.A. and McNeil, B.J., The meaning and use of the area under a receiver operating characteristic (ROC) curve, *Radiology*, 143, 29, 1982.

[68] Hoover, A., Kouznetsova, V., and Goldbaum, M., Locating blood vessels in retinal images by piecewise threshold probing of a matched filter response,

IEEE Transactions on Medical Imaging, 19(3), 203, 2000.

[69] Staal, J., Abramoff, M.D., Niemeijer, M., et al., Ridge-based vessel segmentation in color images of the retina, *IEEE Transactions on Medical Imaging*, 23(4), 501, 2004.

[70] Hellstedt, T. and Immonen, I., Disappearance and formation rates of microaneurysms in early diabetic retinopathy, *British Journal of Ophthalmology*, 80, 135, 1996.

[71] Baudoin, C., Maneshi, F., Quentel, G., et al., Quantitative-evaluation of fluorescein angiograms-microaneurysm counts, *Diabetes*, 32, 8, 1983.

[72] Jalli, P.Y., Hellstedt, T.J., and Immonen, I.J., Early versus late staining of microaneurysms in fluorescein angriography, *Retina*, 17, 211, 1997.

7

Retinal Vascular Changes as Biomarkers of Systemic Cardiovascular Diseases

Ning Cheung, Tien Y. Wong, and Lauren Hodgson

CONTENTS

7.1   Introduction 185
7.2   Early Description of Retinal Vascular Changes 186
7.3   Retinal Vascular Imaging 187
7.4   Retinal Vascular Changes and Cardiovascular Disease 189
7.5   Retinal Vascular Changes and Metabolic Diseases 194
7.6   Retinal Vascular Changes and Other Systemic Diseases 197
7.7   Genetic Associations of Retinal Vascular Changes 200
7.8   Conclusion 201
7.A   Appendix: Retinal Vessel Caliber Grading Protocol 201
      References 207

7.1   Introduction

The retinal vasculature can be viewed directly and noninvasively, offering a unique and easily accessible "window" to study the health of the human microcirculation in vivo. Pathological changes of the retinal vasculature, such as the appearance of microaneurysms, focal areas of arteriolar narrowing, arteriovenous (AV) nicking, and retinal hemorrhages are common fundus findings in older people, even in those without hypertension or diabetes. Recent advances in retinal image analysis have allowed reliable and precise assessment of these retinal vascular changes, as well as objective measurement of other topographic vascular characteristics such as generalized retinal vascular caliber. Using standardized protocols to evaluate retinal photographs, a new series of population-based studies have furthered our understanding of the clinical significance and systemic associations of these retinal vascular features. This chapter provides an overview of the standardized assessment of retinal vascular changes and the role of retinal image analysis as a means to investigate clinical and subclinical systemic diseases.

7.2 Early Description of Retinal Vascular Changes

Cardiovascular disease remains the leading cause of death in developed countries. Clinicians have long been relying on a spectrum of "traditional" cardiovascular risk factors, such as the presence of diabetes, hypertension, hyperlipidemia and cigarette smoking to help identify, monitor, and treat high-risk individuals [1–4]. However, there is a belief that these "traditional" risk factors are inadequate in explaining a substantial proportion of cardiovascular morbidity and mortality [5–7]. To pursue further refinement in cardiovascular risk stratification, there has been increasing interest in searching for other biomarkers of predictors that may provide additional information regarding a person's cardiovascular risk [8–10].

The human retina may provide an ideal platform to hunt for these variables as the retinal vasculature, which can be visualized directly, shares similar anatomical and physiological properties with the cerebral and coronary circulation [11–14]. Retinal vascular damage in essence reflects damage from chronic hypertension, diabetes, and other processes [12; 15–19], and may therefore be a biomarker for cardiovascular disease risk [11; 14].

Recognition of this potential dates back a century ago [20–23] when Keith, Wagener, and Barker showed that the severity of retinal vascular changes was predictive of mortality in patients with hypertension [24]. Subsequent researchers described associations of various retinopathy signs with different cardiovascular diseases and mortality [25–32]. Nevertheless, since the 1960s there has been less interest in this field of research for a number of reasons. First, the association between retinal vascular changes and cardiovascular disease was not consistently demonstrated in all studies [25; 26; 33–38], and the majority of studies had significant limitations, such as lack of control for potential confounders and the use of clinic- or hospital-based patients not representative of the general population. Second, early studies were conducted in populations with untreated hypertension, in which the more severe retinal abnormalities were observed (e.g. Keith, Wagener, and Barker Grade III and IV retinopathy [24].). This degree of retinopathy was felt to be uncommon in the modern setting with better blood pressure control [39–43]. Third, despite many attempts to improve previous grading systems, there was no general consensus regarding a clinically meaningful and standardized classification of retinal vascular signs [44]. Finally, the detection of retinal vascular abnormalities using the direct ophthalmoscope was found to be subjective and unreliable [36–38; 45–47].

These issues have been largely addressed in the last decade with advancements in the field of retinal photography and image-analysis techniques, enabling objective quantification of a range of retinal vascular parameters [48] and large population-based studies to determine clinical significance [49]. Furthermore, more subtle changes in the retinal vasculature (e.g., degree of generalized retinal arteriolar narrowing) are now quantifiable from high-resolution digitized photographs [49–53]. These new approaches to study retinal vascular characteristics have renewed the interest in using digital retinal photography as a potential tool for the prediction of systemic cardiovascular disorders.

7.3 Retinal Vascular Imaging

7.3.1 Assessment of retinal vascular signs from retinal photographs

Modern digital imaging systems have revolutionized the assessment of retinal photographs. Using these newly developed quantitative methods, several studies have demonstrated excellent reproducibility for the detection of well-defined retinopathy signs (kappa values have ranged from 0.80–0.99 for microaneurysms and retinal hemorrhages) and good reproducibility for more subtle retinal arteriolar lesions (0.40–0.79 for focal retinal arteriolar narrowing and arteriovenous nicking) [49; 50].

In addition, objective measurement of historically subjective retinal vascular changes, such as generalized retinal arteriolar narrowing, is now possible with the semi-automated retinal image-analysis software. Parr, Hubbard, and their associates developed formulae to generate summarized measures of retinal arteriolar (central retinal arteriolar equivalent [CRAE]) and venular (central retinal venular equivalent [CRVE]) diameters, as well as their dimensionless quotient (arteriovenous ratio [AVR]) [49; 54; 55]. These retinal vascular indices have been used in several large-scale epidemiological studies [49; 50; 52; 53; 56], which demonstrated substantial reproducibility for these vessel measurements (intra-class correlation coefficient ranged from 0.80–0.99), providing further evidence that retinal photography offers a more sensitive and precise means of assessing architectural changes in the retinal vascular network.

Based on these new standardized assessments of photographs, retinal vascular signs have been found to be fairly common in adult people 40 years and older, even in those without a history of diabetes or hypertension. Prevalence [40; 43; 57] and incidence [41; 58] rates ranging from 2 to 15% have been reported for various retinal vascular lesions.

Other emerging computer imaging systems have features such as automated detection of optic disc, identification and tracking of arterioles and venules, batch processing of retinal images (i.e., analysis of multiple images at a time), and measurement of retinal vessel diameters with greater precision and reproducibility [52; 59]. Whether these systems are superior to existing techniques in cardiovascular risk prediction remains to be seen.

7.3.2 Limitations in current retinal vascular imaging techniques

While retinal image analysis posts exciting possibilities [48], its applicability in clinical settings is yet to be established, partly due to a number of methodological issues concerning its use.

First, the formulae utilized to combine individual retinal vascular diameters into summarized indices are based on theoretical and empiric models. The Parr [54; 55] and Hubbard [49] formulae for CRAE and CRVE were derived from examination of a large number of retinal images with branching points, calculating the relationship between individual trunk vessels and their respective branch vessels using a root mean square deviation model that best fit the observed data. Although used widely in many epidemiological studies of cardiovascular and ocular diseases, there are some drawbacks in using these formulae. Knudtson and associates made an important observation that the Parr-Hubbard formulae were dependent on the number of retinal vessels measured [60]. In addition, since the formulae contained constants within the equations, they were also dependent on the units with which the vessels were measured. Knudtson and colleagues therefore developed a modified formula for summarizing retinal vascular caliber, and demonstrated clear superiority of their formula over the previously used Parr-Hubbard formulae [60]. It is likely that there will be further refinement. Recently, for example, some investigators suggested a revised formula for more accurate estimation of arteriolar branch coefficient [61]. This formula used a linear regression model that incorporated a relationship to the asymmetry index of the vessel branches being measured. However, whether this or other newer formulae can indeed improve the predictive ability to detect associations with systemic cardiovascular diseases is unclear.

Second, existing retinal vascular research has largely focused on differences in retinal vascular changes between groups of people (e.g., people with smaller retinal arteriolar diameter are more likely to develop cardiovascular disease than people with relatively larger arteriolar diameter). To allow the use of retinal vessel measurement as a potential risk stratification tool in a clinic setting, retinal image analysis must produce results that enable an assessment of absolute risk in individual patients. The measurement of absolute retinal vascular caliber, for example, is critical to this development [53; 62]. This requires addressing the issue of magnification effect from retinal photography, either by incorporating an adjusted measurement to compensate for this effect or using dimensionless measurements. While there are already a few methods to adjust for magnification using ocular biometric data (e.g., axial length) [48], most were designed for telecentric cameras. For nontelecentric cameras, Rudnicka and colleagues have described a method to adjust for magnification using plan films [63], but its applicability on digitized retinal photographs is unknown.

To account for magnification effects and allow for comparison of measurements of retinal topographical changes between individuals, studies have sought alternative geometric attributes of retinal vasculature that are dimensionless in nature. These include the retinal AVR, junctional exponents, vascular bifurcation angles, vascular tortuosity, and length-to-diameter ratio [48]. Among these, the AVR has been the most commonly used measure. It is important to note, however, that the AVR has significant limitations, including the inability to capture separately the information of the individual arteriolar and venular caliber component measurements [64; 65]. For example, both narrower arterioles and wider venules may produce a smaller AVR. Thus, AVR cannot differentiate between changes in arteriolar and venular caliber. There is increasing evidence that this differentiation is important, as different systemic diseases appear to be associated with specific caliber changes in arterioles and venules. While smaller retinal arteriolar caliber is associated with hypertension, and may even precede clinical hypertension development, larger retinal venular caliber has been associated with inflammation, smoking, hyperglycemia, obesity and dyslipidemia [56]. These observations suggest that changes in retinal arteriolar and venular caliber may reflect different pathophysiological processes underlying the associated systemic diseases. Combining these two components into one estimate, the AVR, without consideration of separate arteriolar or venular caliber measurements, therefore masks these associations.

Third, researchers have recently discovered another important concept in retinal vascular imaging analysis: the need to adjust for retinal arteriolar caliber in analysis of retinal venular caliber, and vice versa [66; 67]. Liew and colleagues showed that the high correlation between retinal arteriolar and venular caliber means that individuals with narrower arterioles are more likely to have narrower venules [66; 67]. As a result, the confounding effect of arteriolar and venular caliber for individual measurements should be taken into consideration. This is clearly demonstrated in the Rotterdam Study, in which a counterintuitive association between retinal venular narrowing and hypertension was initially reported [68], but after the use of the new analytical approach, modeling retinal arteriolar and venular calibers simultaneously, retinal venular narrowing was shown to have no association with hypertension [69].

Finally, despite the vast amount of data on retinal vessel measures in numerous population-based studies, there is a lack of knowledge about the normative data for these measurements. Defining what is normal and abnormal is crucial for development of a clinical tool. One of the challenges in deriving normative data using studies in the adult population was that it was difficult to completely control for the confounding effect of systemic (e.g., hypertension, diabetes, smoking, medications) and ocular (e.g., diabetic retinopathy, glaucoma) disease processes on retinal vessel measurements. Studying retinal vascular caliber in healthy children, who are generally free of these influences, may provide a better understanding of the reference data for this important vascular variable [70]. Several studies of retinal vascular measurements in children are currently underway.

7.4 Retinal Vascular Changes and Cardiovascular Disease

One of the major advances in retinal vascular imaging research in the last decade has been the clear demonstration that physiological and pathological alterations in the retinal vascular network are associated with a variety of cardiovascular diseases, including hypertension, stroke, coronary heart disease (CHD) and congestive heart failure (Table 7.1).

7.4.1 Hypertension

It has long been known that hypertension exerts a profound effect on the retinal vasculature. The association of retinal vascular changes with blood pressure, in particular, is strong, graded, and consistently seen in both adult [40; 41; 43; 56; 57; 71; 72; 74; 96–98] and child populations [91].

The Beaver Dam Eye Study in Wisconsin has reported increases in both prevalence [40] and 5-year incidence [41] of various retinal arteriolar abnormalities in hypertensive individuals compared to those without hypertension. Among these,

Table 7.1: Retinal Vascular Changes and Cardiovascular Disease, Selected Population-Based Studies

Retinal Vascular Signs	Associations	Strength*	References
Retinopathy	Blood pressure	+++	[40; 41; 71–74]
	Incident hypertension	++	[75]
	Prevalent stroke	+++	[57; 76; 77]
	Incident stroke	+++	[76; 78–81]
	Prevalent CHD	++	[57]
	Incident CHD	+++	[82]
	Incident hear failure	+++	[83]
	Incident renal disease	+++	[84; 85]
Smaller AVR	Blood pressure	+++	[40; 68; 71; 72]
			[74; 86; 87]
	Incident hypertension	++	[75; 88; 89]
	Incident stroke	++	[76; 78; 80]
	Incident CHD	++	[90]
Arteriolar narrowing	Blood pressure	+++	[56; 67; 91; 92]
	Prevalent hypertension	–	[56]
	Incident hypertension	++	[67; 92]
	Prevalent CHD	–	[87]
	Incident CHD	++	[93; 94]
Venular dilatation	Incident CHD	++	[93; 94]
	Incident stroke	++	[93; 95]

CHD = coronary heart disease; AVR = arteriole-to-venule ratio; WESDR = Wisconsin Epidemiological Study of Diabetic Retinopathy.
*Odds ratio or relative risk < 1.5 (+), 1.5–2.0 (++), > 2.0 (+++) and quantified using other measures (–).

generalized retinal arteriolar narrowing has long been regarded as an early characteristic sign of hypertension [12; 44; 45]. Using a new semi-automated computer-based image-analytical technique, the Atherosclerosis Risk in Communities (ARIC) study in the United States reported that retinal arteriolar diameter is strongly and inversely related to higher blood pressure levels [71], a finding subsequently confirmed in four other population-based studies [68; 73; 74; 96]. In the Beaver Dam Eye Study, each 10 mmHg increase in mean arterial blood pressure was associated with a 6 μm (or 3%) decrease in retinal arteriolar diameter, even after adjusting for age, gender, diabetes, smoking, and other vascular risk factors [73]. While these data support the strong link between generalized arteriolar narrowing and hypertension, the subtle degree of arteriolar narrowing also suggests that a clinical examination based on ophthalmoscopy is unlikely to be capable of detecting such small changes. While earlier studies have predominantly used smaller AVR as the only measure of generalized retinal arteriolar narrowing, subsequent studies in both adults [67; 92] and children [91] evaluating retinal arteriolar and venular calibers separately have validated the strong association of hypertension with arteriolar narrowing.

In the last few years, researchers have attempted to answer a key research question: are retinal vascular changes markers of cumulative, long-term blood pressure damage, or do they only reflect a transient effect of acutely elevated blood pressure? Several studies addressed this question by analyzing the association of specific retinopathy signs with both concurrent and past blood pressure levels [71; 74; 86]. These studies found that generalized arteriolar narrowing and AV nicking were independently related to past blood pressure levels, indicating that these signs may reflect persistent structural arteriolar changes from long-term hypertension [71; 74; 86]. In contrast, studies show that focal arteriolar narrowing, retinal hemorrhages, microaneurysms, and cotton wool spots were related to only concurrent but not past blood pressure levels, and therefore may be related more to fleeting, possibly physiological, changes caused by acute blood pressure elevation [71; 74].

Prospective data from four population-based studies have provided new understanding into the relation of generalized retinal arteriolar narrowing to subsequent development of systemic hypertension [75; 88; 89; 92]. In the ARIC study, normotensive participants who had generalized retinal arteriolar narrowing at baseline were 60% more likely to be diagnosed with hypertension over a three year period than individuals without arteriolar narrowing (relative risk 1.62, 95% CI, 1.21 to 2.18) [75]. The severity of arteriolar narrowing also appeared to correlate positively with the degree of change in blood pressure, independent of preexisting blood pressure, body mass index, and other known hypertension risk factors. Similar results were generated from the Beaver Dam, Rotterdam, and the Blue Mountains Eye studies [88; 89; 92], providing strong evidence that generalized arteriolar narrowing, possibly mirroring similar peripheral arteriolar changes elsewhere in the body, is a preclinical marker of hypertension. These observations support the concept that the microcirculation is critical to the pathogenesis of hypertension [99].

There is increasing evidence, albeit from a limited number of clinical reports, that hypertensive retinopathy signs may regress with improved blood pressure control [100–103]. For example, it has been reported that hypertensive retinopathy caused by accelerated hypertension can improve after normalization of blood pressure [100]. In addition, in a clinical study of 51 hypertensive patients, Pose-Reino and colleagues presented objective and quantitative evidence of generalized retinal arteriolar narrowing regression associated with six months of hypertension treatment with losartan, an angiotensin II inhibitor [103]. In another small study of mildly hypertensive patients randomized to treatment with enalapril (an angiotensin converting enzyme inhibitor) or hydrocholorthiazide, retinal arteriolar wall opacification (although not other retinopathy signs) was significantly reduced after 26 weeks of enalapril treatment while hydrochlorothiazide did not seem to have any effect on the retinopathy signs [101]. As yet, however, due to the lack of controlled clinical trials, the important clinical question of whether regression of hypertensive retinopathy signs is also associated with a concurrent reduction in a person's cardiovascular risk remains unanswered.

7.4.2 Stroke and cerebrovascular disease

The retinal and cerebral vasculature share similar embryological origin, anatomical features, and physiological properties [104]. This concept provides strong biological rationale for the use of retinal image analysis to indirectly study the cerebral microvasculature and related diseases. In support of this theory is the strong and consistent evidence that retinal vascular changes are associated with both clinical and subclinical stroke and a variety of cerebrovascular conditions independent of traditional risk factors such as hypertension, diabetes, and cigarette smoking.

Since the 1970s, physicians have reported that in people with hypertension, the presence of retinopathy signs is associated with both subclinical and clinical stroke [34; 105–107]. Newer population-based studies, using standardized grading of digitized retinal photographs, have confirmed these early observations. In the ARIC study, among more than 10 000 individuals without a history of stroke, those with microaneurysms, retinal hemorrhages, and cotton wool spots were two to three times more likely to develop an incident clinical stroke in the next three years than those without these retinopathy signs, even after factoring the effects of multiple vascular risk factors [78]. Similar associations were seen in persons with type 2 diabetes [79]. Among the ARIC participants without clinical cerebrovascular disease, these retinal vascular abnormalities were also related to cognitive decline [108], and magnetic resonance imaging (MRI) detected structural abnormalities including cerebral white matter lesions [80] and atrophy [109]. Furthermore, the ARIC study suggests a possible synergistic interaction between the presence of retinal vascular abnormalities and subclinical white matter lesions on the subsequent risk of clinical stroke. Participants with both retinopathy and white matter lesions had a substantially higher stroke risk than those without either finding (relative risk 18.1, 95% confidence intervals, 5.9 to 55.4) [80]. Thus cerebrovascular pathology may be more severe or extensive in persons with both cerebral and retinal signs of microvascular disease.

The Cardiovascular Health Study, which examined older persons, found similar associations. In a cross-sectional analysis, after controlling for blood pressure and risk factors, participants with retinopathy were twice as likely to have a prevalent stroke as those without retinopathy (odds ratio 2.0, 95% confidence intervals, 1.1 to 3.6) [57]. In this older population, retinal arteriolar abnormalities were also associated with prevalent and incident MRI-defined cerebral infarcts, as well as presence and progression of white matter changes [76]. These observations are consistent with data from the Blue Mountains Eye Study in Australia, in which nondiabetic persons with retinopathy were 70% more likely to suffer stroke-related death than those without retinopathy [81]. Similarly, in a nested case-control study in the Beaver Dam Eye Study cohort, the presence of retinal microaneurysms, retinal hemorrhages, and retinal arteriolar narrowing was associated with an increased 10-year risk of stroke mortality [110]. Finally, there is new evidence that in persons with impaired glucose tolerance, retinopathy signs are associated with prevalent stroke [77].

In addition to retinopathy signs, variations in retinal vascular caliber have also been linked to stroke risk. The ARIC study previously showed that a smaller retinal AVR, interpreted as generalized retinal arteriolar narrowing, might be an independent predictor of incident stroke in middle-aged individuals. Smaller clinical investigations support this finding [111–113]. In a series of patients with symptomatic atherosclerotic disease (recent ischemic stroke, myocardial infarction, or peripheral arterial disease), retinal arteriolar narrowing and sclerosis, defined from retinal photographs, were related to presence of white matter lesions and lacunar infarcts detected on MRI [111]. Other researchers found that retinal microvascular flow is reduced in persons with cerebral small vessel disease [112; 114], and that retinal and cerebral arteriolar histopathology is similar in stroke decedents [113]. Subsequent discovery of the shortfalls relating to the use of retinal AVR prompted newer studies to evaluate the association of retinal arteriolar and venular calibers separately with stroke risk [64; 65]. Using this approach, both the Rotterdam Eye Study [95] and the Cardiovascular Health Study [93] showed that rather than narrower retinal arteriolar caliber, wider retinal venular caliber predicted the future risk of clinical stroke, independent of other stroke-related risk factors. Thus, the relative importance of arteriolar and venular caliber in stroke risk prediction remains to be determined

The importance of the reported associations of retinal vascular signs with stroke, white matter lesions, cerebral atrophy, and cognitive impairment is that it supports a contribution of small vessel disease to the pathogenesis of a wide range of cerebrovascular disorders. In addition, because the retinal signs (e.g., microaneurysms, retinal hemorrhages and cotton wool spots) that are most strongly related to cerebrovascular diseases are usually the result of a disruption in the blood-retinal-barrier, it may be possible to infer that a breakdown of the cerebral blood-brain-barrier may also be a key pathophysiological process in the pathogenesis of cerebrovascular diseases [115].

7.4.3 Coronary heart disease and congestive heart failure

Similar to cerebrovascular disease, the current literature provides increasing evidence that retinal vascular changes are related to CHD and congestive heart failure development. Previous clinical studies based on ophthalmoscopic examinations have linked retinopathy signs with ischemic T-wave changes on electrocardiogram [25; 26], severity of coronary artery stenosis on angiography [116], and more recently, with incident clinical CHD events [117].

Newer population-based studies using retinal imaging techniques have produced stronger evidence supportive of these findings, demonstrating associations of various retinal vascular signs with CHD and CHD mortality. In the ARIC study, smaller AVR (initially interpreted as generalized retinal arteriolar narrowing and subsequently found to be due to generalized retinal venular dilatation) was shown to be an independent predictor of incident CHD in women (relative risk 2.2; 95% confidence intervals: 1.0–4.6), but not in men [90]. This gender difference was also present in the Blue Mountains Eye Study [94] and the National Health Examination Survey [33]. These important observations suggest a more prominent role of microvascular disease in the pathogenesis of CHD in women than in men [118], a theory that has been well described in the past [119]. However, gender difference in the relationship between retinopathy signs and risk of CHD may not be present in high-risk populations. For example, the Lipid Research Clinic's Coronary Primary Prevention Trial provides evidence of an independent association of retinopathy with incident CHD in high-risk men. Additional analysis of the ARIC study data found that in persons with diabetes, CHD risk doubles in those with retinopathy signs as compared to those without retinopathy (relative risk 2.07; 95% confidence intervals: 1.38–3.11), independent of multiple CHD-related risk factors including carotid artery atherosclerosis and nephropathy [82]. This association appears to be graded with retinopathy severity, strongest with CHD mortality (relative risk 3.35; 95% confidence intervals: 1.40–8.01), and present in both men and women [82]. Consistent with these findings, others have reported a positive association of retinopathy with CHD in diabetic populations [120–122].

The finding of a relationship of retinopathy signs with CHD corroborates with observations that retinopathy is associated with subclinical coronary macrovascular and microvascular pathology. Studies have found that individuals with retinopathy were more likely to have myocardial perfusion defects [123–125], poorer coronary flow reserve [126], and a lower coronary collateral score [127] than those without retinopathy. The presence of retinopathy signs has also been associated with a higher degree of coronary artery calcification [128; 129], and more diffuse and severe coronary artery stenosis on angiograms [130], two strong markers of coronary atherosclerotic burden. However, the fundamental question of whether the association of retinopathy with CHD is driven by macrovascular or microvascular disease is unclear. It is likely that the associations are due to a mixture of microvascular and macrovascular processes mediated by common pathogenic pathways. In diabetic populations, these may involve, for example, advanced glycation end products, which are known to cause both micro- and macro-vascular injury in diabetes [131].

Finally, there is evidence that in addition to CHD, retinopathy signs are associated with the development of congestive heart failure. In the ARIC study, participants with retinopathy were found to have a twofold higher risk of incident congestive heart failure than those without retinopathy (relative risk 1.96; 95% confidence intervals: 1.51–2.54) [83]. Interestingly, among those with a lower cardiovascular risk profile (without preexisting CHD, diabetes, or hypertension), the presence of retinopathy was associated with an even higher risk of congestive heart failure (relative risk 2.98; 95% confidence intervals: 1.50–5.92) [83]. The reason for this phenomenon is not apparent, but it suggests that microvascular disease may be a more important risk factor for cardiac pathology in the absence of established risk factors. These findings also underscore the potential of retinopathy signs in identifying people who are more likely to develop heart disease despite having a more favorable cardiovascular risk profile.

7.5   Retinal Vascular Changes and Metabolic Diseases

Retinal vascular signs may reflect the profound adverse effects of metabolic disorders, such as diabetes, metabolic syndrome, and obesity, on the systemic microcirculation (Table 7.2).

Table 7.2: Retinal Vascular Changes and Metabolic Disease, Selected Population-Based Studies

Retinal Vascular Signs	Associations	Strength*	Studies and References
Retinopathy	Prevalent diabetes	+++	WESDR [132; 133] DCCT [134] UKPDS [135]
	Incident diabetes	+++	ARIC [136] (with family history)
	Metabolic syndrome	+	ARIC [137]
	IGT	+	ARIC [137]
	Hyperlipidemia	++	WESDR [138] ETDRS [139] FIELD [140]
	Obesity	–	MESA [141]
	Neuropathy	+++	AusDiab [142]
Smaller AVR	Metabolic syndrome	+	ARIC [137]
	Incident diabetes	++	ARIC [143] BDES [144]
	Hyperlipidemia	–	ARIC [98]
Arteriolar narrowing	Prevalent diabetes	–	MESA [56]
Venular dilatation	Prevalent diabetes	–	MESA [56] Rotterdam [145]
	IGT	+	Rotterdam [145]
	Obesity	+++	BMES [146] MESA [56] SCORM [147] Rotterdam [68] WESDR [87]
	Hyperlipidemia	–	Rotterdam [68] MESA [56]

IGT = impaired glucose tolerance; AVR = arteriole-to-venule ratio; WESDR = Wisconsin Epidemiological Study of Diabetic Retinopathy; ETDRS = Early Treatment Diabetic Retinopathy Study; FIELD = Fenofibrate Intervention and Event Lowering in Diabetes; UKPDS = United Kingdom Prospective Diabetes Study; DCCT = Diabetes Control and Complications Trial.

*Odds ratio or relative risk < 1.5 (+), 1.5–2.0 (++), > 2.0 (+++) and quantified using other measures (–).

7.5.1 Diabetes mellitus

The hypothesis that diabetes may have etiologic links with microvascular disease has been tested in recent studies using retinal vessel measurements. In the ARIC and Beaver Dam Eye studies, nondiabetic individuals with smaller AVR were shown to have about a 50% to 70% higher risk of incidence with diabetes, independent of other diabetes-related risk factor [143; 144]. The Beaver Dam Study showed that this association is noticeably stronger in individuals with hypertension at baseline (relative risk 3.41; 95% confidence intervals: 1.66–6.98) [144]. The Rotterdam Eye Study proposed that this association may be due to retinal venular dilatation instead of arteriolar narrowing and demonstrated an association of larger retinal venular caliber with impaired fasting glucose [145]. This finding is consistent with earlier findings of prevalence data from the ARIC study [137]. While the underlying biological mechanisms for these observations remain to be elucidated, experimental studies have shown that administration of intravenous dextrose can cause dilatation of retinal venules in normoglycemic patients [148]. Moreover, reduced vascular reactivity associated with endothelial dysfunction and inflammatory processes may also play an integral role in the development of wider retinal venules and diabetes [149].

Even though diabetic retinopathy is a classic example in which retinal vascular changes evidently reflect the status of a metabolic disorder, there has been inconsistent evidence to support the hypothesis that early retinopathy signs in nondiabetic persons are preclinical markers of diabetes. Epidemiological data from several cross-sectional studies indicate that retinopathy signs are associated with impaired glucose metabolism [77; 137; 150; 151] and prevalent diabetes [56]. Some investigators speculated that retinopathy development may precede the onset of diabetes [152]. This theory, nevertheless, is unsupported by currently available prospective data. The ARIC study reported that the presence of typical retinopathy signs in persons without diabetes is not associated with subsequent development of diabetes over a period of 3.5 years [136], suggesting that these retinal lesions may reflect pathological conditions other than diabetes (e.g., hypertension). This is in agreement with findings from the Blue Mountain Eye Study [153]. Nonetheless, in stratified analysis, the ARIC study revealed a possible association of retinopathy with twofold increased risk of incident diabetes in those with a family history of diabetes [136]. The significance of this finding awaits further exploration.

7.5.2 The metabolic syndrome

Apart from diabetes, metabolic syndrome, defined by the presence of three out of five clinical or biochemical features (abdominal obesity, hypertriglyceridemia, low high-density lipoprotein cholesterol, high blood pressure, and impaired fasting glucose), has also been associated with retinal vascular changes. The ARIC study found that persons with metabolic syndrome are more likely to have typical signs of retinopathy as well as larger retinal venules [137]. The prevalence of these retinal vascular changes also appears to be higher with an increasing number of metabolic syndrome components. These findings are further reinforced by data from the Multi-

Ethnic Study of Atherosclerosis (MESA), reporting associations of larger retinal venular caliber with a number of metabolic syndrome components in a multi-ethnic population-based cohort [56].

7.5.3 Overweight and obesity

Obesity may have a profound effect on the eye [154], but the retinal vascular manifestations of obesity are poorly understood. There is evidence that obesity increases the risk of retinopathy development in both diabetic and nondiabetic populations [149]. Interestingly, recent studies have shown that variations in retinal vascular caliber may also be associated with obesity correlates. The ARIC and Blue Mountain Eye studies both reported an association of larger retinal venular caliber with body mass index and prevalent obesity [137; 146]. Prospective data from the Blue Mountains Eye Study further indicated that larger retinal venular caliber may even predict the incidence of obesity over a 5-year period, suggesting the existence of altered microvascular function in the pathogenesis of obesity [146]. These findings are in keeping with data from a cohort of young healthy children [147], in which confounding effects of systemic and ocular disease processes are of less concern. Inflammation, oxidative stress, hyperleptinemia, and nitric oxide dysregulation have all been implicated as potential pathways in the link between larger retinal venules and obesity development [146; 147].

7.6 Retinal Vascular Changes and Other Systemic Diseases

7.6.1 Renal disease

Retinopathy and nephropathy are two well known microvascular complications of diabetes [155; 156]. Experimental studies show a high correlation of pathological changes in the retinal vessels with those that occur in the renal vasculature [157]. However, there have been few studies that have explored the independent association of retinal vascular abnormalities with nephropathy, particularly in people without diabetes. An earlier study of individuals with hypertension demonstrated a strong relationship of retinopathy grades with microalbuminuria, a preclinical marker of renal dysfunction [158]. This is supported by more recent studies of clinical renal disease in the general population. In the ARIC study, various retinopathy signs, such as AV nicking, retinal hemorrhages, microaneurysms, and cotton wool spots, were associated with a higher risk of renal dysfunction than those without these retinal lesions [84]. This association was independent of vascular risk factors and was seen in persons with and without diabetes or hypertension. Similarly, in the Cardiovascular Health Study, the presence of retinopathy was independently associated with an increased risk of incident renal dysfunction as well as progression of renal impairment [85]. These findings raise the possibility that retinopathy and nephropathy may share common pathogenic pathways (e.g., endothelial dysfunction, inflammation), even in nondiabetic individuals, and highlight the need to monitor renal function in individuals with retinopathy.

7.6.2   Atherosclerosis

Atherosclerosis, the key pathophysiological disease process of CHD and stroke, has been the focus of interest in studies of retinal vascular measurements (Table 7.3). The evidence of a link between direct measures of atherosclerosis and retinal vascular changes, however, has not been consistently demonstrated. In the ARIC study, factoring the effect of blood pressure and other risk factors, smaller AVR was associated with carotid artery plaque but not intima-media thickness (IMT), whereas AV nicking was associated with carotid artery IMT but not plaque [98]. The Rotterdam Eye Study, on the other hand, found an association of smaller AVR with carotid artery IMT [68]. Moreover, smaller AVR has also been independently associated with increased carotid artery stiffness, an early marker of atherosclerosis [159]. These findings, nevertheless, are contradictory to data from the Cardiovascular Health Study (CHS),which revealed no consistent independent association between smaller AVR and measures of large artery atherosclerosis [57].

Apart from retinal vessel measurements, retinopathy signs (e.g., microaneurysms) have also been related to atherosclerosis. For example, the CHS showed an independent association of retinopathy with carotid artery plaque and increased carotid IMT [57]. This is supported by data from the Chennai Urban Rural Epidemiology Study, which demonstrate independent associations of retinopathy signs with both increased carotid IMT and arterial stiffness in diabetic individuals [165]. Furthermore, newer data from the MESA indicate that retinopathy is positively associated with coronary artery calcification, a robust measure of coronary atherosclerotic burden, independent of blood pressure, diabetes, and other risk factors [129].

These data imply that while changes in retinal vascular caliber may be pathologically distinct from atherosclerotic processes [98], there is need to further understand the link between other retinopathy signs and atherosclerosis.

7.6.3   Inflammation and endothelial dysfunction

Retinal vascular changes in diabetes, hypertension,and other systemic disease processes may be related to inflammation and/or endothelial dysfunction (Table 7.3). This concept is supported by data from three population-based studies, in which various inflammatory markers were demonstrated to be associated with larger retinal venules [56; 68; 164]. In the Beaver Dam Eye Study, indicators of endothelial dysfunction were also shown to be associated with larger retinal venular caliber [164]. These observations agree with findings from experimental studies, which demonstrated an increase in the diameter of retinal venules, but not arterioles, after administration of lipid hydroperoxide into the vitreous of rats with a resultant increase in the number of leukocytes in the retinal microvasculature [166]. Dilatation of retinal venules has been postulated to be a result of increased production of nitric oxide secondary to release of inflammatory mediators [167]. The collective data from these

Table 7.3: Retinal Vascular Changes and Markers of Subclinical Disease Selected Population-Based Studies

Retinal Vascular Signs	Associations	Strength*	Studies and References
Retinopathy	Cerebral abnormalities	+++	ARIC [80; 109; 160]
	Carotid artery disease	+++	ARIC [98] CHS [57]
	Cardiac remodeling	–+	MESA [161]
	Coronary artery disease	–	MESA [129]
	Endothelial dysfunction	+	ARIC [156]
	Inflammation	+	ARIC [156]
Smaller AVR	Carotid artery disease	++	ARIC [98] ARIC [159] Rotterdam [68]
	Inflammation	+	ARIC [98] Rotterdam [68]
Arteriolar narrowing	Preclinical hypertension	++	Rotterdam [92] BMES [67]
	Left ventricular hypertrophy and remodeling	++	ARIC [162] MESA [161]
Venular dilatation	Cerebral abnormalities	++	Rotterdam [163]
	Subclinical atherosclerosis	+	Rotterdam [68]
	Inflammation	+–+	BDES [164] MESA [56] Rotterdam [68]

AVR = arteriole-to-venule ratio.
*Odds ratio or relative risk < 1.5 (+), 1.5–2.0 (++), > 2.0 (+++) and quantified using other measures (–).

studies suggest that both inflammation and endothelial dysfunction may play key mechanistic roles in interlinking retinal venular dilatation with systemic diseases.

7.6.4   Subclinical cardiac morphology

Prospective data from the ARIC study indicate that retinopathy may predict clinical CHD and congestive heart failure events in the general population [83]. There is now evidence that retinal vascular changes may be associated with early geometric alterations in the heart prior to manifestation of clinical heart disease (Table 7.3). Previous studies have demonstrated strong correlations of retinopathy grades with left ventricular hypertrophy (LVH) in persons with hypertension [102; 168; 169]. In the ARIC study, both focal and generalized narrowing of retinal arterioles were associated with increased odds of LVH in middle-aged African-Americans, independent of blood pressure and other risk factors [162]. This is supported by recent analysis of the cross-sectional data from the MESA, showing that in the general population, narrower retinal arteriolar caliber is associated with left ventricular concentric remodeling, determined from cardiac MRI, even after adjusting for traditional risk factors (odds ratio 1.87; 95% confidence intervals: 1.41–2.48) [161]. This association remained significant in those without diabetes, hypertension,or significant coronary calcification, but was strongest in diabetic persons (odds ratio 4.02; 95% confidence intervals: 2.05–7.88) [161]. Therefore narrowing of retinal arterioles may be a marker of early subclinical myocardial abnormalities.

7.7   Genetic Associations of Retinal Vascular Changes

The effects of genetic and environmental factors are intertwined in the development of cardiovascular diseases [170–173]. However, the genetic influence on the microvasculature is unclear. Utilizing new retinal image-analysis technology, emerging studies have begun exploring this important aspect.

For example, the Beaver Dam Eye Study reported that retinal vascular calibers were more highly correlated between relatives than between unrelated individuals, an observation proposed to be due to shared genes [174]. This is in keeping with data from a recent twin study, showing that 70% of the variance in retinal arteriolar caliber and 83% of the variance in retinal venular caliber were attributable to genetic factors [175]. Newer data from the Beaver Dam Eye Study, based on a genome-wide linkage scan, further reinforce the genetic contribution to the variation in retinal vascular calibers, independent of hypertension and other confounders [176]. The investigators showed that the linkage regions for retinal vascular caliber overlap with regions that have been previously associated with essential hypertension, coronary heart disease, endothelial dysfunction, and vasculogenesis [176]. These novel findings provide the first genetic evidence to support the clinical observations, as described in Section 7.4, that changes in retinal arteriolar and venular caliber may precede and contribute to the pathogenesis of cardiovascular disease (e.g., hypertension).

While the currently available data regarding the genetic basis of retinal vascular changes are limited, findings from recent studies clearly demonstrate the usefulness of retinal image analysis in advancing our understanding of the complex genetic-environmental interaction pathways involved in the pathogenesis of cardiovascular disease. The exciting prospect of this expanding field of research opens many possibilities [177].

7.8 Conclusion

There is increasing recognition that retinal vascular image analysis presents great potential to advance our understanding of the role of microvascular disease in the development of various systemic disorders. Retinal vascular changes have now been linked to a spectrum of clinical and subclinical cardiovascular and metabolic outcomes. The mounting evidence generated from recent studies supports the notion that the retinal vasculature may provide a lifetime summary measure of genetic and environmental exposure, and may therefore act as a valuable risk marker for future systemic diseases. Nonetheless, despite an increasing application of retinal image analysis in research settings, its clinical value remains to be determined. Epidemiological evidence that retinal vascular changes are significantly predictive of morbid events does not necessarily translate directly into clinical practice. Further research is clearly required, perhaps with a more directed focus in assessing the ability of retinal imaging to provide clinically useful information above and beyond currently available risk stratification methods to aid prevention and management of cardiovascular and metabolic diseases. Finally, there remain additional novel measures of retinal vascular structure [178–182] that may offer additive value to the existing traditional retinal vascular signs in predicting systemic diseases. The role of these new measures in retinal image analysis remains to be clarified.

7.A Appendix: Retinal Vessel Caliber Grading Protocol

IVAN is a semi-automated system used to measure retinal vessel widths from a digital retinal image. IVAN is operated off of a two-monitor workstation with the image files organized by reading lists. The software opens on the primary monitor with three windows: the image display window, the control window, and the vessel data parameters file.

The image display is viewed on the primary monitor (Figure 7.A.1) and the control panel is moved to the secondary monitor (Figure 7.A.2).

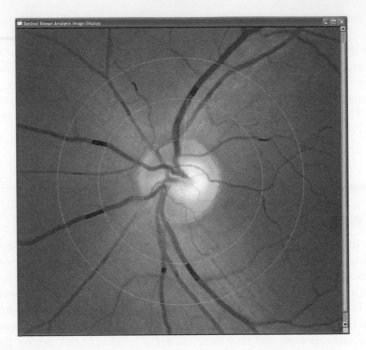

FIGURE 7.A.1
Primary monitor — image display.

The concept of "zone" adopted from the Modified ARIC grid is used in IVAN; it is composed of three concentric circles that demarcate an average optic disc with Zone A defined as the region from the disc margin to $\frac{1}{2}$ disc diameter from the disc, and Zone B defined as the region from $\frac{1}{2}$ disc diameter to 1 disc diameter from the disc. All retinal vessels are measured in Zone B.

7.A.1   Grading an image

Upon opening IVAN, the software automatically places the overlying grid on the brightest point of the image (usually the optic disc), detects vessels, and traces their width. The color blue denotes venules and the color red denotes arterioles. The vessels are automatically assigned as arteriole or venule; in the case of uncertainty, the vessel is assigned as an arteriole. The data table on the control window locates each vessel by its clockwise angle in degrees and displays the mean width and standard deviation (sigma) for each measured vessel (Figure 7.A.2).

The grader is responsible for visual evaluation of the automated display and making any necessary modifications. This includes the option to override any of the initial automated decisions or measurements such as adjusting the placement of the grid, changing the vessel type, deleting vessels, remeasuring vessels, and adding significant vessels missed in the initial automation.

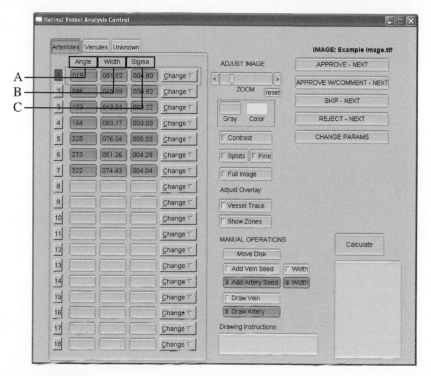

FIGURE 7.A.2

Secondary monitor — control panel (in arteriole view). The labels are: (A) angle of vessel in degrees, (B) mean width, and (C) standard deviation (sigma). **(See color insert following page 174.)**

The grader determines the validity of a measurement by the visual display and the width and standard deviation values. More significance should be given to the visual display.

An acceptable measurement is required to have the following:

- The visual vessel trace should have no obvious outliers from the visible edges of the vessel and must have a sigma value ≤ 8.00.

- The length of the measured segment should be as long as possible through Zone B for each particular vessel. A reasonable length will depend on the branching of the vessel and the photographic quality of the digital image.

All measurements must be taken proximal to all visible branching regardless of the length of the trunk or the length of the measured segment. If the trunk length in Zone B is short, it may be difficult to get a reliable measurement. In this case, a comment should be added to the saved data indicating the location of the possibly suspect vessel width. If the trunk is ungradeable, then both branches should be measured instead of the trunk.

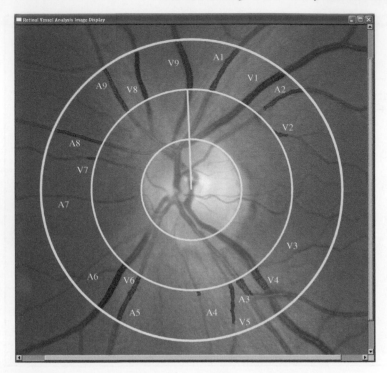

FIGURE 7.A.3
Automated display before grader interaction. **(See color insert.)**

7.A.2 Example of the grading process

The grader performs the following operations (see Figures 7.A.3 and 7.A.4 for pre- and post grader interaction):

A1 — proximal chop (after outliers)

A2 — proximal chop/truncate (outliers)

A3 — proximal chop/truncate (outliers)

A4 — delete/artery seed

A5 — proximal chop

A6 — artery seed

A7 — artery seed

A8 — no change

A9 — proximal chop/truncate (outliers)

V1 — truncate (before outlier)

V2 — change type/proximal chop/truncate

V3 — vein seed

V4 — proximal chop/truncate (outliers)

V5 — change type/proximal chop/truncate (outliers)

V6 — truncate (before branch)

V7 — change type/truncate (outliers)

V8 — truncate (before branch)

V9 — change type/truncate (outliers)

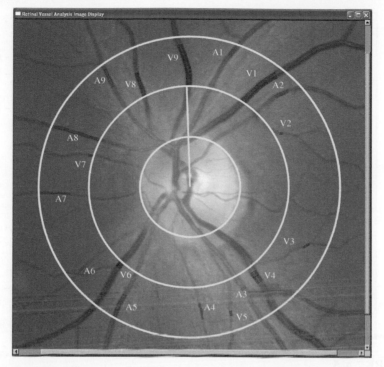

FIGURE 7.A.4
Completed grading with grader interaction. (**See color insert.**)

7.A.3 Obtaining results

When the grader is satisfied that the biggest six arterioles and venules have been traced correctly and are within the acceptable standard deviation, they choose to calculate the image (Figure 7.A.5, label A) to obtain the required results (Figure 7.A.5, label B).

Following Knudtson's revised formula [60] to calculate the Central Retinal Artery Equivalent (CRAE) and the Central Retinal Vein Equivalent (CRVE), only the width data from the six largest venules and six largest arterioles are required. Artery-to-Vein ratio (A/V ratio) is simply calculated as CRAE divided by CRVE.

The algorithm is thus:

$$\text{Arterioles:} \qquad \hat{W} = 0.88\sqrt{w_1^2 + w_2^2} \qquad (7.1)$$

$$\text{Venules:} \qquad \hat{W} = 0.95\sqrt{w_1^2 + w_2^2} \qquad (7.2)$$

where $\hat{W}$ is the estimate of parent trunk arteriole or venule, and w_1 and w_2 are the widths of the narrower branch and the wider branch, respectively.

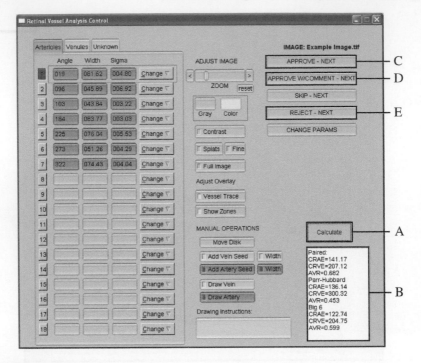

FIGURE 7.A.5
Control panel view after calculation. The labels are: (A) Calculate button, (B) Results panel, (C) APPROVE, (D) APPROVE W/COMMENT, and (E) REJECT. **(See color insert.)**

7.A.4   Saving data

At the completion of grading, there are three options for saving the data:

1. APPROVE (Figure 7.A.5, label C)

2. APPROVE W/COMMENT (Figure 7.A.5, label D)

3. REJECT (Figure 7.A.5, label E)

The APPROVE option is used for images that are gradeable and no comment is necessary. The APPROVE W/COMMENT option is used for images that are gradeable but had grading discrepancies that may affect the consistency of the data. These comments will be evaluated by the statisticians. The REJECT option is used for images that are ungradeable and no comment is necessary. Images that are ungradeable very often will have no acceptable automated vessels on the initial display and the grader will have difficulty discerning any vessels. Eyes that have fewer than four acceptable measurements of either vessel type will be considered ungradeable. Output data will automatically be sent to the specified comma separated values (.csv) file upon selecting one of the three saving options and the grader will be prompted to open the next image for grading.

References

[1] van den Hoogen, P.C., Feskens, E.J., Nagelkerke, N.J., et al., The relation between blood pressure and mortality due to coronary heart disease among men in different parts of the world. Seven Countries Study Research Group, *N Engl J Med*, 342, 1, 2000.

[2] MacMahon, S., Blood pressure and the risk of cardiovascular disease, *N Engl J Med*, 342, 50, 2000.

[3] Stamler, J., Dyer, A.R., Shekelle, R.B., et al., Relationship of baseline major risk factors to coronary and all-cause mortality, and to longevity: findings from long-term follow-up of Chicago cohorts, *Cardiology*, 82, 191, 1993.

[4] Wolf, P.A., D'Agostino, R.B., Kannel, W.B., et al., Cigarette smoking as a risk factor for stroke. the Framingham study, *JAMA*, 259, 1025, 1988.

[5] Langer, R.D., Ganiats, T.G., and Barrett-Connor, E., Paradoxical survival of elderly men with high blood pressure, *BMJ*, 298, 1356, 1989.

[6] Pekkanen, J., Tervahauta, M., Nissinen, A., et al., Does the predictive value of baseline coronary risk factors change over a 30-year follow-up? *Cardiology*, 82, 181, 1993.

[7] Prospective studies collaboration, Cholesterol, diastolic blood pressure, and stroke: 13,000 strokes in 450,000 people in 45 prospective cohorts, *Lancet*, 346, 1647, 1995.

[8] Harjai, K.J., Potential new cardiovascular risk factors: left ventricular hypertrophy, homocysteine, lipoprotein(a), triglycerides, oxidative stress, and fibrinogen, *Ann Intern Med*, 131, 376, 1999.

[9] Oparil, S. and Oberman, A., Nontraditional cardiovascular risk factors, *Am J Med Sci*, 317, 193, 1999.

[10] Pahor, M., Elam, M.B., Garrison, R.J., et al., Emerging noninvasive biochemical measures to predict cardiovascular risk, *Arch Intern Med*, 159, 237, 1999.

[11] Goto, I., Katsuki, S., Ikui, H., et al., Pathological studies on the intracerebral and retinal arteries in cerebrovascular and noncerebrovascular diseases, *Stroke*, 6, 263, 1975.

[12] Tso, M.O. and Jampol, L.M., Pathophysiology of hypertensive retinopathy, *Ophthalmology*, 89, 1132, 1982.

[13] Wendland, J.P., Retinal arteriolosclerosis in age, essential hypertension, and diabetes mellitus, *Trans Am Ophthalmol Soc*, 64, 735, 1966.

[14] Wells, R.E., Herman, M., and Gorlin, R., Microvascular changes in coronary artery disease, *Circulation*, 237, 33, 1966.

[15] Ashton, N. and Harry, J., The pathology of cotton wool spots and cytoid bodies in hypertensive retinopathy and other diseases, *Trans Ophthalmol Soc UK*, 83, 91, 1963.

[16] Ashton, N., Peltier, S., and Garner, A., Experimental hypertensive retinopathy in the monkey, *Trans Ophthalmol Soc UK*, 88, 167, 1969.

[17] Ashton, N., The eye in malignant hypertension, *Trans Am Acad Ophthalmol Otolaryngol*, 76, 17, 1972.

[18] Garner, A., Ashton, N., Tripathi, R., et al., Pathogenesis of hypertensive retinopathy. an experimental study in the monkey, *Br J Ophthalmol*, 59, 3, 1975.

[19] Garner, A. and Ashton, N., Pathogenesis of hypertensive retinopathy: a review, *J R Soc Med*, 72, 362, 1979.

[20] Gunn, R.M., Ophthalmoscopic evidence of (1) arterial changes associated with chronic renal diseases and (2) of increased arterial tension, *Trans Ophthalmol Soc UK*, 12, 124, 1892.

[21] Gunn, R.M., On ophthalmoscopic evidence of general arterial disease, *Trans Ophthalmol Soc UK*, 18, 356, 1898.

[22] O'Hare, J.P. and Walker, W.G., Arteriosclerosis and hypertension, *Arch Intern Med*, 33, 343, 1924.

[23] Friedenwald, H., The Doyne Memorial Lecture: Pathological changes in the retinal blood-vessels in arteriosclerosis and hypertension, *Trans Ophthalmol Soc UK*, 50, 452, 1930.

[24] Keith, N.M., Wagener, H.P., and Barker, N.W., Some different types of essential hypertension: their course and prognosis, *Am J Med Sci*, 197, 332, 1939.

[25] Breslin, D.J., Gifford, Jr., R.W., Fairbairn, 2nd, J.F., et al., Prognostic importance of ophthalmoscopic findings in essential hypertension, *JAMA*, 195, 335, 1966.

[26] Breslin, D.J., Gifford, Jr., R.W., and Fairbairn, 2nd, J.F., Essential hypertension. A twenty-year follow-up study, *Circulation*, 33, 87, 1966.

[27] Scheie, H.G., Evaluation of ophthalmoscopic changes of hypertension and arteriolar sclerosis, *AMA Arch Ophthalmol*, 49, 117, 1953.

[28] Salus, R., A contribution to the diagnosis of arteriosclerosis and hypertension,

Am J Ophthalmol, 45, 81, 1958.

[29] Leishman, R., The eye in general vascular disease: hypertension and arteriosclerosis, *Br J Ophthalmol*, 41, 641, 1957.

[30] Evelyn, K.A., Nicholis, J.V., and Turnbull, W., A method of grading and recording: the retinal changes in essential hypertension, *Am J Ophthalmol*, 45, 165, 1958.

[31] Frant, R. and Groen, J., Prognosis of vascular hypertension; a 9 year follow-up study of 418 cases, *Arch Med Interna*, 85, 727, 1950.

[32] Cohen, M., Lesions of the fundus in essential hypertension and in arterial and renal diseases, *Arch Ophthalmol*, 17, 99401007, 1937.

[33] Gillum, R.F., Retinal arteriolar findings and coronary heart disease, *Am Heart J*, 122, 262, 1991.

[34] Nakayama, T., Date, C., Yokoyama, T., et al., A 15.5-year follow-up study of stroke in a Japanese provincial city. The Shibata Study, *Stroke*, 28, 45, 1997.

[35] Ralph, R.A., Prediction of cardiovascular status from arteriovenous crossing phenomena, *Ann Ophthalmol*, 6, 323, 1974.

[36] Kagan, A., Aureli, E., and Dobree, J., A note on signs in the fundus oculi and arterial hypertension: conventional assessment and significance, *Bull World Health Organ*, 34, 955, 1966.

[37] Dimmitt, S.B., West, J.N., Eames, S.M., et al., Usefulness of ophthalmoscopy in mild to moderate hypertension, *Lancet*, 1, 1103, 1989.

[38] Aoki, N., Horibe, H., Ohno, Y., et al., Epidemiological evaluation of funduscopic findings in cerebrovascular diseases. III. Observer variability and reproducibility for funduscopic findings, *Jpn Circ J*, 41, 11, 1977.

[39] Klein, R., Klein, B.E., Moss, S.E., et al., Blood pressure, hypertension and retinopathy in a population, *Trans Am Ophthalmol Soc*, 91, 207, 1993, discussion 222-6.

[40] Klein, R., Klein, B.E., Moss, S.E., et al., Hypertension and retinopathy, arteriolar narrowing, and arteriovenous nicking in a population, *Arch Ophthalmol*, 112, 92, 1994.

[41] Klein, R., Klein, B.E., and Moss, S.E., The relation of systemic hypertension to changes in the retinal vasculature: the Beaver Dam Eye Study, *Trans Am Ophthalmol Soc*, 95, 329, 1997, discussion 348-50.

[42] Klein, R., Retinopathy in a population-based study, *Trans Am Ophthalmol Soc*, 90, 561, 1992.

[43] Yu, T., Mitchell, P., Berry, G., et al., Retinopathy in older persons without diabetes and its relationship to hypertension, *Arch Ophthalmol*, 116, 83, 1998.

[44] Wong, T.Y. and Mitchell, P., Hypertensive retinopathy, *N Engl J Med*, 351, 2310, 2004.

[45] Walsh, J.B., Hypertensive retinopathy. description, classification, and prognosis, *Ophthalmology*, 89, 1127, 1982.

[46] Schubert, H.D., Ocular manifestations of systemic hypertension, *Curr Opin Ophthalmol*, 9, 69, 1998.

[47] Dodson, P.M., Lip, G.Y., Eames, S.M., et al., Hypertensive retinopathy: a review of existing classification systems and a suggestion for a simplified grading system, *J Hum Hypertens*, 10, 93, 1996.

[48] Patton, N., Aslam, T.M., MacGillivray, T., et al., Retinal image analysis: concepts, applications and potential, *Prog Retin Eye Res*, 25, 99, 2006.

[49] Hubbard, L.D., Brothers, R.J., King, W.N., et al., Methods for evaluation of retinal microvascular abnormalities associated with hypertension/sclerosis in the Atherosclerosis Risk in Communities Study, *Ophthalmology*, 106, 2269, 1999.

[50] Couper, D.J., Klein, R., Hubbard, L.D., et al., Reliability of retinal photography in the assessment of retinal microvascular characteristics: the Atherosclerosis Risk in Communities Study, *Am J Ophthalmol*, 133, 78, 2002.

[51] Sherry, L.M., Wang, J.J., Rochtchina, E., et al., Reliability of computer-assisted retinal vessel measurementin a population, *Clin Experiment Ophthalmol*, 30, 179, 2002.

[52] Li, H., Hsu, W., Lee, M.L., et al., Automatic grading of retinal vessel caliber, *IEEE Trans Biomed Eng*, 52, 1352, 2005.

[53] Wong, T.Y., Knudtson, M.D., Klein, R., et al., Computer-assisted measurement of retinal vessel diameters in the Beaver Dam Eye Study: methodology, correlation between eyes, and effect of refractive errors, *Ophthalmology*, 111, 1183, 2004.

[54] Parr, J.C. and Spears, G.F., General caliber of the retinal arteries expressed as the equivalent width of the central retinal artery, *Am J Ophthalmol*, 77, 472, 1974.

[55] Parr, J.C. and Spears, G.F., Mathematic relationships between the width of a retinal artery and the widths of its branches, *Am J Ophthalmol*, 77, 478, 1974.

[56] Wong, T.Y., Islam, F.M., Klein, R., et al., Retinal vascular caliber, cardiovascular risk factors, and inflammation: the multi-ethnic study of atherosclerosis (MESA), *Invest Ophthalmol Vis Sci*, 47, 2341, 2006.

[57] Wong, T.Y., Klein, R., Sharrett, A.R., et al., The prevalence and risk factors of retinal microvascular abnormalities in older persons: the Cardiovascular Health Study, *Ophthalmology*, 110, 658, 2003.

[58] van Leiden, H.A., Dekker, J.M., Moll, A.C., et al., Risk factors for incident retinopathy in a diabetic and nondiabetic population: the Hoorn study, *Arch Ophthalmol*, 121, 245, 2003.

[59] Lowell, J., Hunter, A., Steel, D., et al., Measurement of retinal vessel widths from fundus images based on 2-D modeling, *IEEE Trans Med Imaging*, 23, 1196, 2004.

[60] Knudtson, M.D., Lee, K.E., Hubbard, L.D., et al., Revised formulas for summarizing retinal vessel diameters, *Curr Eye Res*, 27, 143, 2003.

[61] Patton, N., Aslam, T., Macgillivray, T., et al., Asymmetry of retinal arteriolar branch widths at junctions affects ability of formulae to predict trunk arteriolar widths, *Invest Ophthalmol Vis Sci*, 47, 1329, 2006.

[62] Wong, T.Y., Wang, J.J., Rochtchina, E., et al., Does refractive error influence the association of blood pressure and retinal vessel diameters? The Blue Mountains Eye Study, *Am J Ophthalmol*, 137, 1050, 2004.

[63] Rudnicka, A.R., Burk, R.O., Edgar, D.F., et al., Magnification characteristics of fundus imaging systems, *Ophthalmology*, 105, 2186, 1998.

[64] Liew, G., Mitchell, P., Wang, J.J., et al., Effect of axial length on retinal vascular network geometry, *Am J Ophthalmol*, 141, 597, 2006, author reply 597-8.

[65] Cheung, N. and Wong, T.Y., The retinal arteriole to venule ratio: informative or deceptive? *Graefe's Clinical and Experimental Ophthalmology*, 2007, forthcoming.

[66] Liew, G., Sharrett, A.R., Kronmal, R., et al., Measurements of retinal vascular caliber: issues and alternatives to using the arteriole to venule ratio, *Invest Ophthalmol Vis Sci*, 48, 52, 2007.

[67] Liew, G., Wong, T.Y., Mitchell, P., et al., Are narrower or wider retinal venules associated with incident hypertension? *Hypertension*, 48, e10, 2006, author reply e11.

[68] Ikram, M.K., de Jong, F.J., Vingerling, J.R., et al., Are retinal arteriolar or venular diameters associated with markers for cardiovascular disorders? The Rotterdam Study, *Invest Ophthalmol Vis Sci*, 45, 2129, 2004.

[69] Ikram, M.K., Witteman, J.C., Vingerling, J.R., et al., Response to are narrower or wider retinal venules associated with incident hypertension? *Hypertension*, 2006.

[70] Cheung, N., Islam, F.M., Saw, S.M., et al., Distribution and associations of retinal vascular caliber with ethnicity, gender and birth parameters in young children, *Invest Ophthalmol Vis Sci*, 48, 1018, 2007.

[71] Sharrett, A.R., Hubbard, L.D., Cooper, L.S., et al., Retinal arteriolar diameters and elevated blood pressure: the Atherosclerosis Risk in Communities Study,

Am J Epidemiol, 150, 263, 1999.

[72] Wang, J.J., Mitchell, P., Leung, H., et al., Hypertensive retinal vessel wall signs in a general older population: the Blue Mountains Eye Study, *Hypertension*, 42, 534, 2003.

[73] Wong, T.Y., Klein, R., Klein, B.E., et al., Retinal vessel diameters and their associations with age and blood pressure, *Invest Ophthalmol Vis Sci*, 44, 4644, 2003.

[74] Wong, T.Y., Hubbard, L.D., Klein, R., et al., Retinal microvascular abnormalities and blood pressure in older people: the Cardiovascular Health Study, *Br J Ophthalmol*, 86, 1007, 2002.

[75] Wong, T.Y., Klein, R., Sharrett, A.R., et al., Retinal arteriolar diameter and risk for hypertension, *Ann Intern Med*, 140, 248, 2004.

[76] Longstreth, Jr., W.T., Larsen, E.K., Klein, R., et al., Associations between findings on cranial magnetic resonance imaging and retinal photography in the elderly, *Am J Epidemiol*, 2006.

[77] Wong, T.Y., Barr, E.L., Tapp, R.J., et al., Retinopathy in persons with impaired glucose metabolism: the Australian Diabetes Obesity and Lifestyle (AusDiab) Study, *Am J Ophthalmol*, 140, 1157, 2005.

[78] Wong, T.Y., Klein, R., Couper, D.J., et al., Retinal microvascular abnormalities and incident stroke: the Atherosclerosis Risk in Communities Study, *Lancet*, 358, 1134, 2001.

[79] Cheung, N., Rogers, S., Couper, D.J., et al., Is diabetic retinopathy an independent risk factor for ischemic stroke? *Stroke*, 38, 398, 2007.

[80] Wong, T.Y., Klein, R., Sharrett, A.R., et al., Cerebral white matter lesions, retinopathy, and incident clinical stroke, *JAMA*, 288, 67, 2002.

[81] Mitchell, P., Wang, J.J., Wong, T.Y., et al., Retinal microvascular signs and risk of stroke and stroke mortality, *Neurology*, 65, 1005, 2005.

[82] Cheung, N., Wang, J.J., Klein, R., et al., Diabetic retinopathy and risk of coronary heart disease: The Atherosclerosis Risk in Communities Study, *Diabetes Care*, 30, 1742, 2007.

[83] Wong, T.Y., Rosamond, W., Chang, P.P., et al., Retinopathy and risk of congestive heart failure, *JAMA*, 293, 63, 2005.

[84] Wong, T.Y., Coresh, J., Klein, R., et al., Retinal microvascular abnormalities and renal dysfunction: the atherosclerosis risk in communities study, *J Am Soc Nephrol*, 15, 2469, 2004.

[85] Edwards, M.S., Wilson, D.B., Craven, T.E., et al., Associations between retinal microvascular abnormalities and declining renal function in the elderly population: the Cardiovascular Health Study, *Am J Kidney Dis*, 46, 214, 2005.

[86] Leung, H., Wang, J.J., Rochtchina, E., et al., Impact of current and past blood pressure on retinal arteriolar diameter in an older population, *J Hypertens*, 22, 1543, 2004.

[87] Klein, R., Klein, B.E., Moss, S.E., et al., Retinal vascular abnormalities in persons with type 1 diabetes: the Wisconsin Epidemiologic Study of Diabetic Retinopathy: XVIII, *Ophthalmology*, 110, 2118, 2003.

[88] Wong, T.Y., Shankar, A., Klein, R., et al., Prospective cohort study of retinal vessel diameters and risk of hypertension, *BMJ*, 329, 79, 2004.

[89] Smith, W., Wang, J.J., Wong, T.Y., et al., Retinal arteriolar narrowing is associated with 5-year incident severe hypertension: the Blue Mountains Eye Study, *Hypertension*, 44, 442, 2004.

[90] Wong, T.Y., Klein, R., Sharrett, A.R., et al., Retinal arteriolar narrowing and risk of coronary heart disease in men and women. the Atherosclerosis Risk in Communities Study, *JAMA*, 287, 1153, 2002.

[91] Mitchell, P., Cheung, N., de Haseth, K., et al., Blood pressure and retinal arteriolar narrowing in children, *Hypertension*, 49, 1156, 2007.

[92] Ikram, M.K., Witteman, J.C., Vingerling, J.R., et al., Retinal vessel diameters and risk of hypertension: the Rotterdam Study, *Hypertension*, 47, 189, 2006.

[93] Wong, T.Y., Kamineni, A., Klein, R., et al., Quantitative retinal venular caliber and risk of cardiovascular disease in older persons: the cardiovascular health study, *Arch Intern Med*, 166, 2388, 2006.

[94] Wang, J.J., Liew, G., Wong, T.Y., et al., Retinal vascular caliber and the risk of coronary heart disease-related mortality, *Heart*, 2006.

[95] Ikram, M.K., de Jong, F.J., Bos, M.J., et al., Retinal vessel diameters and risk of stroke: the Rotterdam Study, *Neurology*, 66, 1339, 2006.

[96] Leung, H., Wang, J.J., Rochtchina, E., et al., Relationships between age, blood pressure, and retinal vessel diameters in an older population, *Invest Ophthalmol Vis Sci*, 44, 2900, 2003.

[97] Sharp, P.S., Chaturvedi, N., Wormald, R., et al., Hypertensive retinopathy in Afro-Caribbeans and Europeans. Prevalence and risk factor relationships, *Hypertension*, 25, 1322, 1995.

[98] Klein, R., Sharrett, A.R., Klein, B.E., et al., Are retinal arteriolar abnormalities related to atherosclerosis?: the Atherosclerosis Risk in Communities Study, *Arterioscler Thromb Vasc Biol*, 20, 1644, 2000.

[99] Feihl, F., Liaudet, L., Waeber, B., et al., Hypertension: a disease of the microcirculation? *Hypertension*, 48, 1012, 2006.

[100] Strachan, M.W. and McKnight, J.A., Images in clinical medicine. improvement in hypertensive retinopathy after treatment of hypertension, *N Engl J*

Med, 352, e17, 2005.

[101] Bock, K.D., Regression of retinal vascular changes by antihypertensive therapy, *Hypertension*, 6, III158, 1984.

[102] Dahlof, B., Stenkula, S., and Hansson, L., Hypertensive retinal vascular changes: relationship to left ventricular hypertrophy and arteriolar changes before and after treatment, *Blood Press*, 1, 35, 1992.

[103] Pose-Reino, A., Rodriguez-Fernandez, M., Hayik, B., et al., Regression of alterations in retinal microcirculation following treatment for arterial hypertension, *J Clin Hypertens (Greenwich)*, 8, 590, 2006.

[104] Wong, T.Y., Is retinal photography useful in the measurement of stroke risk? *Lancet Neurol*, 3, 179, 2004.

[105] Okada, H., Horibe, H., Yoshiyuki, O., et al., A prospective study of cerebrovascular disease in Japanese rural communities, Akabane and Asahi. Part 1: evaluation of risk factors in the occurrence of cerebral hemorrhage and thrombosis, *Stroke*, 7, 599, 1976.

[106] Tanaka, H., Hayashi, M., Date, C., et al., Epidemiologic studies of stroke in Shibata, a Japanese provincial city: preliminary report on risk factors for cerebral infarction, *Stroke*, 16, 773, 1985.

[107] Svardsudd, K., Wedel, H., Aurell, E., et al., Hypertensive eye ground changes. prevalence, relation to blood pressure and prognostic importance. the study of men born in 1913, *Acta Med Scand*, 204, 159, 1978.

[108] Wong, T.Y., Klein, R., Sharrett, A.R., et al., Retinal microvascular abnormalities and cognitive impairment in middle-aged persons: the Atherosclerosis Risk in Communities Study, *Stroke*, 33, 1487, 2002.

[109] Wong, T.Y., Mosley, Jr., T.H., Klein, R., et al., Retinal microvascular changes and MRI signs of cerebral atrophy in healthy, middle-aged people, *Neurology*, 61, 806, 2003.

[110] Wong, T.Y., Klein, R., Nieto, F.J., et al., Retinal microvascular abnormalities and 10-year cardiovascular mortality: a population-based case-control study, *Ophthalmology*, 110, 933, 2003.

[111] Kwa, V.I., van der Sande, J.J., Stam, J., et al., Retinal arterial changes correlate with cerebral small-vessel disease, *Neurology*, 59, 1536, 2002.

[112] Schneider, R., Rademacher, M., and Wolf, S., Lacunar infarcts and white matter attenuation. Ophthalmologic and microcirculatory aspects of the pathophysiology, *Stroke*, 24, 1874, 1993.

[113] Dozono, K., Ishii, N., Nishihara, Y., et al., An autopsy study of the incidence of lacunes in relation to age, hypertension, and arteriosclerosis, *Stroke*, 22, 993, 1991.

[114] Hiroki, M., Miyashita, K., Yoshida, H., et al., Central retinal artery doppler flow parameters reflect the severity of cerebral small-vessel disease, *Stroke*, 34, e92, 2003.

[115] Wardlaw, J.M., Sandercock, P.A., Dennis, M.S., et al., Is breakdown of the blood-brain barrier responsible for lacunar stroke, leukoaraiosis, and dementia? *Stroke*, 34, 806, 2003.

[116] Michelson, E.L., Morganroth, J., Nichols, C.W., et al., Retinal arteriolar changes as an indicator of coronary artery disease, *Arch Intern Med*, 139, 1139, 1979.

[117] Duncan, B.B., Wong, T.Y., Tyroler, H.A., et al., Hypertensive retinopathy and incident coronary heart disease in high risk men, *Br J Ophthalmol*, 86, 1002, 2002.

[118] Maguire, M.G., Explaining gender differences in coronary heart disease: hunting for clues with the ophthalmoscope, *Arch Ophthalmol*, 121, 1328, 2003.

[119] Cannon, 3rd, R.O. and Balaban, R.S., Chest pain in women with normal coronary angiograms, *N Engl J Med*, 342, 885, 2000.

[120] Miettinen, H., Haffner, S.M., Lehto, S., et al., Retinopathy predicts coronary heart disease events in NIDDM patients, *Diabetes Care*, 19, 1445, 1996.

[121] Klein, B.E., Klein, R., McBride, P.E., et al., Cardiovascular disease, mortality, and retinal microvascular characteristics in type 1 diabetes: Wisconsin Epidemiologic Study of Diabetic Retinopathy, *Arch Intern Med*, 164, 1917, 2004.

[122] Faglia, E., Favales, F., Calia, P., et al., Cardiac events in 735 type 2 diabetic patients who underwent screening for unknown asymptomatic coronary heart disease: 5-year follow-up report from the Milan Study on Atherosclerosis and Diabetes (MiSAD), *Diabetes Care*, 25, 2032, 2002.

[123] Giugliano, D., Acampora, R., De Rosa, N., et al., Coronary artery disease in type-2 diabetes mellitus: a scintigraphic study, *Diabete Metab*, 19, 463, 1993.

[124] Ioannidis, G., Peppa, M., Rontogianni, P., et al., The concurrence of microalbuminuria and retinopathy with cardiovascular risk factors; reliable predictors of asymptomatic coronary artery disease in type 2 diabetes, *Hormones (Athens)*, 3, 198, 2004.

[125] Yoon, J.K., Lee, K.H., Park, J.M., et al., Usefulness of diabetic retinopathy as a marker of risk for thallium myocardial perfusion defects in non-insulin-dependent diabetes mellitus, *Am J Cardiol*, 87, 456, 2001, a6.

[126] Akasaka, T., Yoshida, K., Hozumi, T., et al., Retinopathy identifies marked restriction of coronary flow reserve in patients with diabetes mellitus, *J Am Coll Cardiol*, 30, 935, 1997.

[127] Celik, T., Berdan, M.E., Iyisoy, A., et al., Impaired coronary collateral vessel development in patients with proliferative diabetic retinopathy, *Clin Cardiol*, 28, 384, 2005.

[128] Yoshida, M., Takamatsu, J., Yoshida, S., et al., Scores of coronary calcification determined by electron beam computed tomography are closely related to the extent of diabetes-specific complications, *Horm Metab Res*, 31, 558, 1999.

[129] Wong, T.Y., Cheung, N., Islam, F.M.A., et al., Microvascular retinopathy is associated with coronary artery calcified plaque: the Multi-Ethnic Study of Atherosclerosis, 2006, unpublished data.

[130] Norgaz, T., Hobikoglu, G., Aksu, H., et al., Retinopathy is related to the angiographically detected severity and extent of coronary artery disease in patients with type 2 diabetes mellitus, *Int Heart J*, 46, 639, 2005.

[131] Goldin, A., Beckman, J.A., Schmidt, A.M., et al., Advanced glycation end products: sparking the development of diabetic vascular injury, *Circulation*, 114, 597, 2006.

[132] Klein, R., Klein, B.E., Moss, S.E., et al., The Wisconsin Epidemiologic Study of Diabetic Retinopathy. II. prevalence and risk of diabetic retinopathy when age at diagnosis is less than 30 years, *Arch Ophthalmol*, 102, 520, 1984.

[133] Klein, R., Klein, B.E., Moss, S.E., et al., Glycosylated hemoglobin predicts the incidence and progression of diabetic retinopathy, *JAMA*, 260, 2864, 1988.

[134] The Diabetes Control and Complications Trial Research Group, The effect of intensive treatment of diabetes on the development and progression of long-term complications in insulin-dependent diabetes mellitus, *N Engl J Med*, 329, 977, 1993.

[135] UK Prospective Diabetes Study (UKPDS) Group, Intensive blood-glucose control with sulphonylureas or insulin compared with conventional treatment and risk of complications in patients with type 2 diabetes (UKPDS 33), *Lancet*, 352, 837, 1998.

[136] Wong, T.Y., Mohamed, Q., Klein, R., et al., Do retinopathy signs in non-diabetic individuals predict the subsequent risk of diabetes? *Br J Ophthalmol*, 90, 301, 2006.

[137] Wong, T.Y., Duncan, B.B., Golden, S.H., et al., Associations between the metabolic syndrome and retinal microvascular signs: the Atherosclerosis Risk in Communities Study, *Invest Ophthalmol Vis Sci*, 45, 2949, 2004.

[138] Klein, B.E., Moss, S.E., Klein, R., et al., The Wisconsin Epidemiologic Study of Diabetic Retinopathy. XIII. relationship of serum cholesterol to retinopathy and hard exudate, *Ophthalmology*, 98, 1261, 1991.

[139] Chew, E.Y., Klein, M.L., Ferris, 3rd, F.L., et al., Association of elevated serum

lipid levels with retinal hard exudate in diabetic retinopathy. Early Treatment Diabetic Retinopathy Study (ETDRS) Report 22, *Arch Ophthalmol*, 114, 1079, 1996.

[140] Keech, A., Simes, R.J., Barter, P., et al., Effects of long-term fenofibrate therapy on cardiovascular events in 9795 people with type 2 diabetes mellitus (the FIELD study): randomised controlled trial, *Lancet*, 366, 1849, 2005.

[141] Wong, T.Y., Klein, R., Islam, F.M., et al., Diabetic retinopathy in a multiethnic cohort in the united states, *Am J Ophthalmol*, 141, 446, 2006.

[142] Barr, E.L., Wong, T.Y., Tapp, R.J., et al., Is peripheral neuropathy associated with retinopathy and albuminuria in individuals with impaired glucose metabolism? The 1999–2000 AusDiab, *Diabetes Care*, 29, 1114, 2006.

[143] Wong, T.Y., Klein, R., Sharrett, A.R., et al., Retinal arteriolar narrowing and risk of diabetes mellitus in middle-aged persons, *JAMA*, 287, 2528, 2002.

[144] Wong, T.Y., Shankar, A., Klein, R., et al., Retinal arteriolar narrowing, hypertension, and subsequent risk of diabetes mellitus, *Arch Intern Med*, 165, 1060, 2005.

[145] Ikram, M.K., Janssen, J.A., Roos, A.M., et al., Retinal vessel diameters and risk of impaired fasting glucose or diabetes: the Rotterdam Study, *Diabetes*, 55, 506, 2006.

[146] Wang, J.J., Taylor, B., Wong, T.Y., et al., Retinal vessel diameters and obesity: a population-based study in older persons, *Obesity (Silver Spring)*, 14, 206, 2006.

[147] Cheung, N., Saw, S.M., Islam, F.M.A., et al., Body mass index and retinal vascular caliber in children, *Obesity*, 15(1), 209, 2007.

[148] Falck, A. and Laatikainen, L., Retinal vasodilation and hyperglycaemia in diabetic children and adolescents, *Acta Ophthalmol Scand*, 73, 119, 1995.

[149] Nguyen, T.T. and Wong, T.Y., Retinal vascular manifestations of metabolic disorders, *Trends Endocrinol Metab*, 17, 262, 2006.

[150] Rajala, U., Laakso, M., Qiao, Q., et al., Prevalence of retinopathy in people with diabetes, impaired glucose tolerance, and normal glucose tolerance, *Diabetes Care*, 21, 1664, 1998.

[151] Singleton, J.R., Smith, A.G., Russell, J.W., et al., Microvascular complications of impaired glucose tolerance, *Diabetes*, 52, 2867, 2003.

[152] Harris, M.I., Klein, R., Welborn, T.A., et al., Onset of NIDDM occurs at least 4–7 yr before clinical diagnosis, *Diabetes Care*, 15, 815, 1992.

[153] Cugati, S., Mitchell, P., and Wang, J.J., Do retinopathy signs in non-diabetic individuals predict the subsequent risk of diabetes? *Br J Ophthalmol*, 90, 928, 2006.

[154] Cheung, N. and Wong, T.Y., Obesity and eye diseases, *Survey of Ophthalmology*, 2007, forthcoming.

[155] Chavers, B.M., Mauer, S.M., Ramsay, R.C., et al., Relationship between retinal and glomerular lesions in iddm patients, *Diabetes*, 43, 441, 1994.

[156] Klein, R., Klein, B.E., Moss, S.E., et al., The 10-year incidence of renal insufficiency in people with type 1 diabetes, *Diabetes Care*, 22, 743, 1999.

[157] Nag, S., Robertson, D.M., and Dinsdale, H.B., Morphological changes in spontaneously hypertensive rats, *Acta Neuropathol (Berl)*, 52, 27, 1980.

[158] Pontremoli, R., Cheli, V., Sofia, A., et al., Prevalence of micro- and macroalbuminuria and their relationship with other cardiovascular risk factors in essential hypertension, *Nephrol Dial Transplant*, 10(Suppl 6), 6, 1995.

[159] Liao, D., Wong, T.Y., Klein, R., et al., Relationship between carotid artery stiffness and retinal arteriolar narrowing in healthy middle-aged persons, *Stroke*, 35, 837, 2004.

[160] Cooper, L.S., Wong, T.Y., Klein, R., et al., Retinal microvascular abnormalities and MRI-defined subclinical cerebral infarction: the Atherosclerosis Risk in Communities Study, *Stroke*, 37, 82, 2006.

[161] Cheung, N., Bluemke, D.A., Klein, R., et al., Relation of retinal arteriolar caliber to left ventricular mass and remodeling: the Multi-Ethnic Study of Atherosclerosis, 2006.

[162] Tikellis, G., Arnett, D.K., Skelton, T., et al., Retinal arteriolar signs and left ventricular hypertrophy in African-Americans, 2006, unpublished data.

[163] Ikram, M.K., De Jong, F.J., Van Dijk, E.J., et al., Retinal vessel diameters and cerebral small vessel disease: the Rotterdam Scan Study, *Brain*, 129, 182, 2006.

[164] Klein, R., Klein, B.E., Knudtson, M.D., et al., Are inflammatory factors related to retinal vessel caliber? The Beaver Dam Eye Study, *Arch Ophthalmol*, 124, 87, 2006.

[165] Rema, M., Mohan, V., Deepa, R., et al., Association of carotid intima-media thickness and arterial stiffness with diabetic retinopathy: the Chennai Urban Rural Epidemiology Study (CURES-2), *Diabetes Care*, 27, 1962, 2004.

[166] Tamai, K., Matsubara, A., Tomida, K., et al., Lipid hydroperoxide stimulates leukocyte-endothelium interaction in the retinal microcirculation, *Exp Eye Res*, 75, 69, 2002.

[167] Chester, A.H., Borland, J.A., Buttery, L.D., et al., Induction of nitric oxide synthase in human vascular smooth muscle: interactions between proinflammatory cytokines, *Cardiovasc Res*, 38, 814, 1998.

[168] Shigematsu, Y., Hamada, M., Mukai, M., et al., Clinical evidence for an asso-

ciation between left ventricular geometric adaptation and extracardiac target organ damage in essential hypertension, *J Hypertens*, 13, 155, 1995.

[169] Saitoh, M., Matsuo, K., Nomoto, S., et al., Relationship between left ventricular hypertrophy and renal and retinal damage in untreated patients with essential hypertension, *Intern Med*, 37, 576, 1998.

[170] Tournier-Lasserve, E., New players in the genetics of stroke, *N Engl J Med*, 347, 1711, 2002.

[171] Nabel, E.G., Cardiovascular disease, *N Engl J Med*, 349, 60, 2003.

[172] Kupper, N., Willemsen, G., Riese, H., et al., Heritability of daytime ambulatory blood pressure in an extended twin design, *Hypertension*, 45, 80, 2005.

[173] McCaffery, J.M., Pogue-Geile, M.F., Debski, T.T., et al., Genetic and environmental causes of covariation among blood pressure, body mass and serum lipids during young adulthood: a twin study, *J Hypertens*, 17, 1677, 1999.

[174] Lee, K.E., Klein, B.E., Klein, R., et al., Familial aggregation of retinal vessel caliber in the Beaver Dam Eye Study, *Invest Ophthalmol Vis Sci*, 45, 3929, 2004.

[175] Taarnhoj, N.C., Larsen, M., Sander, B., et al., Heritability of retinal vessel diameters and blood pressure: a twin study, *Invest Ophthalmol Vis Sci*, 47, 3539, 2006.

[176] Xing, C., Klein, B.E., Klein, R., et al., Genome-wide linkage study of retinal vessel diameters in the Beaver Dam Eye Study, *Hypertension*, 47, 797, 2006.

[177] Wang, J.J. and Wong, T.Y., Genetic determinants of retinal vascular caliber: additional insights into hypertension pathogenesis, *Hypertension*, 47, 644, 2006.

[178] Witt, N., Wong, T.Y., Hughes, A.D., et al., Abnormalities of retinal microvascular structure and risk of mortality from ischemic heart disease and stroke, *Hypertension*, 47, 975, 2006.

[179] Hughes, A.D., Martinez-Perez, E., Jabbar, A.S., et al., Quantification of topological changes in retinal vascular architecture in essential and malignant hypertension, *J Hypertens*, 24, 889, 2006.

[180] Gould, D.B., Phalan, F.C., van Mil, S.E., et al., Role of COL4A1 in small-vessel disease and hemorrhagic stroke, *N Engl J Med*, 354, 1489, 2006.

[181] Gekeler, F., Shinoda, K., Junger, M., et al., Familial retinal arterial tortuosity associated with tortuosity in nail bed capillaries, *Arch Ophthalmol*, 124, 1492, 2006.

[182] Muiesan, M.L. and Grassi, G., Assessment of retinal vascular changes in hypertension: new perspectives, *J Hypertens*, 24, 813, 2006.

8

Segmentation of Retinal Vasculature Using Wavelets and Supervised Classification: Theory and Implementation

João V. B. Soares and Roberto M. Cesar Jr.

CONTENTS

8.1 Introduction 221
8.2 Theoretical Background 224
8.3 Segmentation Using the 2-D Gabor Wavelet and Supervised Classification . 235
8.4 Implementation and Graphical User Interface 245
8.5 Experimental Results 249
8.6 Conclusion 258
     Acknowledgments 260
     References 261

8.1 Introduction

Inspection of the optic fundus vasculature can reveal signs of hypertension, diabetes, arteriosclerosis, cardiovascular disease, and stroke [1]. Retinal vessel segmentation is a primary step towards automated analysis of the retina for detection of anomalies and image registration. Automated assessment of the retinal vasculature morphology can be used as part of a screening tool for early detection of diabetic retinopathy, while retinal image registration is of interest in detecting retinal changes, mosaic synthesis, and real-time tracking and spatial referencing for assistance in laser surgeries.

Different techniques are used for acquiring retinal images. Most common are colored or monochromatic photography and angiography using fluorescent dyes. In monochromatic photography, color filters are used to select light wavelengths that enhance the visibility of various fundus structures. Lighting using wavelengths close to the green region of the spectrum (known as red-free lighting) is frequently employed, as it leaves vessels, hemorrhages, and exudates more apparent. Angiographies, on the other hand, require the injection of a small amount of fluorescent dye into the patient, usually sodium fluorescein or indocyanine green. Fluorescence angiography permits recording of blood vessels and flow and also the detection of eventual leakages, of interest for diagnostic purposes. However, it is inadequate for screening programs, as angiograms can only be obtained by specialists in ophthalmology clinics, and is invasive, presenting a certain risk of side effects to the patient.

In face of the different forms of image acquisition, it is desirable that segmentation methods be able to work on images from different modalities. As an additional difficulty, even images of the same modality present large variability depending on the patient, presence of pathologies, camera model, illumination, and focus adjustment. Images with strong illumination variation or deficiency, light reflexes from the cornea, and inadequate focus are common and, depending on the application at hand, must be treated appropriately, posing an additional challenge in the development of segmentation methods [2].

The retinal vasculature is comprised of two complex networks — one of veins, the other of arteries — that spread out from the optic disc and branch successively to occupy different regions of the fundus. Retinal blood vessels are locally continuous with respect to position, curvature, and width, with vessel width gradually decreasing with distance from the optic disc [3–5]. These properties are specially important during the design of tracking algorithms [3; 6; 7]. Additionally, vessels are defined by a pair of parallel borders in which the image derivative presents opposite signs [3; 8; 9] in such a manner that the shapes of vessel cross-sections can be locally approximated by Gaussian functions [10]. These properties provide for vessel models that are usually as valid for retinal photographs as for angiograms, with vessels appearing as lighter than the background in angiograms and darker in colored and red-free photographs.

Diabetic retinopathy screening involves assessment of the optic fundus with attention to a series of indicative features. Of great importance is the detection of changes in blood vessel structure and flow, due to either vessel narrowing, complete occlusion or neovascularization [11–13]. Neovascularization is a condition associated with proliferative diabetic retinopathy (PDR), an advanced stage of the disease in which new vessels are formed emerging from the area of the optic disc or from peripheral vessels [1]. Prior to neovascularization, it is common to note vessel narrowing/dilation and increases in tortuosity. These changes can be detected by morphological analysis techniques through quantitative measures, such as vessel width and length [14], tortuosity [15], and fractal dimension [16].

Another major application of retinal vessel segmentation is registration of images captured at various instants of time or under different angles. Branching and crossing points or the skeletonized vasculature may be used as spatial landmarks that provide for registration of images, even from different modalities [17; 18]. Temporal registration assists in the detection of diseases and assessing effects of treatment. It may also be used for analysis of blood flow in angiographic video sequences, as the fluorescent dye reaches the optic fundus and retinal vessels. Partial views of the retina taken at different angles can also be combined to synthesize retinal mosaics. The mosaics can then be used for taking accurate morphological measurements or planning and assistance during laser surgeries, through real-time tracking and spatial referencing [2]. Finally, registration of images from different modalities allows visualizing superpositions of clinically important elements that previously appeared separately.

The retinal and choroidal vessel structures are used in biometrics for identification/verification of persons in security systems. Among many possible biometric features used, the optic fundus vascular patterns possess possibly the lowest error rate, besides being very stable through time and practically impossible to counterfeit. However, its use has limited reach due to high cost and a slight discomfort to the user during image acquisition. These disadvantages could possibly be surpassed, but with the variety of available biometrics, it is hard to predict the future of this particular application [19].

An automated assessment for pathologies of the optic fundus initially requires the precise segmentation of the vessels from the background, so that suitable feature extraction and processing may be performed. Several methods have been developed for vessel segmentation, but visual inspection and evaluation by receiver operating characteristic (ROC) analysis have shown that there is still room for improvement: human observers are significantly more accurate than the methods, which show flaws around the optic disc and in detection of the thinnest vessels [20; 21]. In addition, it is important to have segmentation algorithms that are fast and do not critically depend on configuring several parameters, so that untrained community health workers may utilize this technology. This motivates the use of the supervised classification framework that only depends on manually segmented images and can be implemented efficiently.

The method and some of the results presented in this chapter were previously published in a journal paper [22]. Here, the method is presented in greater detail, including a denser theoretical review, new tests, and analysis of results. An open-source prototype of an interactive software implementation is also described, including details on the most important steps of the segmentation process. The method developed uses the 2-D continuous wavelet transform (CWT) coupled with supervised pixel classification into classes *vessel* and *nonvessel*. Wavelet detection works similarly to matched filters, while at the same time incorporating the scale-angle representation, especially suited for the detection of blood vessels. A significant problem discussed in some works is the choice of an adequate scale for local detection filters. Filters of different scales have been combined empirically [23], while many other algorithms work off only one scale [10; 24; 25]. The approach presented here combines wavelet responses from different scales in feature vectors, allowing for pixel classification based on the statistical training of classifiers.

An essential property of many methods is their foundation on sets of rules that deal with specific situations, leading to complex algorithms that are parameter dependent (for example, [10; 25–27]). Even with a large number of rules, situations such as central vessel reflexes and branching/crossing points usually fail to be dealt with satisfactorily. In turn, the pixel classification approach is conceptually simple and allows the classifier to handle more specific situations, avoiding the formulation of rules and need for parameter adjustment. The approach takes into account only information local to each pixel, leaving space for improvement through the addition of a global inference phase. Even so, it is capable of segmenting the complete vascular networks and does not depend on user interaction, but on available manual segmentation for training.

Algorithm efficiency must be taken into account in practical and real-time applications, leading to specific considerations during method design [3]. Feature generation and classification of all image pixels may turn out to be a slow process depending on the choice of classifier [28]. In the method described in this chapter, a Bayesian classifier using Gaussian mixture models for class likelihoods was evaluated. The classifier showed good results with respect to ROC analysis, as it allows for complex decision surfaces, while at the same time providing a fast classification phase.

This chapter begins reviewing the theoretical foundations of the segmentation method (Section 8.2), including properties of the 2-D CWT and the 2-D Gabor wavelet, as well as the supervised classifiers evaluated. Section 8.3 describes the approach adopted, which combines wavelet features generation with supervised pixel classification. The same section also lays out the experimental evaluation performed, covering the description of image databases and a brief review of ROC analysis. An overview of the open-source implementation and graphical user interface developed for tests is given in Section 8.4. Experimental results are presented in Section 8.5, followed by the conclusion in Section 8.6, containing a discussion and directions for future work.

8.2   Theoretical Background

8.2.1   The 1-D CWT

Signal analysis may be carried out using transforms capable of emphasizing a signal's relevant properties, allowing processing tasks such as parameter estimation, noise filtering, and feature detection to be performed on the transformed signal. The wavelet transform is an example of such a signal processing tool, that is based on the Fourier transform, and is, as the latter, linear and invertible. Fourier analysis extracts global frequencies from a signal and is therefore appropriate for signals whose properties do not evolve with time (stationary signals). However, it is incapable of locating or analyzing frequencies of limited time duration (present in nonstationary signals). One of the first attempts to overcome this problem was the *short-time Fourier transform* (STFT), also known as Gabor transform [29; 30], in which a sliding window function delimits the signal portion to be analyzed by the Fourier transform. Notwithstanding, the STFT is restricted, as a constant resolution is used for analyzing all frequencies, given by the window's size.

The wavelet transform varies the size of the limiting window when analyzing different frequencies, giving rise to a multiresolution analysis. As observed by Gabor [29], the product between the time and frequency resolutions is lower bounded.

This implies that there is a trade-off between time and frequency resolution: increasing time precision leads to decreasing frequency precision and vice versa. The wavelet transform is defined to maintain a constant relative bandwidth during analysis. This means that low frequencies are observed through large windows (i.e., low time precision, high frequency precision), whereas high frequencies are observed through small windows (i.e., high time precision, low frequency precision). This type of frequency varying behavior is encountered in a great variety of signals, thus explaining the success of the wavelet transform. In fact, the development of the CWT theory was motivated by the problem of analyzing microseismic signals derived from oil prospecting, which present this type of behavior [31; 32]. Accordingly, the wavelet transform is specially suitable for detecting singularities and analyzing instantaneous frequencies [33; 34].

The CWT is defined as

$$U(b,a) = |a|^{-1/2} \int \psi^*(a^{-1}(x-b))f(x)\,dx, \tag{8.1}$$

where $a \in \mathbb{R}$ is the scale parameter, which relates the analyzing window size to the frequency; $b \in \mathbb{R}$ is the central time position being analyzed; ψ is the *analyzing wavelet* (also called *mother wavelet*); and ψ^* denotes the complex conjugate of ψ. The transform may be seen as a linear decomposition of the signal as projections onto basis functions $\psi_{b,a}(x) = \psi(a^{-1}(x-b))$, each one associated to a given location in time b and scale a. The domain of the transform $U(b,a)$ is referred to as the *time-scale* plane.

There are various analyzing wavelets that may be used depending on the kind of information to be extracted from the signal. The Morlet wavelet is defined as a Gaussian modulated by a complex exponential of frequency k_0,

$$\psi(x) = g(x)\exp(-ik_0 x) + \text{correction}, \tag{8.2}$$

where $g(x)$ is a Gaussian function, $i = \sqrt{-1}$ and the correction term is included to guarantee the wavelet admissibility condition (zero mean). The wavelet's definition shows a strong relation to the STFT, also minimizing the time-frequency joint uncertainty [30].

Wavelet theory represents a unified view of various signal processing techniques developed independently in fields such as pure mathematics, physics, and engineering. Being a versatile tool, it is applied to a wide range of applications, such as problems arising in physics [35]; audio, image, and video coding [30]; fractal and shape analysis [36]; and biomedical applications [37] (e.g., to detect brain activity in fMRI [38]).

8.2.2 The 2-D CWT

The CWT may be extended to higher dimensional spaces, allowing, for instance, the analysis of images (2-D signals) and video sequences (time-varying 2-D signals). This extension of the CWT preserves the fundamental properties of the 1-D case, being founded on coherent states and group theory. The theoretical framework allows the definition of operations over the wavelet space that preserve notions of symmetry. For the 1-D case, the natural operations are translation and dilation, being extended to the 2-D case as translation, dilation, and rotation [39; 40].

The CWT is mostly used for signal analysis and feature detection, in contrast to the *discrete wavelet transform* (DWT), preferable for data synthesis and compression, yielding very efficient algorithms. The 2-D DWT provides orthogonal and biorthogonal bases, thus allowing efficient signal representation, while the CWT necessarily leads to a redundant representation. However, the 2-D DWT is formulated as a tensor product of two 1-D schemes. It is therefore restricted to the Cartesian geometry, where directional analysis is much more difficult. In contrast, the introduction of the rotation operation in the 2-D CWT is specially suited for the analysis of oriented image structures by using the so called directional wavelets. This fact explains the adoption of the 2-D CWT with the Gabor wavelet to analyze the blood vessels, as proposed in Section 8.2.3.

The 2-D CWT has been used in a variety of applications in computer vision and image processing, such as analysis of medical and astronomical images [41], texture identification [42], edge detection [34; 43; 44], and fractal analysis [45; 46]. There are also imaging applications in physical problems such as analysis of geological faults and turbulence in fluids [47] or detection of dilation and rotation symmetries [48]. The main 2-D CWT concepts and properties used in this chapter are presented in the following.

The real plane $\mathbb{R} \times \mathbb{R}$ is denoted as $\mathbb{R}^2$ and 2-D vectors are represented as bold letters, e.g., $\mathbf{x}, \mathbf{b}, \mathbf{k} \in \mathbb{R}^2$. Images are taken as finite energy functions (i.e., square integrable) $f \in L^2(\mathbb{R}^2)$. The vector $\mathbf{x}$ is used to represent a spatial position in the image, while $\mathbf{k}$ is associated to a given spatial frequency. The spatial frequency domain is defined by the 2-D Fourier transform $\hat{f}$ of a given image f as

$$\hat{f}(\mathbf{k}) = (2\pi)^{-1} \int \exp(-i\mathbf{k}\mathbf{x}) f(\mathbf{x}) \, d^2\mathbf{x}. \qquad (8.3)$$

An analyzing wavelet $\psi \in L^2(\mathbb{R}^2)$ may take on complex values and must satisfy the admissibility condition, described below. A family of wavelets $\{\psi_{\mathbf{b},a,\theta}\}$ of same shape is defined by translations, dilations, and rotations (by $\mathbf{b}$, a and θ, respectively) of the analyzing wavelet:

$$\psi_{\mathbf{b},a,\theta}(\mathbf{x}) = a^{-1} \psi(a^{-1} r_{-\theta}(\mathbf{x} - \mathbf{b})), \qquad (8.4)$$

$$\hat{\psi}_{\mathbf{b},a,\theta}(\mathbf{k}) = a \exp(-i\mathbf{b}\mathbf{k}) \hat{\psi}(a r_{-\theta}(\mathbf{k})), \qquad (8.5)$$

where $a > 0$ and r_θ denotes the usual 2-D rotation,

$$r_\theta(\mathbf{x}) = (x\cos\theta - y\sin\theta, x\sin\theta + y\cos\theta), \quad 0 \le \theta < 2\pi. \qquad (8.6)$$

The translation, dilation, and rotation operations generate the 2-D Euclidean group with dilations acting over $L^2(\mathbb{R}^2)$, denoted G [39].

The CWT $T_\psi \in L^2(G)$ is defined as the scalar product between f and each wavelet $\psi_{\mathbf{b},a,\theta}$, as a function of $(\mathbf{b}, a, \theta) \in G$:

$$T_\psi(\mathbf{b}, a, \theta) = \langle \psi_{\mathbf{b},a,\theta} | f \rangle \tag{8.7}$$

$$= a^{-1} \int \psi^*(a^{-1} r_{-\theta}(\mathbf{x} - \mathbf{b})) f(\mathbf{x}) d^2\mathbf{x}, \tag{8.8}$$

$$= a \int \exp(i\mathbf{b}\mathbf{k}) \hat{\psi}^*(a r_{-\theta}(\mathbf{k})) \hat{f}(\mathbf{k}) d^2\mathbf{k}. \tag{8.9}$$

The transform is thus a local representation in each of the four dimensions of G, capable of revealing dilation and rotation symmetries [41; 48]. The wavelet transform may be viewed as a series of correlation operations, presenting stronger responses whenever the transformed wavelet $\psi_{\mathbf{b},a,\theta}$ matches the signal portion.

If ψ and $\hat{\psi}$ are well localized, the transform acts at constant relative bandwidth, i.e., the bandwidth of the filter is always proportional to the analyzing frequency. Thus, as in the 1-D case, the transform presents high frequency precision in low frequencies and high spatial precision in high frequencies. This explains why the wavelet transform is suitable for detecting image singularities, such as edges in images [34; 43]. The wavelet transform conserves energy and provides a linear decomposition of f in terms of the wavelet family $\{\psi_{\mathbf{b},\theta,a}\}$ with coefficients $T_\psi(\mathbf{b}, \theta, a)$. The transform can be inverted, providing a reconstruction of the original signal from the coefficients as

$$f(\mathbf{x}) = c_\psi^{-1} \iiint T(\mathbf{b}, a, \theta) \psi_{\mathbf{b},a,\theta}(\mathbf{x}) a^{-3} d^2\mathbf{b} da d\theta, \tag{8.10}$$

where c_ψ is the normalization constant. For the above formula to hold, the wavelet *admissibility condition* must be met,

$$c_\psi = (2\pi)^2 \int |\hat{\psi}(\mathbf{k})|^2 |\mathbf{k}|^{-2} d^2\mathbf{k} < \infty. \tag{8.11}$$

If ψ satisfies $\psi \in L^1(\mathbb{R}^2) \cap L^2(\mathbb{R}^2)$, then the admissibility condition reduces to requiring that the analyzing wavelet have zero mean,

$$\hat{\psi}(\mathbf{0}) = 0 \iff \int \psi(\mathbf{x}) d^2\mathbf{x} = 0. \tag{8.12}$$

Besides the admissibility condition, additional desirable properties may be defined, such as that ψ and $\hat{\psi}$ be well localized and that ψ present a certain number of vanishing moments, thus being blind to polynomials up to the corresponding degree.

The CWT can be implemented efficiently employing the Fast Fourier Transform (FFT) [49] and its Fourier domain definition (Equation 8.9). Otherwise, for analyzing only small scales, the analyzing wavelet may be cropped off in the spatial domain so that the standard correlation implementation might actually become faster. The CWT information is highly redundant and, in practice, it is generally calculated over a discrete family of wavelets $\{\psi_{\mathbf{b}_i,a_j,\theta_k}\}$. An approximate reconstruction formula can then be given by

$$\tilde{f}(\mathbf{x}) = \sum_{ijk} \psi_{\mathbf{b}_i,a_j,\theta_k} T_\psi(\mathbf{b}_i, a_j, \theta_k), \tag{8.13}$$

where $\tilde{f}$ is the reconstructed version of f. The parameters $\mathbf{b}_i, a_j, \theta_k$ should be chosen to provide a stable reconstruction, defining the so called *frame*. The precision of the analyzing wavelet is studied in order to provide directives for defining a suitable sampling, so that the frames may satisfactorily cover the spatial and frequency domains [39; 50; 51]. Even so, the resulting representation will necessarily be redundant, in contrast to the DWT, which allows for deriving orthogonal bases.

8.2.3 The 2-D Gabor wavelet

The 2-D Gabor wavelet has been extensively used within the computer vision community, with special attention to its relevance to studies of the human visual system. One of its most important properties is its capability of detecting and analyzing directional structures. It is also optimal in the sense of minimizing the inherent uncertainty in the spatial and frequency domains. The 2-D version of the Gabor filter was probably introduced in [52], which, together with [53], showed that the filter represents a good model for simple cells of the visual cortex. In a subsequent paper [54], Daugman suggested the generalization of the filter to a wavelet, which was then called the Gabor wavelet. On the other hand, Antoine, Murenzi, and collaborators [39; 40] introduced the generalization of the CWT to two or more dimensions based on coherent states and group theory, in which the same wavelet was called Morlet wavelet, being the natural generalization of the 1-D Morlet wavelet. The name most commonly adopted in the computer vision community is Gabor wavelet, which is therefore also used in this work. Applications of the 2-D Gabor wavelet in computer vision include object representation [51; 55] (particularly, faces [56]), texture detection and segmentation [42; 57], and oriented structure analysis [41; 58]. The 2-D Gabor wavelet has also been shown to outperform other linear filters for detection of oriented features [59].

The 2-D Gabor wavelet is defined as

$$\psi_G(\mathbf{x}) = \exp(i\mathbf{k}_0\mathbf{x}) \exp\left(-\frac{1}{2}(\mathbf{x}A\mathbf{x})\right) + \text{correction}, \tag{8.14}$$

$$\hat{\psi}_G(\mathbf{k}) = (\det B)^{1/2} \exp\left(-\frac{1}{2}((\mathbf{k}-\mathbf{k}_0)B(\mathbf{k}-\mathbf{k}_0))\right) + \text{correction}, \tag{8.15}$$

where A is a 2×2 positive definite matrix that defines the wavelet anisotropy, $B = A^{-1}$ and $\mathbf{k}_0 \in \mathbb{R}^2$ defines the complex exponential basic frequency. The anisotropy matrix is taken as

$$A = \begin{bmatrix} \varepsilon^{-1} & 0 \\ 0 & 1 \end{bmatrix}, \tag{8.16}$$

with elongation given by $\varepsilon \geq 1$.

The 2-D Gabor wavelet is therefore simply an elongated Gaussian modulated by a complex exponential, which clarifies its relationship to the 1-D Morlet wavelet. The wavelet smoothes the signal in all directions, but detects sharp transitions in the direction of $\mathbf{k}_0$. In spatial frequencies, the Gabor wavelet is given by a Gaussian function centered at $\mathbf{k}_0$ and elongated by ε in the k_y direction. It is thus well localized both in position space, around the origin, and in the spatial frequency space, around $\mathbf{k}_0$. Angular selectivity increases with $|\mathbf{k}_0|$ and ε. These effects can be combined choosing $\mathbf{k}_0 = [0, k_y]$ and $\varepsilon \gg 1$. Figure 8.1 shows the effects of changing the wavelet's parameters (both in space and spatial frequencies).

The correction term is necessary to enforce the admissibility condition ($\hat{\psi}_G(\mathbf{0}) = 0$) [39]. However, it is worth noting that the term is numerically negligible for $|\mathbf{k}_0| \geq 5.6$ and in many situations can be simply dropped. We do not use the correction term, since it implies a loss in spatial localization ($|\psi_G|^2$ becomes bimodal [60]), and this problem should be addressed in future studies, as discussed in Section 8.6.2.

The definition of a directional wavelet is stated in terms of its spatial frequency domain support [50]. An analyzing wavelet is said to be *directional* if its effective support in the spatial frequency domain is contained within a convex cone with apex at the origin. Wavelets with directional support only in the spatial domain may not be able to detect directional structures, as is the case with the anisotropic Mexican hat [50], which does not satisfy the previously given definition. The Gabor wavelet is thus said to be directional, as its spatial frequency domain support is an ellipse given by the elongated Gaussian of Equation 8.15, as can be seen in the examples of Figure 8.1. If the definition is to be strictly observed, the Gabor wavelet is only approximately directional, given the Gaussian tails that are outside the ellipse, but are numerically negligible. The resolving power of the Gabor wavelet has been analyzed in terms of its scale and angular selectivity, helping define wavelet frames that tile the spatial frequency domain [39; 50; 51]. Many other 2-D analyzing wavelets have been proposed in the literature, designed for specific problems, and the reader is referred to [50] for a review.

In the case of vessel segmentation, the Gabor wavelet should be tuned to a suitable frequency, so that vessels may be emphasized while noise and other undesirable structures are filtered out. For the methods presented in this chapter (see Section 8.3.2), the parameters were set to $\varepsilon = 4$, resulting in an elongated wavelet, and $\mathbf{k}_0 = [0, 3]$, providing a low frequency complex exponential with transitions in the direction of its smaller axis, as shown on the bottom row of Figure 8.1. The Gabor wavelet's capability of detecting oriented features is fundamental in blood vessel detection. It is interesting to note that the wavelet's shape is locally similar to that of a blood vessel and is preserved across different orientations and scales. Therefore, stronger wavelet responses are produced when the wavelet is found at the same position, orientation, and scale as a vessel in the image.

8.2.4 Supervised classification

In the proposed vessel segmentation approach, image pixels are seen as objects represented by feature vectors, so that statistical classifiers might be applied for segmentation. In this case, each pixel is classified as *vessel* or *nonvessel*, using previously trained classifiers (supervised classification). The training sets for the classifiers are derived from manual segmentations of training images: pixels that were manually segmented out are labeled as *vessel*, while the remaining receive the *nonvessel* label. The approach allows the use of different responses of the wavelet transform to characterize pixels, as well as application to different image modalities, provided a

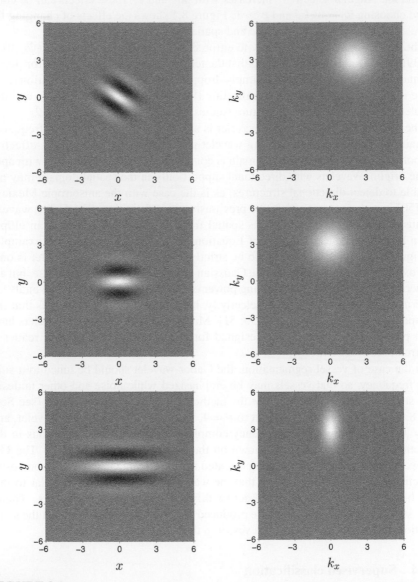

FIGURE 8.1

The Gabor wavelet in the spatial domain (represented by its real part) is shown in the left column, while the frequency domain counterpart is shown in the right column. Different configurations of the parameters are shown to illustrate the corresponding effects. Light and dark gray levels correspond to positive and negative coefficients, respectively. The parameters for the three rows are, from top to bottom: $\mathbf{k}_0 = [2,3]$, $\varepsilon = 1$; $\mathbf{k}_0 = [0,3]$, $\varepsilon = 1$; and $\mathbf{k}_0 = [0,3]$, $\varepsilon = 4$.

corresponding training set is available. The rest of this section contains descriptions pointing out important qualities of three classifiers: the Bayesian classifier using the Gaussian mixture model (Sections 8.2.5 and 8.2.6), the k-nearest neighbor classifier (Section 8.2.7), and the linear minimum squared error classifier (Section 8.2.8).

8.2.5   Bayesian decision theory

Bayesian decision theory is one of the main approaches adopted in pattern recognition problems. It is based on associating costs (or losses) to classification decisions, which are then chosen using the probability distributions of the objects being classified. In most cases, the probability distributions are unknown and must be estimated, which can be done using prior knowledge of the problem structure along with the available training data. *Bayes's decision rule* for an observed feature vector $\mathbf{v}$ in a two class problem (classes C_1 and C_2) can be written in terms of posterior probabilities as:

$$\text{decide } C_1 \text{ if } P(C_1|\mathbf{v}) > P(C_2|\mathbf{v});$$
$$\text{otherwise, decide } C_2. \tag{8.17}$$

The decision follows natural intuition and is shown to minimize the average probability of error [61].

Bayes's formula is written as

$$P(C_i|\mathbf{v}) = \frac{p(\mathbf{v}|C_i)P(C_i)}{p(\mathbf{v})}, \tag{8.18}$$

where $p(\mathbf{v}|C_i)$ is the class-conditional probability density function, also known as likelihood, $P(C_i)$ is the prior probability of class C_i, and $p(\mathbf{v})$ is the probability density function of $\mathbf{v}$, also known as evidence. To obtain a decision rule based on estimates from the training data (as will be needed in Section 8.2.6), Bayes's formula is applied to Equation 8.17, resulting in the equivalent decision rule:

$$\text{decide } C_1 \text{ if } p(\mathbf{v}|C_1)P(C_1) > p(\mathbf{v}|C_2)P(C_2);$$
$$\text{otherwise, decide } C_2. \tag{8.19}$$

8.2.6   Bayesian Gaussian mixture model classifier

According to Bayesian decision theory, classification decisions can be made using estimates of prior probabilities and likelihood functions. In the experiments performed by us, prior probabilities $P(C_i)$ were estimated as N_i/N, the ratio of class C_i samples in the training set. The class likelihoods, in turn, were described using the *Gaussian mixture model* (GMM), which consists of a linear combination of Gaussian functions [61; 62]. The Bayesian classifier using the GMM for class likelihoods will be called the GMM classifier. The procedure for estimating the model's parameters was applied separately for each class likelihood. To simplify notation, suppose the class C_i whose likelihood will be estimated is fixed. The likelihood of the class (earlier denoted $p(\mathbf{v}|C_i)$) is then simply denoted $p(\mathbf{v}|\boldsymbol{\phi})$, being modeled by

$$p(\mathbf{v}|\boldsymbol{\phi}) = \sum_{j=1}^{c} P_j \, p(\mathbf{v}|\boldsymbol{\phi}_j), \qquad (8.20)$$

where c Gaussians are used, given by $p(\mathbf{v}|\boldsymbol{\phi}_j)$ and weights P_j. Each $\boldsymbol{\phi}_j$ describes the parameters of Gaussian j, while the complete set of parameters that describe the model is denoted $\boldsymbol{\phi} \equiv \{\boldsymbol{\phi}_1, \ldots, \boldsymbol{\phi}_c, P_1, \ldots, P_c\}$. The Gaussian functions are

$$p(\mathbf{v}|\boldsymbol{\phi}_j) = \frac{1}{\sqrt{\det(2\pi\Sigma_j)}} \exp\left(-\frac{1}{2}(\mathbf{v}-\boldsymbol{\mu}_j)^T \Sigma_j^{-1}(\mathbf{v}-\boldsymbol{\mu}_j)\right). \qquad (8.21)$$

where $\boldsymbol{\phi}_j = \{\boldsymbol{\mu}_j, \Sigma_j\}$, $\boldsymbol{\mu}_j$ is the mean and Σ_j the covariance matrix that describe the Gaussian. In order for $p(\mathbf{v}|\boldsymbol{\phi})$ to be a probability density function, it is necessary that

$$\sum_{j=1}^{c} P_j = 1 \qquad \text{and} \qquad \int p(\mathbf{v}|\boldsymbol{\phi}_j)d\mathbf{v} = 1, \quad j = 1, \ldots, c. \qquad (8.22)$$

GMMs are extensively used for clustering in unsupervised learning problems. In that context, each Gaussian models the likelihood of a class with previously unknown distribution, with each Gaussian weight representing a prior class probability. Here, the GMM is used with a different purpose, in the description of class likelihoods from samples with known labels. The GMM allows likelihoods to be represented with arbitrary precision, being a flexible model applicable to complex and multi-modal distributions. In both applications, there is the need to estimate the Gaussians' parameters and weights from the available data.

The GMM parameters $\boldsymbol{\phi}$ are estimated so as to maximize the likelihood of the training samples. The parameters enter the likelihood in a nonlinear fashion, requiring nonlinear optimization techniques. In the experiments performed, the parameters were estimated using the *Expectation-Maximization* (EM) algorithm [61–63]. EM is an iterative process usually chosen for the estimation of mixture model parameters. It guarantees a local maximum of the function being optimized and can be applied to maximize likelihoods or posterior probabilities.

A difficulty in estimating the GMMs is the choice of the number of Gaussians c to use. It can be shown that GMMs can approximate with arbitrary precision any continuous probability density function, given a sufficiently large number of Gaussians. However, large values of c may cause models to adjust excessively to the data (a phenomenon known as over-fitting), while too small a c might not permit flexibility enough to properly describe the probability function. Experiments were performed varying the values of c for both classes, leading to different results. Finally, EM guarantees only a local maximum of the likelihood, being dependent on initialization. EM has received a good amount of attention in the last years, being used in a variety of applications. Many methods were developed to overcome the above mentioned problems [64], but were not explored in this work.

GMMs fall between purely nonparametric and parametric approaches, providing a fast classification phase at the cost of a more expensive training algorithm. Nonparametric methods (as k-nearest neighbor classification presented in Section 8.2.7) are computationally demanding for large numbers of training samples, though they do not impose restrictions on the underlying probability distributions. On the other hand, GMMs guarantee a fast classification phase that depends only on the chosen c (i.e., independent of the number of training samples), while still allowing for modeling complex distributions.

8.2.7 k-nearest neighbor classifier

A simple and popular classification approach is given by the *k-nearest neighbor* (*k*NN) *rule*. Let N be the total number of labeled training samples. Given an odd number k of neighbors, a distance measure, and a feature vector $\mathbf{v}$, the k-nearest neighbor classification rule can be summarized in the following steps:

1. out of the N training samples, identify the k-nearest neighbors of $\mathbf{v}$ using the given distance measure;

2. out of the k nearest samples identified, count the number of samples k_i that belong to each class C_i;

3. classify $\mathbf{v}$ as belonging to the class C_i with the largest number k_i of samples.

Various distance measures may be used, such as Euclidean or Mahalanobis distances, leading to different outcomes [61]. The Euclidean distance was used in this work for all experiments. The kNN classifier is nonparametric (independent of a probability distribution model) and capable of producing complex nonlinear decision boundaries. Theoretical superior limits on the classifier's error probability can be established, which decrease with N, so that when $k \rightarrow \infty$, the error tends to the optimal Bayesian error [61].

The classification rule may be interpreted as a decision taken based on estimates of the posterior probabilities $P(C_i|\mathbf{v})$ — simply estimated as k_i/k — from the data. From this perspective, as k increases, so does the confidence on the estimates, but spatial precision is lost, as samples that are far from $\mathbf{v}$ start being considered. The greater the number of samples N, the smaller the effect of loss in spatial precision, allowing for larger values of k to be used. In this study, many training samples are available, allowing for good estimates, but demanding a large computational effort. A problem with nearest neighbor techniques is the computational complexity of the search for nearest neighbors among the N training samples. If the dimension of the feature space is fixed, exhaustive search of the nearest neighbors of one sample takes time at least $O(N)$, necessary for the calculation of distances. Being so, strategies have been studied to improve performance, including efficient searches and reduction of the number of training samples used [61; 62]. Only the exhaustive search was implemented for the results shown in this chapter.

8.2.8 Linear minimum squared error classifier

The *linear minimum squared error classifier* [61; 62], denoted LMSE, was also tested. Linear classifiers are defined by a linear decision function g in the d-dimensional feature space:

$$g(\mathbf{v}) = \mathbf{w}^T \mathbf{v} + w_0, \tag{8.23}$$

where $\mathbf{v}$ is a feature vector, $\mathbf{w}$ is the weight vector, and w_0 is the threshold. The classification rule is to decide C_1 if $g(\mathbf{v}) > 0$ and C_2 otherwise. To simplify the formulation, the threshold w_0 is accommodated by defining the extended $(d+1)$-dimensional vectors $\mathbf{v}' \equiv [\mathbf{v}^T, 1]^T$ and $\mathbf{w}' \equiv [\mathbf{w}^T, w_0]^T$, so that $g(\mathbf{v}) = \mathbf{w}'^T \mathbf{v}'$.

The classifier is determined by finding $\mathbf{w}'$ that minimizes the *sum of squared error* criterion on the training set, defined as

$$J(\mathbf{w}') = \sum_{i=1}^{N} (\mathbf{v}_i'^T \mathbf{w}' - y_i)^2, \tag{8.24}$$

where N is the total number of training samples, $\mathbf{v}_i'$ is the extended i^{th} training sample, and y_i is its desired output. The criterion measures the sum of squared errors between the output of the classifier $\mathbf{v}_i'^T \mathbf{w}'$ and the desired output y_i. The desired outputs were arbitrarily set to $y_i = 1$ for $\mathbf{v}_i \in C_1$ and $y_i = -1$ for $\mathbf{v}_i \in C_2$.

Defining

$$V = \begin{bmatrix} \mathbf{v}_1'^T \\ \mathbf{v}_2'^T \\ \vdots \\ \mathbf{v}_N'^T \end{bmatrix}, \qquad \mathbf{y} = \begin{bmatrix} y_1 \\ y_2 \\ \vdots \\ y_N \end{bmatrix}, \tag{8.25}$$

the gradient of the criterion function can be written as

$$\nabla J(\mathbf{w}') = \sum_{i=1}^{N} 2(\mathbf{v}_i'^T \mathbf{w}' - y_i)\mathbf{v}_i' \tag{8.26}$$

$$= 2V^T(V\mathbf{w}' - \mathbf{y}). \tag{8.27}$$

The criterion function is minimized by calculating $\hat{\mathbf{w}}'$ where the gradient equals zero, resulting in

$$(V^T V)\hat{\mathbf{w}}' = V^T \mathbf{y} \Rightarrow \hat{\mathbf{w}}' = (V^T V)^{-1} V^T \mathbf{y}. \tag{8.28}$$

$(V^T V)^{-1} V^T$ is called the *pseudoinverse* of V and exists only if $V^T V$ is invertible. $V^T V$ is the *correlation matrix* of the training samples and will be invertible when V has full rank $d+1$. Given the nature of the data used in tests and the large number of training samples, this always occurred.

In comparison to the previously described kNN and GMM classifiers, the LMSE classifier has faster training and test phases, but is restricted in the sense that it is linear, while the others allow for complex decision boundaries. However, as will be shown, the results obtained using LMSE are comparable to those using GMMs (see Section 8.5), representing a reasonable trade-off.

8.3 Segmentation Using the 2-D Gabor Wavelet and Supervised Classification

Initially, promising results of vessel detection using the 2-D Gabor wavelet were shown [11; 65]. The segmentation method evolved with the introduction of supervised pixel classification, allowing wavelet responses from different scales to be combined [66]. Finally, the Bayesian Gaussian mixture model classifier showed to be specially appropriate for the segmentation task and was quantitatively evaluated using ROC analysis. A diagram illustrating the training of a classifier is presented in Figure 8.2(a). After training, the classifier can be applied to pixels of test images as shown in Figure 8.2(b). The process presented in the diagrams is described in greater detail throughout this section. The supervised learning approach combining different wavelet scale responses simplifies method use, minimizing the need for interaction and parameter configuration.

The GMM classifier is shown to provide good results, while at the same time guaranteeing a fast classification phase. For comparison, tests were performed in which the GMM classifier is substituted by the kNN and LMSE classifiers (see Section 8.2). Performance of the 2-D Gabor wavelet in enhancing blood vessels is demonstrated by comparing results of filtering using a single wavelet scale with results of the 2-D Gaussian matched filter of Chaudhuri et al. [24]. Quantitative performance evaluation is performed using ROC analysis, which has been previously used for evaluation and comparison of retinal vessel segmentation methods on publicly available image databases [25–28; 67].

8.3.1 Preprocessing

When the red-green-blue (RGB) components of colored images are visualized separately, the green channel shows the best vessel to background contrast, whereas the red and blue channels usually present low vessel contrast and are noisy [10]. Hence, for colored images, only the green channel is used for the generation of the wavelet features, as well as to compose the feature vector itself, i.e., the green channel intensity of each pixel is taken as one of its features. The green channel is inverted before the application of the wavelet transform to it, so that the vessels appear brighter than the background. Accordingly, the inversion is also applied to red-free, gray-scale images and fluorescein angiograms do not require inversion (see Section 8.1).

The Gabor wavelet responds strongly to high contrast edges, which may lead to false detection of the borders of the camera's aperture. In order to reduce this effect, an iterative algorithm has been developed. The intent is to remove the strong contrast between the retinal fundus and the region outside the camera's field-of-view (FOV) (see Figure 8.3).

The preprocessing algorithm starts with a region of interest (ROI) determined by the camera's aperture and iteratively grows this ROI. Each step of the algorithm consists of the following: first, the set of pixels of the exterior border of the ROI is deter-

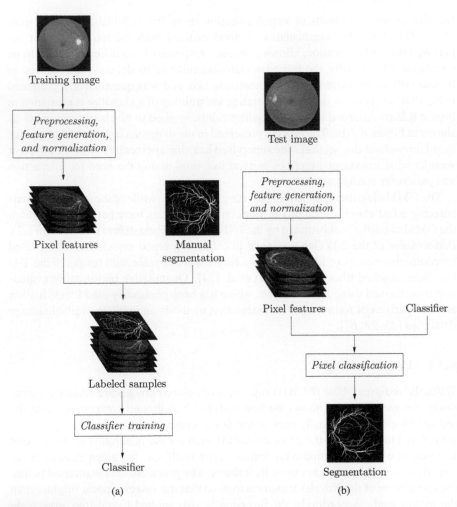

FIGURE 8.2

Supervised pixel classification approach. The left diagram illustrates the supervised training of a classifier. The trained classifier can then be applied to the segmentation of test images, as illustrated in the right diagram.

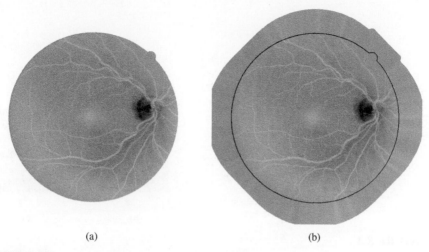

(a)   (b)

FIGURE 8.3
Image preprocessing for removing undesired border effects. The inverted green channel of the image presented in Figure 8.6 appears on the left. The inverted green channel after preprocessing, presenting the extended border, appears on the right (the original image limit is presented for illustration).

mined, i.e., pixels that are outside the ROI and are neighbors (using 4-neighborhood) to pixels inside it; then, each pixel value of this set is replaced with the mean value of its neighbors (this time using 8-neighborhood) inside the ROI; finally, the ROI is expanded by inclusion of this set of changed pixels. This process is repeated and may be seen as artificially increasing the ROI, as shown in Figure 8.3(b).

8.3.2   2-D Gabor wavelet features

Among several available 2-D analyzing wavelets, the Gabor wavelet was adopted for vessel detection here and in previous works [65], based on the following properties. The wavelet is capable of detecting directional structures and of being tuned to specific frequencies (see Section 8.2.3), which is specially important for filtering out the background noise present in retinal images. Furthermore, it has been shown to outperform other oriented feature detectors [59].

The Gabor wavelet parameters must be configured in order to enhance specific structures or features of interest. In the tests performed, the elongation parameter was set to $\varepsilon = 4$, making the filter elongated and $\mathbf{k_0} = [0,3]$, i.e., a low frequency complex exponential with few significant oscillations perpendicular to the large axis of the wavelet, as shown in Figure 8.4. These two characteristics are specially suited for the detection of directional features and have been chosen in order to enable the transform to present stronger responses for pixels associated with vessels. Note that the wavelet's shape is similar to the vessels', so that the transform yields strong

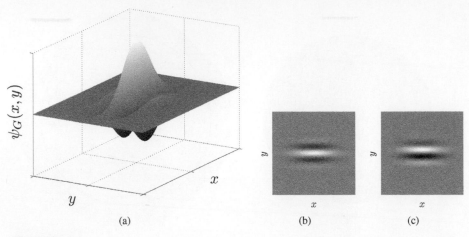

(a)   (b)   (c)

FIGURE 8.4

Different representations for the 2-D Gabor wavelet (ψ_G) with parameters $\varepsilon = 4$ and $\mathbf{k}_0 = [0,3]$: (a) surface representation of the real part; (b) real part; (c) imaginary part. Darker and lighter shades represent, respectively, positive and negative values.

coefficients when at the same position, scale, and orientation as a vessel, by means of the scalar product in $L^2(\mathbb{R}^2)$ (see Section 8.2.2).

In order to detect vessels in any orientation, for each considered position and scale, the response with maximum modulus over all possible orientations is kept, i.e.,

$$M_\psi(\mathbf{b}, a) = \max_\theta |T_\psi(\mathbf{b}, a, \theta)|. \tag{8.29}$$

Thus, for each pixel position and chosen scale, the Gabor wavelet transform is computed for θ spanning from 0 up to 170 degrees at steps of 10 degrees and the maximum is taken (this is possible because $|T_\psi(\mathbf{b}, a, \theta)| = |T_\psi(\mathbf{b}, a, \theta + 180)|$). The maximum moduli of the wavelet transform over all angles for various scales are then taken as pixel features. $M_\psi(\mathbf{b}, a)$ is shown in Figure 8.5 for $a = 2$ and $a = 5$ pixels.

8.3.3   Feature normalization

The measures used as features may have ranges spanning different orders of magnitude. This can lead to errors in the classification process because of the disparity of each feature's influence in the calculation of feature space distances. A strategy to obtain a new random variable with zero mean and unit standard deviation, compensating for eventual magnitude differences, is to apply the normal transformation to each feature. The normal transformation is defined as [36]

$$\hat{v}_i = \frac{v_i - \mu_i}{\sigma_i}, \tag{8.30}$$

where v_i is the ith feature of each pixel, μ_i is the average value of the feature, and σ_i is its standard deviation.

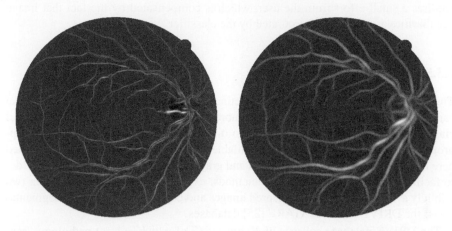

FIGURE 8.5

Maximum modulus of the Gabor wavelet transform over angles, $M_\psi(\mathbf{b}, a)$ (Equation 8.29), for scale values of $a = 2$ (left) and $a = 5$ (right) pixels.

The normal transformation was applied separately to each image, i.e., each image's feature space was normalized using its own means and standard deviations, helping to compensate for intrinsic variation between images, such as global illumination variation.

8.3.4 Supervised pixel classification

After feature generation and normalization, segmentations were obtained through supervised classification of image pixels into the classes $C_1 = \{vessel\ pixels\}$ and $C_2 = \{nonvessel\ pixels\}$. Supervised classification involves using labeled training samples (samples with known classes) to compose a training set, that then serves as a basis for future classification. Manual image segmentations (see Section 8.3.5) can be used to provide these labels. Many classifiers then go through a training phase, involving, for example, parameter estimation on the training set, preparing them for classification of new, unlabeled, pixel samples (see Figure 8.2).

In the experiments performed, the training sets were composed of labeled pixels from several manually segmented retinal images. Due to the computational cost of training the classifier and the large number of samples, subsets of the available labeled samples were randomly selected to actually be used for training.

Another approach for image segmentation through supervised classification, that showed interesting results, is to form the training set with labeled samples taken from a portion of the image to be segmented [68]. Using this approach, a semi-automated fundus segmentation software could be developed, in which the user only has to draw a small portion of the vessels over the input image or simply click on several pixels associated with vessels. The remaining image would then be automatically segmented based on this specific training set. This approach is interesting since it requires a small effort from the user, which is compensated by the fact that image peculiarities are directly incorporated by the classifier.

8.3.5 Public image databases

There are different ways of obtaining retinal images, such as with colored digital cameras or through angiography using fluorescent dyes (see Section 8.1). The pixel classification approach can be applied to different image modalities, provided appropriate manual segmentations are available for training. The approach described here has been tested on colored images and gray-scale angiograms [65; 66]. In order to facilitate comparisons with other methods, experiments are presented using two publicly available databases of colored images and corresponding manual segmentations: the DRIVE [28] and STARE [25] databases.

The DRIVE database consists of 40 images (7 of which present pathology), randomly selected from a diabetic retinopathy screening program in the Netherlands, along with manual segmentations of the vessels. They were captured in digital form from a Canon CR5 nonmydriatic 3CCD camera at 45° FOV. The images are of size 768×584 pixels, 8 bits per color channel and have an FOV of approximately 540 pixels in diameter. The images are in compressed JPEG-format, which is unfortunate for image processing, but is commonly used in screening practice.

The authors of this database divided the 40 images into fixed training and test sets, each containing 20 images (the training set has 3 images with pathology and the test set, 4) [21; 28]. The images have been manually segmented by three observers trained by an ophthalmologist. Images in the training set were segmented once, while images in the test set were segmented twice, resulting in sets A and B of manual segmentations. The observers of sets A and B produced similar segmentations: in set A, 12.7% of pixels where marked as vessel, against 12.3% vessel for set B. A normal image from the test set and its respective manual segmentations are illustrated in Figure 8.6. Performance is measured on the test set using the segmentations of set A as ground truth. The segmentations of set B are tested against those of A, serving as a human observer reference for performance comparison.

The STARE database consists of 20 digitized slides captured by a TopCon TRV-50 fundus camera at 35° FOV. The slides were digitized to 700×605 pixels, 8 bits per color channel. The FOV in the images is approximately 650×550 pixels in diameter. Images were selected so that ten of them contained pathologies, which complicates vessel detection. This choice was made so that the performance difference on normal and pathological images could be assessed. Two observers manually segmented all 20 images. The first observer segmented 10.4% of pixels as vessel, against 14.9% vessels for the second observer. The segmentations of the two observers are fairly different in that the second observer consistently segmented much more of the thinner vessels than the first. Figure 8.6 shows an image from the database and its respective manual segmentations. Previous tests using this database [20; 25–28] calculated performance using segmentations from the first observer as ground truth, with the second observer's segmentations being tested against the first. There is no predefined

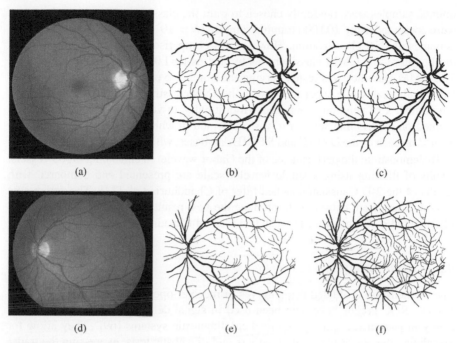

(a)   (b)   (c)

(d)   (e)   (f)

FIGURE 8.6

Images from the DRIVE and STARE databases and their respective manual segmentations: (a) normal image from the test set of the DRIVE database; (b) manual segmentation from set A; (c) manual segmentation from set B; (d) normal image from the STARE database; (e) manual segmentation by the first observer; and (f) manual segmentation by the second observer. **(See color insert following page 174.)**

separation into training and test sets, therefore leave-one-out tests are performed for supervised method performance evaluation.

8.3.6 Experiments and settings

The methods described were tested on the DRIVE and STARE databases with the following settings. The pixel features used for classification were the inverted green channel and its maximum Gabor wavelet transform response over angles $M_\psi(\mathbf{b}, a)$ (Equation 8.29) for scales $a = 2, 3, 4, 5$ pixels (see Subsection 8.3.2). These scales were chosen to span the possible widths of vessels throughout the images, so that all vessels could be detected.

For the DRIVE database, the training set was formed by pixel samples from the 20 labeled training images. For the STARE database, leave-one-out tests were performed, i.e., every image was segmented using samples from the other 19 images for the training set (see Section 8.3.5). The three classifiers presented in Section 8.2 were evaluated to allow their comparison. Due to the large number of pixels, in all experiments, samples were randomly chosen to train the classifiers. The three classifiers were compared using 100 000 training samples ($N = 10^5$), because of computational demands of kNN classification. However, for comparison with other methods from the literature, the GMM classifier was trained using 1 000 000 samples ($N = 10^6$). The GMM classifier was tested varying the number c of Gaussians modeling each class likelihood, while experiments with the kNN classifier used different values for the number k of neighbors analyzed. Additionally, to verify the dependence of the method on the training set, a test was performed in which the GMM classifier was trained on each of the DRIVE and STARE databases, while being tested on the other.

To demonstrate the performance of the Gabor wavelet in enhancing blood vessels, results of filtering using a single wavelet scale are presented and compared with results of the 2-D Gaussian matched filter of Chaudhuri et al. [24]. The parameters of both filters were chosen as to produce the best results: $a = 4$ pixels for wavelet filtering and $\sigma = 1$ pixel for the matched filter of Chaudhuri et al.

8.3.7   ROC analysis

The methods are evaluated using curves in receiver operating characteristic (ROC) graphs. ROC graphs have long been used in signal detection theory and more recently in pattern recognition and medical diagnostic systems [69]. They allow for visualizing the performance of classifiers and diagnostic tests, expressing the trade-off between increased detection and false alarm rates.

ROC curves are formed by ordered pairs of true positive and false positive fractions. Different fractions are established varying each method's parameters [25–27] or thresholds on posterior probabilities [28]. For each configuration of parameters or threshold value, a pair formed by a true positive and a false positive fraction corresponding to the method's outcome is marked on the graph, producing a curve as in Figure 8.7. In the scenario of evaluating vessel segmentations, true positives are pixels marked as vessel (positive) in both the segmentation given by a method and the manual segmentation used as ground truth. False positives are pixels marked as vessel by the method, but are actually negative in the ground truth. Classification measures are summarized in the *confusion matrix* (also known as contingency table), illustrated in Table 8.1. The total of positives and negatives in the ground truth are denoted P and N; the total number of true and false positives are TP and FP; and true and false negatives are denoted TN and FN, as shown in the confusion matrix. Metrics used in evaluation can then be derived from the matrix elements. True positive and false positive fractions, denoted TPF and FPF, are given by

$$\mathrm{TPF} = \frac{\mathrm{TP}}{\mathrm{P}} \qquad \mathrm{FPF} = \frac{\mathrm{FP}}{\mathrm{N}}. \tag{8.31}$$

The accuracy (fraction of correctly classified pixels) of the methods and human observers tested against the ground truth are also measured during performance evaluation. Accuracy is given by $(\mathrm{TP} + \mathrm{TN})/(\mathrm{P} + \mathrm{N})$, simply measuring the fraction of correct classification. Contrasting with ROC measures, accuracy does not express

Table 8.1: Confusion matrix.

		Ground Truth	
		Positive (P)	Negative (N)
Method result	Positive	True positive (TP)	False positive (FP)
	Negative	False negative (FN)	True negative (TN)

the relation between quantities of true positives and false positives, being sensitive to skews in class distribution.

Some points on the ROC graph help give an intuitive idea of the representation (see Figure 8.7). The lower left point $(0,0)$ represents an extremely conservative method that assigns only negative to all samples. Thus, it is incapable of producing true positives, though it also does not produce false positives. The opposite strategy, which is to assign positive to all samples, corresponds to the upper right point $(1,1)$. The closer an ROC curve is to the upper left corner, the better the method's performance, with the point $(0,1)$ representing a perfect agreement with the ground truth. Accordingly, an ROC curve is said to dominate another if it is completely above and to the left of it. The diagonal line in which TPF = FPF represents a random assignment strategy, with different points of the line corresponding to different fractions of random assignment of negatives and positives.

A very important property of ROC graphs is their invariance to changes in prior class distributions, represented by the proportion of positive and negative samples. This is possible because the fractions analyzed are relative to the total of samples in each class. The same does not apply to other measures, such as accuracy, described previously. In an analogous manner, ROC graphs are also invariant to changes in costs associated with classification decisions [70].

The area under an ROC curve (A_z) is used as a single scalar measure of a method's performance. A_z values, being fractions of a unitary square, necessarily lie between 0 and 1. Nevertheless, as a random classifier would produce a diagonal line connecting $(0,0)$ and $(1,1)$ with $A_z = 0.5$, in practice, methods should always have $A_z \geq 0.5$. A method that agreed completely with the manual segmentations used as ground truth would yield an $A_z = 1$. It is possible for a method with larger area under the curve to have a worse performance in a given region of the graph than one with smaller area, as illustrated in Figure 8.7. However, the area serves as good estimate of a method's overall performance. The areas under the ROC curves have an important statistical property: they are equivalent to the Wilcoxon statistic [71], the probability that a method assign a larger chance or rank to a randomly chosen positive sample than that assigned to a randomly chosen negative sample.

In order to draw conclusions about method superiority, it is not sufficient that a method's ROC curve calculated over a given dataset dominate that of another, as variances must be taken into account. These variances can be estimated using approaches such as cross-validation and bootstrapping [69]. The same principle applies for comparison of accuracy and A_z measures. In [27; 28; 67], these measures were

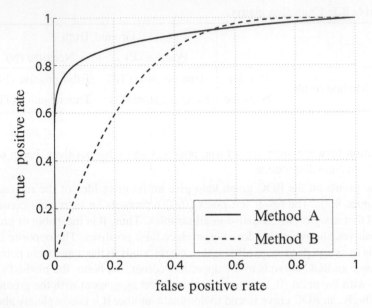

FIGURE 8.7

Example of an ROC graph with two curves. The area under the curve (A_z) of method
A is larger than that of method *B*, though *B* should be preferred for false positive
fractions larger than approximately 0.5.

taken for different methods and compared in paired statistical hypothesis tests, with
the accuracy and A_z of each image segmentation result representing an observation.
Here, the evaluation does not include significance tests, though that may provide for
a stronger statement.

In the experiments performed, measures were taken over all test images, considering only pixels inside the FOV defined by the camera aperture. For the GMM and
*k*NN classifiers, ROC curves are produced by varying the thresholds on posterior
pixel probability estimates, while the LMSE ROC curve is produced by varying the
threshold w_0 applied to the scalar product between the classifier's weight vector and
pixel feature vectors (Equation 8.23). Finally, the ROC curves for filtering using a
single wavelet scale and the matched filter of Chaudhuri et al. are produced varying the threshold on the filters' responses. For the DRIVE database, performance is
calculated using manual segmentations from set A as ground truth and human observer performance is estimated from manual segmentations from set B, which only
provides one true/false positive fraction pair, appearing as a point in the ROC graph
(Figure 8.13). For the STARE database, the first observer's manual segmentations are
used as ground truth and the second observer's true/false positive rate pair is plotted
on the graph (Figure 8.14). It is important to point out that the manual segmentations
evaluated do not present perfect true/false positive fractions, as they disagree on several pixels with the segmentations used as ground truth. Thus, the variance between
observers can be estimated, helping set a goal for method performance.

8.4 Implementation and Graphical User Interface

8.4.1 Overview

The implentation of the method for performing experiments led to a package of MATLAB [72] scripts, that now also includes a graphical user interface (GUI) for preliminary testing. The package, named mlvessel, is available as open-source code under the GNU General Public License (GPL) [73] at the project's collaborative development Web site, http://retina.iv.fapcsp.br. The Web site also contains some of the results presented here, allowing researchers to evaluate them in new and diverse manners. Experiments can be executed through function calls, with the specification of options and parameters in configuration files. Results are then presented as images and tables organized in HTML pages, as illustrated in Figure 8.8. Most of the package's functionality is also accessible through the GUI, outlined in Section 8.4.4.

To facilitate testing, a pipeline architecture was used, in which intermediate results are saved on disc for reutilization. In this manner, pixel features, training sets, and classifiers can be reused in different tests, saving up the computational effort necessary for their creation. Components of the pipeline, such as feature generation or classifier training (refer to Figure 8.2), can then be substituted for comparative tests. The software implementation is organized as the modules listed below, each corresponding to a directory inside the src/ directory.

- **tests**: examples of tests, which manipulate other modules. For complete examples, see scripts testmixed.m and testleaveoneout.m.

- **gui**: The GUI is initialized through its main window in guimain.m, which provides access to all others.

- **ftrs**: feature generation and manipulation, including creation of training sets. The createfeatures functions produce raw pixel features from images. The createlabelled functions receive the raw features and also manual segmentations, saving everything as labeled pixel features. Finally, the function createprocessed normalizes the labeled features, forming a training set that can then be fed to the classifiers.

- **gmm**: This module contains the GMM classifier. gmmcreatemodel receives a processed training set in order to create and save a classifier. gmmclassify receives a saved classifier and raw pixel features, producing each pixel's class as output.

- **knn**: an exhaustive implementation of the kNN classifier.

- **lmse**: This module contains the LMSE classifier. Creation and application of the classifier is analogous to that of the **gmm** module.

- **stats**: statistics generation from results. ROC graphs and statistics are organized in HTML pages, as illustrated in Figure 8.8.

- **html**: functions for formatting and saving HTML pages.

- **skel**: postprocessing and scale-space skeletonization [36] for application to vasculature segmentations. Part of the module is written in C with a MATLAB® programming interface.

MATLAB is a software extensively used for tasks such as image processing and includes an environment that provides for fast, prototypical software development. However, it is a commercial program and its use requires a license that is usually paid for. A new implementation of the method and interface is being developed in C++, which should be faster, have better usability, and be independent of MATLAB.

8.4.2 Installation

Installation should be simple, consisting of the following steps.

1. Download the mlvessel package, version 1.2 or later, from the project's Web site (http://retina.iv.fapesp.br).

2. Unpack the package (mlvessel.zip or mlvessel.tar.gz), using unzip or gnuzip and tar. Move the unzipped files to the directory where you wish the package to be installed.

3. Run the mlvesselinstall.m script from within MATLAB.

The mlvesselinstall.m script compiles the C code in the **skel** module, records the installation directory for future use, adds the **gui** and **tests** modules to the MATLAB path, and creates shortcut files for starting the software. You might want to add the **gui** and **tests** modules permanently to the paths in startup.m. Alternatively, the software may be started through the shortcuts mlvessel.bat and mlvesselgui.bat on Windows or mlvessel.sh and mlvesselgui.sh on Unix platforms, which should add the paths appropriately on startup. It is important to note that the package requires standard MATLAB toolboxes to run properly, such as the image processing toolbox.

8.4.3 Command line interface

All of the package's features are available through functions accessible from the command prompt of the MATLAB environment. Some of the features, such as the **stats** module for generation of statistics from results, are currently only available through function invocation, as the GUI has not yet been developed for them. The tests' outputs are saved as images, .mat files, and HTML pages as illustrated in Figure 8.8. The major experiments listed below serve as good starting points and examples of use:

>> testmixed(someconfig): experiments for separate train and test sets, as used here for the DRIVE database;

>> testleaveoneout(someconfig): leave-one-out experiments, as used here for the STARE database.

someconfig describes a structure containing all experimental configurations, including testing and training image file names, classifier specifications, and pixel features to be used. Examples of configuration structures are in src/tests/driveconfig.m and src/tests/stareconfig.m. Images for tests were not included in the package, but can be downloaded directly from the DRIVE and STARE databases.

8.4.4 Graphical user interface

A GUI has been implemented in MATLAB for preliminary testing by users. It can be initialized through its main window (Figure 8.9(a)) in guimain.m, which provides access to all others. The interface currently comprehends:

- visualizing and saving images composed of pixel features;

- specifying, configuring, training, and saving classifiers;

- opening and visualizing classifiers and applying them for image segmentation.

Following is a brief description of GUI use, which illustrates the supervised classification framework, from feature generation and classifier training to image segmentation.

8.4.4.1 Visualizing Pixel Features

Images can be opened through the main window menu at **File → Image → Open**. After opening an image, pixel features are generated and viewed by accessing **Image → View Features** from the image window menu (Figure 8.9(b)). The **Choose features** dialogue will then appear so that features may be specified. First, the image type must be informed. Depending on image type, possible pixel feature choices are the inverted green channel (colored images), inverted gray-scale channel (red-free images), or original gray-scale channel (fluorescein angiograms) and each of these processed by the Gabor wavelet ($M_\psi(\mathbf{b}, a)$, as in Equation 8.29) for different possible choices of the parameters: vertical basic frequency k_y, elongation ε, and scale a (see Equation 8.14). After confirming feature selection, they are generated (feature generation may take a few minutes), after which a window for visualization will appear, providing the option of saving pixel feature images.

8.4.4.2 Creating and Saving a Classifier

Figure 8.9(c) illustrates a classifier window in which a set of classifier options has been chosen. The following steps should be followed in order to create a classifier.

1. In the main program window menu, choose **File → Classifier → New**. This will open a new classifier window.

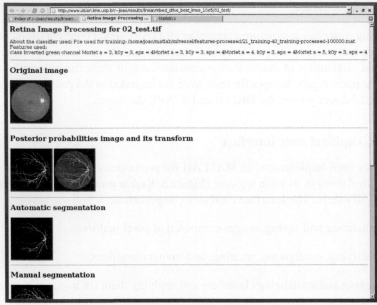

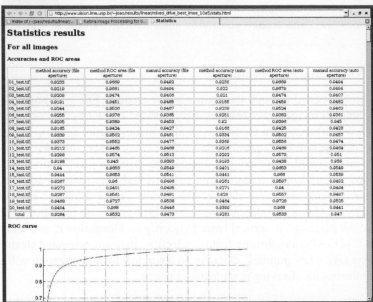

FIGURE 8.8

Examples of HTML outputs produced using the mlvessel package. Top: segmentation results for an image from the DRIVE database. Bottom: statistics and ROC graphs for results on the DRIVE database. **(See color insert.)**

2. Specify the classifier properties: type of classifier (GMM, kNN, or LMSE), its parameters, and number of training samples.

3. Choose the image type (colored, red-free, or fluorescein angiogram) for the classifier and specify pixel features to be used.

4. Indicate training images and respective manual segmentations.

5. Click on **Create classifier**. Depending on the previous choices, the classifier creation process may take from minutes to hours.

Once the classifier is created, it is ready to be used to segment new images. Classifiers can be saved for future use through their menu at **Classifier** → **Save as** and should be loaded through the main window menu at **File** → **Classifier** → **Open**, which also allows all of the classifier's properties to be viewed.

8.4.4.3 Applying a Classifier for Image Segmentation

In order to segment an image, a suitable classifier must be chosen. The **Segment image** dialogue, shown in Figure 8.9(d), is used to match an image with a classifier for segmentation. It can be reached through the image window menu at **Image** → **Segment Image** or the classifier window at the **Segment Image** button. The image chosen to be segmented should match the modality and approximate resolution of the images used to train the classifier, as the features generated for segmentation will be the same as specified during classifier creation. In this manner, the segmentation step does not require choosing features or any kind of parameter configuration. The result will then appear as a gray-scale image representing posterior probabilities, along with the final segmentation (see Figure 8.9(e)), both of which can then be saved.

8.5 Experimental Results

Illustrative segmentation results for a pair of images from each of the DRIVE and STARE databases (produced by the GMM classifier with $c = 20$ and $N = 10^6$), along with corresponding manual segmentations, are shown in Figures 8.10 and 8.11. Figure 8.12 presents results for the same images and settings, but with the GMM classifier being trained on each of the DRIVE and STARE databases, while tested on the other. The results shown are images formed by estimated posterior probabilities of each pixel belonging to class C_1 (vessel), as well as the final segmentation, produced by thresholding the posterior probabilities at $p(C_1|\mathbf{v}) > 0.5$.

Table 8.2 presents comparative results for the three different classifiers tested. Areas under the ROC curves (A_z) and accuracies are presented for the GMM classifier with different values of c; kNN classifier with different values of k and the LMSE classifier. The results for this table were produced with classifiers trained

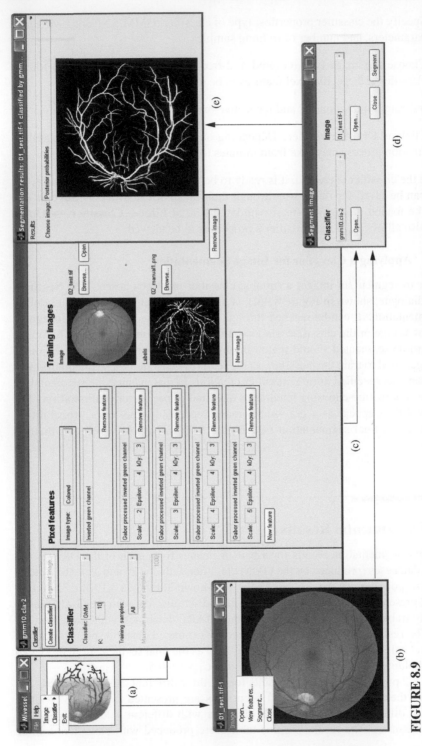

FIGURE 8.9

Windows and dialogues from the GUI illustrating the supervised image segmentation process: (a) main window; (b) image window; (c) classifier window; (d) image segmentation dialogue; and (e) segmentation result window. **(See color insert.)**

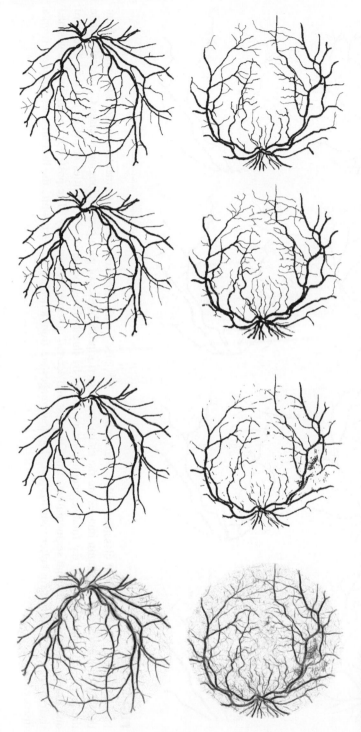

FIGURE 8.10

Results produced by the GMM classifier with $c = 20$ and $N = 10^6$, along with respective manual segmentations, for two images from the DRIVE database. First column images are the estimated posterior probabilities of each pixel belonging to class C_1 (vessel), while the second column images are the final segmentations, produced by thresholding posterior probabilities at $p(C_1|\mathbf{v}) > 0.5$. The third and fourth columns are manual segmentations from sets A and B, respectively. The posterior probability images had their histograms modified for better visualization.

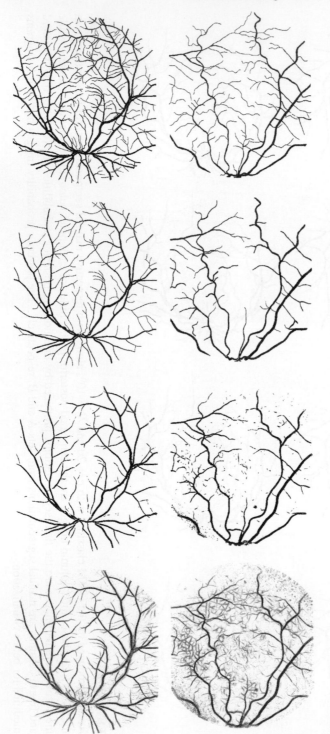

FIGURE 8.11

Results produced by the GMM classifier with $c = 20$ and $N = 10^6$, along with respective manual segmentations, for two images from the STARE database. First column images are the estimated posterior probabilities of each pixel belonging to class C_1 (vessel), while the second column images are the final segmentations, produced by thresholding posterior probabilities at $p(C_1|\mathbf{v}) > 0.5$. The third and fourth columns are manual segmentations from the first and second observer, respectively. The posterior probability images had their histograms modified for better visualization. Top row images are from a healthy subject, while the bottom ones originate from a diseased subject.

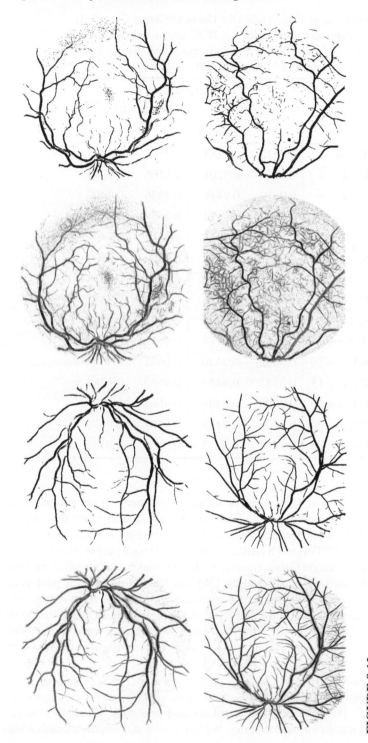

FIGURE 8.12

Results produced by training the GMM classifier with $c = 20$ and $N = 10^6$ on each of the DRIVE and STARE databases, with testing on the other, for images presented in Figures 8.10 and 8.11. First and third column images are the estimated posterior probabilities of each pixel belonging to class C_1 (vessel), while the second and fourth column images are the final segmentations, produced by thresholding posterior probabilities at $p(C_1|\mathbf{v}) > 0.5$. The posterior probability images had their histograms modified for better visualization.

Table 8.2: A_z and Accuracies for Using Different Classifiers (A_z indicates the area under the ROC curve, while the accuracy is the fraction of correctly classified pixels. All classifiers were trained using 100 000 samples ($N = 10^5$).)

Classifier used	Database			
	DRIVE		STARE	
	A_z	Accuracy	A_z	Accuracy
LMSE	0.9532	0.9284	0.9602	0.9365
kNN, $k = 1$	0.8220	0.9201	0.8166	0.9273
kNN, $k = 8$	0.9339	0.9446	0.9336	0.9460
kNN, $k = 32$	0.9529	0.9473	0.9558	0.9480
kNN, $k = 64$	0.9568	0.9475	0.9612	0.9482
kNN, $k = 128$	0.9591	0.9479	0.9636	0.9480
kNN, $k = 256$	0.9605	0.9478	0.9653	0.9478
kNN, $k = 512$	0.9609	0.9476	0.9658	0.9472
GMM, $c = 1$	0.9287	0.9227	0.9409	0.9244
GMM, $c = 5$	0.9549	0.9419	0.9616	0.9437
GMM, $c = 10$	0.9582	0.9446	0.9657	0.9474
GMM, $c = 15$	0.9592	0.9454	0.9657	0.9469
GMM, $c = 20$	0.9600	0.9468	0.9666	0.9478
GMM, $c = 30$	0.9609	0.9468	0.9661	0.9476
GMM, $c = 40$	0.9610	0.9473	0.9665	0.9479

with 100 000 samples ($N = 10^5$). Diverse segmentation methods are compared in Table 8.3, that presents areas under the ROC curves and accuracies for the following methods: GMM classifier with $c = 20$ and $N = 10^6$; the same classifier being trained on each of the DRIVE and STARE databases and tested on the other (crossed test); filtering using a single Gabor wavelet scale; the matched filter of Chaudhuri et al. [24]; and the methods of Jiang et al. [26] and Staal et al. [28], as published in [28]. Accuracies are also presented for manual segmentations from human observers. ROC curves for the DRIVE and STARE databases produced using the GMM classifier with $c = 20$ and $N = 10^6$, filtering using a single Gabor wavelet scale, the matched filter of Chaudhuri et al., as well as points representing human observer performance, are shown in Figures 8.13 and 8.14.

The Expectation-Maximization training process for the GMMs is computationally more expensive as c increases, but can be done off-line, while the classification phase is fast. The kNN classifier, implemented in a straightforward exhaustive manner, does not go through training, but has a very demanding classification

Table 8.3: A_z and Accuracies for Different Segmentation Methods and a Second Human Observer (A_z indicates the area under the ROC curve, while the accuracy is the fraction of correctly classified pixels.)

	Database			
Classifier used	DRIVE		STARE	
	A_z	Accuracy	A_z	Accuracy
GMM, $c = 20$, $N = 10^6$	0.9614	0.9466	0.9671	0.9480
Crossed test, GMM, $c = 20$, $N = 10^6$	0.9522	0.9404	0.9601	0.9328
$M_\psi(\mathbf{b}, 4)$	0.9312		0.9351	
Chaudhuri et al. [24]	0.9103		0.8987	
Jiang et al. [26]	0.9327	0.8911	0.9298	0.9009
Staal et al. [28]	0.9520	0.9441	0.9614	0.9516
Second observer		0.9473		0.9349

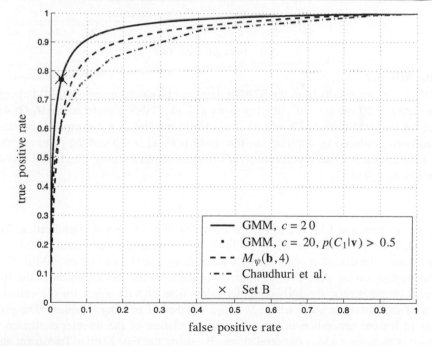

FIGURE 8.13

ROC curves for results from the DRIVE database produced using the GMM classifier with $c = 20$ and $N = 10^6$, filtering using a single Gabor wavelet scale ($M_\psi(\mathbf{b}, 4)$) and the matched filter of Chaudhuri et al. Point marked as • corresponds to classifications produced by applying the threshold $p(C_1|\mathbf{v}) > 0.5$ and the point marked as × corresponds to set B, the second set of manual segmentations. The GMM classifier has $A_z = 0.9614$.

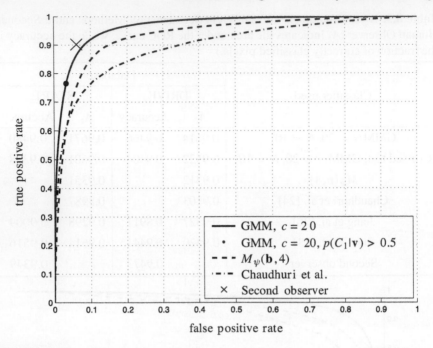

FIGURE 8.14
ROC curves for results from the STARE database produced using the GMM classi-
fier with $c = 20$ and $N = 10^6$, filtering using a single Gabor wavelet scale ($M_\psi(\mathbf{b}, 4)$)
and the matched filter of Chaudhuri et al. Point marked as ● corresponds to clas-
sifications produced by applying the threshold $p(C_1|\mathbf{v}) > 0.5$ and the point marked
as × corresponds to the second observer's manual segmentations. The GMM classifier has $A_z = 0.9671$.

phase. In turn, the LMSE classifier is both fast in training and classification, but
provides poorer results, as shown in Table 8.2. Fixing the dimension of the feature space, classification of an image's pixel feature vectors using the GMM classifier is fast, taking time $O(cP)$, where P is the total number of pixels in the image. Comparatively, the kNN classifier takes time $O(NP)$ solely for the calculation of the distances used, where N is the number of training samples. The process of feature generation is basically the calculation of the wavelet coefficients,
which is done by a series of correlations. By using the Fast Fourier Transform and
the Fourier definition of the wavelet transform (Equation 8.15), these are done in
$O(P\log_2 P)$ [49]. A nonoptimized MATLAB implementation was used for these
tests. On an AMD Athlon XP 2700+ PC (2167 MHz clock) with 1 GB memory,
feature generation for typical images from the DRIVE and STARE databases takes
about 3 minutes. Estimation of the GMM parameters with $c = 20$ and $N = 10^5$
takes up to 2 hours (though this would speed up considerably with an optimized
implementation), while the classification of an image's pixels using this classifier

takes less than 10 seconds. On the other hand, classification of an image's pixels with the kNN classifier with the same number of training samples takes about 4 hours.

Note that the A_z and accuracy for the GMM classifier increased with c (Table 8.2). After some value of c, though, it is expected that the performance declines, since the model will probably be excessively adjusted (over-fit) to the training data (see Section 8.2.6). In a similar fashion, the A_z of the kNN classifier increased with k, but after a certain value a loss in the spatial precision of estimates is expected, which would also lead to performance decline (see Section 8.2.7). This kind of behavior is observed by the decrease in accuracy of the kNN classifier for $k \geq 128$. The decrease is caused by the small number of training samples coupled with high values of k, leading to an excessive amount of test samples being attributed to the nonvessel class. As ROC analysis is invariant to skews in class distribution, the A_z values were not affected, though it is still expected they decrease for larger values of k.

The manual segmentations help give an estimate of the variance between human observers. On the DRIVE database, the GMM classifier ROC curve is very close to the point representing the second set of manual segmentations (Figure 8.13). The method presents very good results on normal, well-behaved images, but pathological or poorly illuminated images (as discussed below) lower the overall performance. It is curious to note that, on the STARE database, the accuracy of some methods is higher than that of the second observer (Table 8.3). The second observer's manual segmentations contain much more of the thinnest vessels than the first observer (lowering their accuracy), while the method, trained by the first observer, is able to segment the vessels at a similar fraction. Nevertheless, the ROC graph (Figure 8.14) still reflects the higher precision of the second observer, due to some difficulties found by the method, as discussed below.

Visual inspection reveals typical problems that must be solved by future work. The major errors are in false detection of noise and other artifacts. False detection occurs in some images at the border of the optic disc, hemorrhages, microaneurysms, exudates, and other types of pathologies that present strong contrast. Another difficulty is the detection of the thinnest vessels that are barely perceived by human observers. Also, the method did not perform well for very large variations in lighting throughout an image, but this occurred for only one image out of the 40 tested from both databases.

The crossed test, in which images from each database were segmented by a classifier trained on the other, presented slightly worse results than the standard experiments (Table 8.3 and Figure 8.12). Though the databases are similar, there is a difference in the typical vessel widths found in each database's images, which contributed significantly to the performance loss. In the results from the DRIVE database, the thinner vessels are poorly detected and there is an increase in noise appearing as false positives. Results from the STARE database present much more noise and also pathologies detected as false positives. While the performance difference is not large, this shows that even for the simple vessel structures there is a certain dependence of the method on the training set. The classifier is capable of adjusting to specific acquisition conditions, but not able to generalize perfectly to others.

8.6   Conclusion

8.6.1   Summary

The Gabor wavelet shows itself efficient in enhancing vessel contrast while filtering out noise, giving better performance than the matched filter of Chaudhuri et al. [24]. Information from wavelet responses at different scales is combined through the supervised classification framework, allowing proper segmentation of vessels of various widths. Of the three classifiers tested, the LMSE gave the worst performance, but with fast training and classification phases. The kNN classifier showed good performance, but with a slow classification phase, complicating its use in interactive applications. Finally, the GMM classifier has a demanding training process, but guarantees a fast classification phase and good performance, similar to that of the kNN. Feature generation consists of computing a series of wavelet coefficients and can be implemented efficiently, resulting in an approach that can be included in an interactive tool. An open-source prototype of an interactive software for vessel segmentation — based on a graphical user interface that assists the process of classifier training and vessel segmentation — was described, including details on the most important steps.

The supervised classification framework demands use of manual labelings, but allows classifiers to be trained for different image modalities, possibly adjusted to specific camera or lighting conditions but are otherwise automatic, i.e., adjustment of parameters or user interaction is not necessary. The experiments in which the GMM classifier was trained on each of the DRIVE and STARE databases and tested on the other showed the dependence of the method on the training set. As an alternative training process, labeled samples from the image to be segmented provided by a user may be used, allowing image peculiarities to be incorporated [68]. Recent supervised methods have shown good results with respect to ROC analysis, even though they are restricted to local vessel detection [21; 28]. Supervised classification avoids formulation of complex rules that deal with specific situations, as the complexity can be directly incorporated by the classifier. Given the conceptual simplicity of the approach presented here, it could easily be applied to the segmentation of other oriented structures, such as neurons or roads in aerial photography, in spite of no experiment having been performed in this sense.

8.6.2   Future work

The work performed here can be improved. In particular, visual inspection of results reveals difficulties that suggest ideas for the future evolution of methods.

The method did not respond well to large lighting variations within images. These variations could be compensated in a preprocessing step or otherwise somehow incorporated into pixel feature vectors. The Gabor wavelet presented in Equation 8.14, when adjusted to low frequencies, does not present zero mean. Thus, in the implementation evaluated, it was not totally insensitive to background variations. This could be corrected with the introduction of the wavelet's correction term [39]. The term, however, when added to low frequency wavelets, leads to loss in spatial precision, being prejudicial when analyzing the modulus. To overcome this, it is possible to separately analyze the real and imaginary parts of the coefficients (or equivalently, modulus and phase) or modify the wavelet appropriately, as was done in [60].

In order to distinguish borders and other artifacts from vessels, information about the presence of edges could be explicitly incorporated, possibly through the inclusion of new wavelet coefficients in the feature vectors. The wavelet transform is capable of providing a local representation of the image, revealing directional structures as the vessels in this work. Representation using the Gabor wavelet is done by deriving frames that provide complete but redundant representations [39; 51]. It is worth noting that there are fast algorithms for calculation of 2-D CWT frames, which could speed up considerably the application of the method [74].

The training approach that uses samples from the image being segmented provided by an operator may present better results, since image peculiarities are incorporated by the classifier. It can be difficult or tiresome for a user to interactively supply a representative sampling. Being so, it would be interesting to study a strategy to take advantage of both the available samples from other images as well as those from the image to be segmented. In this manner, with minimal user effort, information about specific image conditions and the large number of examples from other images can be taken into account.

A drawback of the approach presented here is that it only takes into account information local to each pixel through the wavelet transform, ignoring useful information from image shapes and structures. The segmentation results can be slightly improved through a post-processing of the segmentations for removal of noise and inclusion of missing vessel pixels as in [66]. An intermediate result of the method is the intensity image of posterior probabilities to which global vessel segmentation algorithms could be applied, providing more precise results. Many approaches have been studied that take into account shape and structure for vessel segmentation, such as tracking [3; 6; 7], threshold probing [25; 26], region growing [23], and deformable models [75; 76].

Depending on the application, different evaluation methods become more appropriate [77]. For example, the evaluation of the vasculature skeleton or tracings would not take into account vessel widths, but could measure other qualities such as the presence of gaps and detection of branching and crossing points. Vessel widths are fundamental in change and pathology detection, but can be discarded in applications like image registration or morphological analysis of the vasculature. In [78], true and false positives are defined from skeletons in the following manner: if a pixel from some method's skeleton is at a distance inferior to three pixels to a pixel from a manual segmentation, it is counted as a true positive; otherwise, it is a false positive. In [67], a similar approach is presented, in which thinned versions of the manual segmentations are used and, additionally, true and false negatives are defined. ROC analysis using complete vessel segmentations, on the other hand, takes vessel widths into account in such a manner that wide vessels have a much larger influence than thin ones. Another interesting form of evaluation would be directly through an application, such as in detection of neovascularization by means of analysis and classification of the vessel structure [11]. Qualitative visual assessment is still very important for segmentation evaluation, allowing the identification of strengths and weaknesses of each method and localizing specific regions in which a given method performs better or worse. Still, it is a laborious and subjective analysis. Though very good ROC results are presented, visual inspection (as discussed in Section 8.5) shows typical difficulties of the method to be worked on.

A major difficulty in evaluating the results is the establishment of a reliable ground truth [2]. Human observers are subjective and prone to errors, resulting in large variability between observations. Thus, it is desirable that multiple human-generated segmentations be combined to establish a ground truth, which was not the case in the analysis presented. Moreover, in an ideal scenario, manual segmentations would be provided by ophthalmologists, so that the classifier be calibrated accordingly. As an alternative to manually segmenting several images, synthetic images might be used. The images would then have segmentations known beforehand and problems of human observers such as subjectivity, errors, and workload would be avoided. The problem with synthetic images is that it is practically impossible to faithfully reproduce the complexity of retinal image formation, yielding this approach inadequate for a complete evaluation. Nonetheless, it could be applied in partial experiments, such as in measuring the adequacy of vessel models or robustness under different kinds of noise. For future work, a more complete evaluation is desirable: it would be interesting to evaluate performance on different image modalities; hypothesis tests could be performed for method comparison (as done in [27; 28; 67]); and confidence bands for ROC curves could also be presented [69].

Properties of the retinal vasculature can be quantified through morphological analysis techniques, assisting in the diagnosis of diabetic retinopathy. Fractal [11] and multifractal [12] analysis provide numeric indicators of the extent of neovascularization, while vessel lengths, widths [14], and curvature [15] have been identified as important characteristics for diagnosing diabetic retinopathy. The segmentation method presented shows good results and large potential for improvement, being theoretically founded on the 2-D CWT and statistical classification. It is capable of producing results in reasonable time and lessens the need for user interaction, representing an effort towards automated retinal assessment. A new implementation of the method is being developed that will be faster, have better usability, and be independent of the MATLAB platform, avoiding the need for licenses. It is expected that the software and graphical user interfaces developed evolve while being tested by final users, including nonspecialized health workers, ophthalmologists, and researchers.

Acknowledgments

The authors are extremely grateful to H. F. Jelinek and M. J. Cree for their long-lasting collaboration. The authors would also like to thank J. J. Staal and colleagues and A. Hoover for making their databases publicly available, Dr. A. Luckie and C. McQuellin from the Albury Eye Clinic for providing fluorescein images used during research, and P. Mani for running the tests of the Chaudhuri et al. method as part of her B. E. degree final year project. JVBS is grateful to CNPq (131403/2004-4) and FAPESP (2006/56128-1). RMC is also grateful to CNPq (300722/98-2, 474596/2004-4 and 491323/2005-0) and FAPESP (2005/00587-5).

References

[1] Kanski, J.J., *Clinical Ophthalmology: A systematic approach*, Butterworth-Heinemann, London, 1989.

[2] Fritzsche, K.H., Can, A., Shen, H., et al., Automated model-based segmentation, tracing, and analysis of retinal vasculature from digital fundus images, in *Angiography and Plaque Imaging: Advanced Segmentation Techniques*, J. Suri and S. Laxminarayan, eds., CRC Press, 225–297, 2003.

[3] Can, A., Shen, H., Turner, J.N., et al., Rapid automated tracing and feature extraction from retinal fundus images using direct exploratory algorithms, *IEEE Transactions on Information Technology in Biomedicine*, 3(2), 125, 1999.

[4] Chutatape, O., Zheng, L., and Krishnan, S.M., Retinal blood vessel detection and tracking by matched Gaussian and Kalman filters, in *Proc. of the 20th Annual International Conference of the IEEE Engineering in Medicine and Biology Society (EMBS)*, 1998, vol. 20, 3144–3149.

[5] Zhou, L., Rzeszotarski, M.S., Singerman, L.J., et al., The detection and quantification of retinopathy using digital angiograms, *IEEE Transactions on Medical Imaging*, 13(4), 619, 1994.

[6] Gang, L., Chutatape, O., and Krishnan, S.M., Detection and measurement of retinal vessels in fundus images using amplitude modified second-order Gaussian filter, *IEEE Transactions on Biomedical Engineering*, 49(2), 168, 2002.

[7] Tolias, Y.A. and Panas, S.M., A fuzzy vessel tracking algorithm for retinal images based on fuzzy clustering, *IEEE Transactions on Medical Imaging*, 17, 263, 1998.

[8] Lalonde, M., Gagnon, L., and Boucher, M.C., Non-recursive paired tracking for vessel extraction from retinal images, in *Proc. of the Conference Vision Interface 2000*, 2000, 61–68.

[9] Pinz, A., Bernogger, S., Datlinger, P., et al., Mapping the human retina, *IEEE Transactions on Medical Imaging*, 17, 606, 1998.

[10] Zana, F. and Klein, J.C., Segmentation of vessel-like patterns using mathemat-

ical morphology and curvature evaluation, *IEEE Transactions on Image Processing*, 10, 1010, 2001.

[11] Cesar, Jr., R.M. and Jelinek, H.F., Segmentation of retinal fundus vasculature in non-mydriatic camera images using wavelets, in *Angiography and Plaque Imaging: Advanced Segmentation Techniques*, J. Suri and T. Laxminarayan, eds., CRC Press, 193–224, 2003.

[12] McQuellin, C.P., Jelinek, H.F., and Joss, G., Characterisation of fluorescein angiograms of retinal fundus using mathematical morphology: A pilot study, in *5th International Conference on Ophthalmic Photography*, Adelaide, 2002, 152.

[13] Wong, T.Y., Rosamond, W., Chang, P.P., et al., Retinopathy and risk of congestive heart failure, *Journal of the American Medical Association*, 293(1), 63, 2005.

[14] Pedersen, L., Ersbøll, B., Madsen, K., et al., Quantitative measurement of changes in retinal vessel diameter in ocular fundus images, *Pattern Recognition Letters*, 21(13-14), 1215, 2000.

[15] Hart, W.E., Goldbaum, M., Côté, B., et al., Measurement and classification of retinal vascular tortuosity, *International Journal of Medical Informatics*, 53, 239, 1999.

[16] Jelinek, H.F., Leandro, J.J.G., Cesar, Jr., R.M., et al., Classification of pathology in diabetic eye disease, in *WDIC2005 ARPS Workshop on Digital Image Computing*, Brisbane, Australia, 2005, 9–13.

[17] Yang, G. and Stewart, C.V., Covariance-driven mosaic formation from sparsely-overlapping image sets with application to retinal image mosaicing, in *IEEE Computer Society Conference on Computer Vision and Pattern Recognition (CVPR)*, 2004, vol. 1, 804–810.

[18] Zana, F. and Klein, J.C., A multimodal registration algorithm of eye fundus images using vessels detection and hough transform, *IEEE Transactions on Medical Imaging*, 18, 419, 1999.

[19] Hill, R., Retina identification, in *Biometrics: Personal Identification in Networked Society*, A.K. Jain, R. Bolle, and S. Pankanti, eds., Kluwer Academic Publishers, 123–141, 1998.

[20] Cree, M.J., Leandro, J.J.G., Soares, J.V.B., et al., Comparison of various methods to delineate blood vessels in retinal images, in *Proc. of the 16th National Congress of the Australian Institute of Physics*, Canberra, Australia, 2005, available from: http://aipcongress2005.anu.edu.au/index.php?req=CongressProceedings. Cited May 2006.

[21] Niemeijer, M., Staal, J.J., van Ginneken, B., et al., Comparative study of retinal vessel segmentation methods on a new publicly available database, in *Medical*

Imaging 2004: Image Processing, J.M. Fitzpatrick and M. Sonka, eds., San Diego, CA, 2004, vol. 5370 of *Proc. SPIE*, 648–656.

[22] Soares, J.V.B., Leandro, J.J.G., Cesar, Jr., R.M., et al., Retinal vessel segmentation using the 2-D Gabor wavelet and supervised classification, *IEEE Transactions on Medical Imaging*, 25, 1214, 2006.

[23] Martínez-Pérez, M.E., Hughes, A.D., Stanton, A.V., et al., Retinal blood vessel segmentation by means of scale-space analysis and region growing, in *Medical Image Computing and Computer-assisted Intervention (MICCAI)*, 1999, 90–97.

[24] Chaudhuri, S., Chatterjee, S., Katz, N., et al., Detection of blood vessels in retinal images using two-dimensional matched filters, *IEEE Transactions on Medical Imaging*, 8, 263, 1989.

[25] Hoover, A., Kouznetsova, V., and Goldbaum, M., Locating blood vessels in retinal images by piecewise threshold probing of a matched filter response, *IEEE Transactions on Medical Imaging*, 19, 203, 2000.

[26] Jiang, X. and Mojon, D., Adaptive local thresholding by verification-based multithreshold probing with application to vessel detection in retinal images, *IEEE Transactions on Pattern Analysis and Machine Intelligence*, 25(1), 131, 2003.

[27] Mendonça, A.M. and Campilho, A., Segmentation of retinal blood vessels by combining the detection of centerlines and morphological reconstruction, *IEEE Transactions on Medical Imaging*, 25, 1200, 2006.

[28] Staal, J.J., Abràmoff, M.D., Niemeijer, M., et al., Ridge based vessel segmentation in color images of the retina, *IEEE Transactions on Medical Imaging*, 23(4), 501, 2004.

[29] Gabor, D., Theory of communication, *Journal of the IEE*, 93, 429, 1946.

[30] Rioul, O. and Vetterli, M., Wavelets and signal processing, *IEEE Signal Processing Magazine*, 8, 14, 1991.

[31] Goupillaud, P., Grossmann, A., and Morlet, J., Cycle-Octave and related transforms in seismic signal analysis, *Geoexploration*, 23, 85, 1984.

[32] Grossmann, A. and Morlet, J., Decomposition of hardy functions into square integrable wavelets of constant shape, *SIAM Journal on Mathematical Analysis*, 15, 723, 1984.

[33] Grossmann, A., Wavelet transforms and edge detection, in *Stochastic Processes in Physics and Engineering*, S. Albeverio, P. Blanchard, M. Hazewinkel, and L. Streit, eds., D. Reidel Publishing Company, 1988, 149–157.

[34] Mallat, S. and Hwang, W.L., Singularity detection and processing with wavelets, *IEEE Transactions on Information Theory*, 38(2), 617, 1992.

[35] Daubechies, I., *Ten lectures on wavelets*, Society for Industrial and Applied Mathematics, Philadelphia, PA, 1992.

[36] Costa, L.F. and Cesar, Jr., R.M., *Shape analysis and classification: Theory and practice*, CRC Press, 2001.

[37] Unser, M. and Aldroubi, A., A review of wavelets in biomedical applications, *Proceedings of the IEEE*, 84, 626, 1996.

[38] Van De Ville, D., Blu, T., and Unser, M., Integrated wavelet processing and spatial statistical testing of fMRI data, *NeuroImage*, 23(4), 1472, 2004.

[39] Antoine, J.P., Carette, P., Murenzi, R., et al., Image analysis with two-dimensional continuous wavelet transform, *Signal Processing*, 31, 241, 1993.

[40] Murenzi, R., *Ondelettes multidimensionelles et application à l'analyse d'images*, PhD thesis, Université Catholique de Louvain, 1990.

[41] Ferrari, R.J., Rangayyan, R.M., Desautels, J.E.L., et al., Analysis of asymmetry in mammograms via directional filtering with Gabor wavelets, *IEEE Transactions on Medical Imaging*, 20, 953, 2001.

[42] Manjunath, B.S. and Ma, W.Y., Texture features for browsing and retrieval of image data, *IEEE Transactions on Pattern Analysis and Machine Intelligence*, 18(8), 837, 1996.

[43] Mallat, S. and Zhong, S., Characterization of signals from multiscale edges, *IEEE Transactions on Pattern Analysis and Machine Intelligence*, 14(7), 710, 1992.

[44] Marr, D. and Hildreth, E., Theory of edge detection, *Proceedings of the Royal Society of London. Series B, Biological Sciences*, 207, 187, 1980.

[45] Argoul, F., Arnéodo, A., Elezgaray, J., et al., Wavelet analysis of the self-similarity of diffusion-limited aggregates and electrodeposition clusters, *Physical Review A*, 41(10), 5537, 1990.

[46] Arnéodo, A., Decoster, N., and Roux, S.G., A wavelet-based method for multifractal image analysis. I. Methodology and test applications on isotropic and anisotropic random rough surfaces, *The European Physical Journal B*, 15, 567, 2000.

[47] Farge, M., Wavelet transforms and their applications to turbulence, *Annual Review of Fluid Mechanics*, 24, 395, 1992.

[48] Antoine, J.P., Murenzi, R., and Vandergheynst, P., Directional wavelets revisited: Cauchy wavelets and symmetry detection in patterns, *Applied and Computational Harmonic Analysis*, 6, 314, 1999.

[49] Gonzalez, R.C. and Woods, R.E., *Digital Image Processing*, Addison-Wesley, 2nd ed., 2002.

[50] Antoine, J.P. and Murenzi, R., Two-dimensional directional wavelets and the scale-angle representation, *Signal Processing*, 52, 259, 1996.

[51] Lee, T.S., Image representation using 2D Gabor wavelets, *IEEE Transactions on Pattern Analysis and Machine Intelligence*, 18(10), 959, 1996.

[52] Daugman, J.G., Two-dimensional spectral analysis of cortical receptive field profiles, *Vision Research*, 20, 847, 1980.

[53] Marčelja, S., Mathematical description of the responses of simple cortical cells, *Journal of the Optical Society of America*, 70(11), 1297, 1980.

[54] Daugman, J.G., Complete discrete 2-D Gabor transforms by neural networks for image analysis and compression, *IEEE Transactions on Acoustics, Speech, and Signal Processing*, 36(7), 1169, 1988.

[55] Krueger, V. and Sommer, G., Gabor wavelet networks for face processing, *Journal of the Optical Society of America*, 19, 1112, 2002.

[56] Feris, R.S., Krueger, V., and Cesar, Jr., R.M., A wavelet subspace method for real-time face tracking, *Real-Time Imaging*, 10, 339, 2004.

[57] Sagiv, C., Sochen, N.A., and Zeevi, Y.Y., Gabor features diffusion via the minimal weighted area method, in *Energy Minimization Methods in Computer Vision and Pattern Recognition (EMMCVPR)*, 2002.

[58] Chen, J., Sato, Y., and Tamura, S., Orientation space filtering for multiple orientation line segmentation, *IEEE Transactions on Pattern Analysis and Machine Intelligence*, 22, 417, 2000.

[59] Ayres, F.J. and Rangayyan, R.M., Performance analysis of oriented feature detectors, in *Proc. of the 18th Brazilian Symposium on Computer Graphics and Image Processing (SIBGRAPI)*, IEEE Computer Society, 2005, 147–154.

[60] Harrop, J.D., Taraskin, S.N., and Elliott, S.R., Instantaneous frequency and amplitude identification using wavelets: Application to glass structure, *Physical Review E*, 66(2), 026703, 2002.

[61] Duda, R.O., Hart, P.E., and Stork, D.G., *Pattern Classification*, John Wiley and Sons, 2001.

[62] Theodoridis, S. and Koutroumbas, K., *Pattern Recognition*, Academic Press, San Diego, CA, 1st ed., 1999.

[63] Dempster, A.P., Laird, N.M., and Rubin, D.B., Maximum likelihood from incomplete data via the EM algorithm, *Journal of the Royal Statistical Society, Series B*, 39(1), 1, 1977.

[64] Figueiredo, M.A.T. and Jain, A.K., Unsupervised learning of finite mixture models, *IEEE Transactions on Pattern Analysis and Machine Intelligence*, 24, 381, 2002.

[65] Leandro, J.J.G., Cesar, Jr., R.M., and Jelinek, H.F., Blood vessels segmentation in retina: Preliminary assessment of the mathematical morphology and of the wavelet transform techniques, in *Proc. of the 14th Brazilian Symposium on Computer Graphics and Image Processing (SIBGRAPI)*, IEEE Computer Society, 2001, 84–90.

[66] Leandro, J.J.G., Soares, J.V.B., Cesar, Jr., R.M., et al., Blood vessels segmentation in non-mydriatic images using wavelets and statistical classifiers, in *Proc. of the 16th Brazilian Symposium on Computer Graphics and Image Processing (SIBGRAPI)*, IEEE Computer Society Press, 2003, 262–269.

[67] Sofka, M. and Stewart, C.V., Retinal vessel centerline extraction using multiscale matched filters, confidence and edge measures, *IEEE Transactions on Medical Imaging*, 25, 1531, 2006.

[68] Cornforth, D.J., Jelinek, H.F., Leandro, J.J.G., et al., Development of retinal blood vessel segmentation methodology using wavelet transforms for assessment of diabetic retinopathy, *Complexity International*, 11, 2005, cited May 2006, http://www.complexity.org.au/ci/vol11/.

[69] Fawcett, T., An introduction to ROC analysis, *Pattern Recognition Letters*, 27, 861, 2006.

[70] Provost, F. and Fawcett, T., Robust classification for imprecise environments, *Machine Learning*, 42(3), 203, 2001.

[71] Hanley, J.A. and McNeil, B.J., The meaning and use of the area under a receiver operating characteristic (ROC) curve, *Radiology*, 143, 29, 1982.

[72] MATLAB, MATLAB website at MathWorks, 2006, cited May 2006, http://www.mathworks.com/products/matlab.

[73] Free Software Foundation, GNU general public license, 1991, cited July 2006, http://www.gnu.org/copyleft/gpl.html.

[74] Vandergheynst, P. and Gobbers, J.F., Directional dyadic wavelet transforms: design and algorithms, *IEEE Transactions on Image Processing*, 11(4), 363, 2002.

[75] Malladi, R., Sethian, J.A., and Vemuri, B.C., Shape modeling with front propagation: A level set approach, *IEEE Transactions on Pattern Analysis and Machine Intelligence*, 17(2), 158, 1995.

[76] McInerney, T. and Terzopoulos, D., T-snakes: Topology adaptive snakes, *Medical Image Analysis*, 4, 73, 2000.

[77] Bowyer, K.W. and Phillips, P.J., eds., *Empirical Evaluation Techniques in Computer Vision*, IEEE Computer Society, 1998.

[78] Lowell, J., Hunter, A., Steel, D., et al., Measurement of retinal vessel widths from fundus images based on 2-D modeling, *IEEE Transactions on Medical Imaging*, 23(10), 1196, 2004.

9

Determining Retinal Vessel Widths and Detection of Width Changes

Kenneth H. Fritzsche, Charles V. Stewart, and Bardrinath Roysam

CONTENTS

9.1 Identifying Blood Vessels 270
9.2 Vessel Models... 270
9.3 Vessel Extraction Methods 271
9.4 Can's Vessel Extraction Algorithm..................................... 271
9.5 Measuring Vessel Width... 276
9.6 Precise Boundary Detection 278
9.7 Continuous Vessel Models with Spline-Based Ribbons 279
9.8 Estimation of Vessel Boundaries Using Snakes.......................... 288
9.9 Vessel Width Change Detection.. 294
9.10 Conclusion... 298
    References 299

Detection of width changes in blood vessels of the retina may be indicative of eye or systemic disease. However, all fundus images, even those taken during a single sitting, are acquired at different perspective geometries, have different scales, and are difficult to manually compare side by side. This problem is increased for images acquired over time and is in no way lessened when different cameras are used as technology improves or patients change doctors. Indeed, even the method of image recording media has changed. In order to compare two images acquired at different times, automated techniques must be used to detect vessels, register images, and identify potential regions of blood vessel width change.

In order to detect vessel width change, vessels must first be identified in available digital images. Several methods for automated vessel detection exist, and this chapter discusses several and presents a method for parameterizing blood vessels in ribbon-like objects that provide continuous boundaries along the entire length of a vessel.

Once blood vessels are identified, these vessels can then be used to identify vessel intersections and bifurcations that are the basis for performing image registration. Once two images are registered and the blood vessels are continuously defined in each, a method for finding common vessels in the image and performing change detection is presented.

9.1 Identifying Blood Vessels

The processes of separating the portions of a retinal image that are vessels from the rest of the image are known as vessel extraction (or tracing) and vessel segmentation. These processes are similar in goal but typically are distinct in process. Each have complications due to such factors as poor contrast between vessels and background; presence of noise; varying levels of illumination and contrast across the image; physical inconsistencies of vessels such as central reflex [1–5]; and the presence of pathologies. All these factors yield different results, both in terms of how the results are modeled and the actual regions identified. Different methods yield distinctly different results and even the same method will yield different results for images taken from the same patient in a single session. These differences become significant for images taken at different points in time as they could be mistaken as change. Methods used to determine the vessel boundaries should strive to lessen the frequency and severity of these inconsistencies.

9.2 Vessel Models

Many models are used to describe and identify vessels in images. Most are based on detectable image features such as edges, cross-sectional profiles, or regions of uniform intensity. Edge models use algorithms that work by identifying vessel boundaries typically by applying an edge detection operator such as differential or gradient operators [6–8]; Sobel operators [9; 10]; Kirsch operators [11]; or first order Gaussian filters [12]. Cross-sectional models employ algorithms that attempt to find regions of the image that closely approximate a predetermined shape such as a half ellipse [13]; Gaussian [1; 14–19]; or 6th degree polynomial [20]. Algorithms that use local areas of uniform intensity generally employ thresholding [21; 22], relaxation [23], morphological operators [16; 24–26], or affine convex sets to identify ridges and valleys [27].

Blood vessel models can more generally be characterized as those that are boundary detection (or edge detection) based or those that are cross section or matched-filter based. Depending on the intended application for the vessels detected, different aspects of the model may be more important. For vessel change detection, we decided that the most important aspect of the vessel model is the accurate and precise location of vessel boundaries.

9.3   Vessel Extraction Methods

Algorithms for identifying blood vessels in a retina image generally fall into two classes — those that segment vessel pixels and those that extract vessel information. Generally, segmentation is referred to as a process in which, for all pixels, certain characteristics of each pixel and its neighbors are examined. Then, based on some criteria, each pixel is determined to belong to one of several groups or categories. In retinal image segmentation, the simplest set of categories is binary — vessel or nonvessel (background). This is what we refer to as "vessel segmentation." Techniques for segmentation include thresholding [21], morphological operations [16; 24–26; 28], matched filters [9; 15–17; 22; 29; 30], neural nets [31–33], FFTs [34], and edge detectors [6; 9; 11; 35; 36]. Segmentation algorithms generally produce binary segmentations, are computationally expensive and typically require further analysis to calculate morphometric information such as vessel width.

Extraction algorithms [1; 8; 12; 14; 18; 36–39] on the other hand, generally use exploratory techniques. They are faster computationally and usually determine useful morphometric information as part of the discovery process. They work by starting on known vessel points and "tracing" or "tracking" the vasculature structure in the image based on probing for certain vessel characteristics such as the vessel boundaries. Since the vessel boundaries are part of the discovery process, these algorithms generally contain information such as vessel widths, center points, and local orientation that can be used later in the change detection process. Many of these methods employ edge-centric models and are well suited for vessel change detection. For these reasons, we selected the exploratory algorithm in Section 9.4 as the basis for the change detection algorithm described in Section 9.9.

9.4   Can's Vessel Extraction Algorithm

Can's vessel extraction (or "tracing") algorithm [8] uses an iterative process of tracing the vasculature based on a localized model. The model is based on two physical properties of vessels — that vessels are locally straight and consist of two parallel sides. As such, it works by searching for two parallel vessel boundaries, found based on detection of two parallel, locally straight edges. The entire algorithm consists of two stages.

Stage 1 (seed point initialization): The algorithm analyzes the image along a coarse grid to gather samples for determining greyscale statistics (contrast and brightness levels) and to detect initial locations of blood vessels using greyscale minima. These minima are considered as "seed points" at which a tracing algorithm will be initiated. False seed points are filtered out by testing for the existence of a pair of sufficiently strong parallel edges around the minima. A seed point is filtered out if the two strongest edges do not both exceed a contrast threshold (generated from the greyscale statistics) or if the directions of the two strongest edges are not sufficiently similar (within 22.5 degrees). On average, about 40% of the initial points are filtered out by this procedure.

Stage 2 (recursive tracing): The second stage is a sequence of recursive tracing steps initiated at each of the filtered seed points. For each filtered seed, the tracing process proceeds along vessel centerlines by searching for vessel edges. These edges are sought starting from a known vessel center point in a direction orthogonal to the local vessel direction. The search stops at a distance of one half the maximum expected vessel width. Vessel boundaries are searched by checking for edges over a discrete set of angles, usually 16 angles, with an interval of 22.5 degrees. Three angles are tested (the previous center point direction ± 1) and the angle of the strongest edge is estimated. The next trace point is determined by taking a step from the current trace point along the direction of the strongest edge. The resulting point is then refined by applying a correction that is calculated based upon how far the new point is from the center of the points at which the left and right boundaries are found. This new point is kept only if (a) it does not intersect any previously detected vessels, (b) it is not outside the image frame, and (c) the sum of edge strengths is greater than the global contrast threshold calculated during seed point detection.

Can's algorithm was created as a means to extract vessels to identify landmarks (vessel bifurcation and crossover points) as a basis for registration. While effective at producing landmarks, it often identified vessel boundaries that are not smooth and entire vessel segments are often missed. Further examination of the algorithm identified several modifications that could improve the suitability of the algorithm for use in the application of the detection of width change.

9.4.1 Improving Can's algorithm

In order to overcome some of the limitations in Can's algorithm, several modifications were implemented that incorporated all of the basic features of the original algorithm, but added several innovations aimed at improving both the accuracy of the results and the efficiency of the algorithm. They are summarized in the following sections. Throughout the remainder of this chapter, the improved version of Can's original algorithm will be referred to as "vessel tracer" and the output will be referred to as "vessel tracing" results.

9.4.1.1 Smoothing vessel boundaries

As discussed in Section 9.4, in order to find the vessel boundaries, Can applied templates iteratively from a point known to be a vessel center point outwards to some distance $M/2$ where M is the expected maximum width of a blood vessel. The point at which the template has the maximum response is determined to be the edge. This technique allows vessel boundaries for adjacent vessel segments to vary significantly. In an attempt to produce smoother boundaries, this search strategy was modified to only search for a vessel edge at a predicted edge location $\pm d/2$, where d is the maximum allowable change in width of a vessel at each step of the tracing algorithm.

Taking into account that there are two boundaries, at each step of the algorithm the largest possible difference in width between adjacent vessel segments is d. Note that the search space is also constrained in that the predicted edge location plus $d/2$ must be less than $M/2$, and the predicted edge location minus $d/2$ must be on the correct side of the predicted center.

9.4.1.2 Local thresholds

The next modification of Can's base algorithm is the implementation of local thresholds. Can's original algorithm computes and uses two global thresholds for different portions of his algorithm. The first threshold was used in initial seed point detection. Its value was computed as the mean intensity of selected sample points from the gridlines used in stage one of his tracing algorithm described in 9.4. The second was called "sensitivity" (denoted as S) and was used for determining the existence of vessel boundaries. The value of this threshold was originally estimated based on the difference between the average intensity of the background (B_{av}) and the average intensity of a vessel (L_{av}). L_{av} was calculated based on the intensity of the seeds discovered in stage one. B_{av} was calculated using samples found elsewhere on the gridlines. S is calculated using the following equation:

$$S = 36(1 + \sigma|L_{av} - B_{av}|).$$

In the above equation, the value of 36 represents the response of a pair of templates (of length 6) to a vessel that was one intensity level lower than the background and σ was empirically set to 0.21.

These thresholds were both modified in the methods used to arrive at their values and the region in which the are applicable. In Can's algorithm, the thresholds were applied globally. Now, thresholds are calculated for each individual point in an image. This is done by calculating threshold values for centers of individual regions. For points in between the centers, bi-linear interpolation is used to determine the appropriate threshold. An example of how thresholds calculated in this manner vary across an image can be seen in Figure 9.1.

In calculating the thresholds, the first threshold is modified to use the median intensity of samples from within a given region. For "sensitivity," it is now defined based on the mean and standard deviation of a directional derivative applied at each sample in a region oriented in four directions 0°, 45 deg, 90°, and 135 deg. These derivatives are descriptive of the contrast for neighboring pixels or potential edge sites within the region. They are used to develop the minimum edge strength threshold referred to as "sensitivity," S, for an edge within a region R, as follows:

$$S(R) = \mu_d(R) + \alpha\sigma_d(R), \tag{9.1}$$

where $\mu_d(R)$ is the mean of the all the derivatives in the region, $\sigma_d(R)$ is the standard deviation of the derivatives in the region, and α is some weighting factor applied to the standard deviation. In this research, a value for α of 1.5 is used.

Using the local thresholds described above, vessel tracing results are improved. The global thresholds in Can's algorithm often resulted in missed vessels, particularly in images with a large degree of variation caused by uneven illumination or the

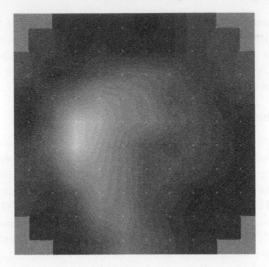

FIGURE 9.1

This image illustrates how a local threshold for an indicator of contrast varies across the entire image and is more appropriate for use than a single global threshold. The "×" points mark the region centers and the threshold at all points between are calculated by bi-linear interpolation.

presence of pathologies. By breaking the image into smaller regions and calculating thresholds for each region, more appropriate thresholds are used and better results achieved.

9.4.1.3 Vessel graph

A third modification concerns breaking vessels into segments. In order to identify vessel crossings and bifurcations and identify associated vessel segments, it is necessary to present the results of the vessel extraction algorithm in a manner that is consistent in all images. To accomplish this, a simple graph structure of the vasculature is built by treating all landmarks (i.e., bifurcation and cross-over points) as nodes and all traces as edges. Vessel segments are defined as starting and ending at either a landmark or at nothing. This requires that detected vessels be split into multiple segments (i.e., graph edges) at each landmark. While this seems to be a trivial distinction, the original algorithm was not concerned with building a vessel graph or with identifying segments. As such it made no effort to organize traces into individual vessel segments. So, in the original algorithm it was possible for a vessel that contained a bifurcation to be represented by only two traces. In the modified version it is now always represented by three.

9.4.1.4　Other modifications to Can's algorithm

Several other modifications improving the accuracy or efficiency of the tracing algorithm were implemented:

1. better initial seed point determination;

2. use of multiple lengths of templates to detect vessel boundaries;

3. use of a binning structure to cache results;

4. interpolation of vessel points to sub-pixel accuracy;

5. better accuracy and repeatability in determining landmark location;

6. inclusion of a momentum strategy to allow tracing to trace through noisy parts of an image;

7. merging of similarly aligned vessels with termination points in close proximity;

8. decision criteria to split traces based on angle of convergence between vessels.

Can's original algorithm with the mentioned modifications was implemented using an open source, multi-platform, computer vision and understanding collection of C++ libraries called VXL [40]. The algorithm is implemented in both a command line and graphical user interface (GUI) version, with results being generated in both text and in any of multiple image formats. Both are easily configurable with parameters in both versions being set at run time as either command line options or, in the GUI version, using dialog boxes. Sample output of the modified vessel tracing algorithm can be seen in Figure 9.2.

9.4.2　Limitations of the modified Can algorithm

While the above techniques have improved Can's original algorithm, there are still some limitations, particularly in two areas. First is in the area of detecting extremely small vessels, particularly neovascular membranes. This is primarily caused by lower contrast of the thin vessels (typically 1-2 pixels in width) and their highly tortuous nature. Thus, the locally straight parallel edge model fails.

The second limitation is in the area of precise location of the vessel boundaries. This is vital for detection of changes in vessel width. It is influenced by factors in the image (such as poor contrast and noise) and by the methodology used to estimate vessel boundaries. Inaccuracies are caused by modeling the boundary with a set of boundary points found by using a discrete set of edge detectors oriented over a discrete set of directions. Additionally, poor contrast and noise affect the response of the edge detection templates and result in yet more errors. These types of errors are illustrated in the results shown in Figure 9.3. This degree of error may be acceptable in certain applications such as low-resolution segmentation or feature extraction for registration, but it is not tolerable at the level of resolution desired for change

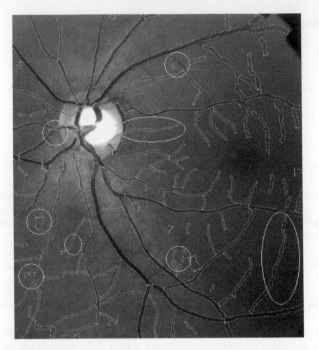

FIGURE 9.2
Figure illustrating an example of the results generated by the vessel-tracing algorithm. Circled areas highlight the areas of poor smoothness or erroneous vessel
detection. **(See color insert following page 174.)**

detection. A method that utilizes Can's results but provides further refinement and
accuracy is described in Section 9.5.

9.5   Measuring Vessel Width

Two potential issues arise when measuring a vessel's width. First, as mentioned in
the preceding section, is the orientation at which to measure the width. The second
is the determination of the points at which to begin and end measurement (i.e., the
vessel boundaries).

Most methods attempt to measure width in a direction perpendicular to the longitudinal orientation of the vessel (also referred to as the "normal" direction). However, these methods suffer from errors induced when the orientations are discretized
into a limited number of directions or when the longitudinal direction is determined
by a human operator. Additionally most methods measure the width directly as the
distance between edges determined by a vessel cross section (that is in the normal

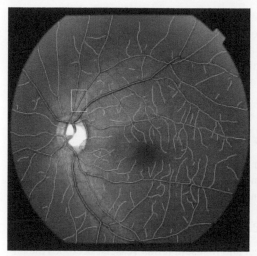
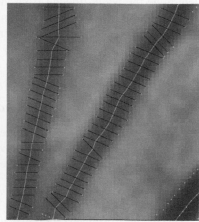

FIGURE 9.3

Illustrating the inaccuracy in the boundaries. The figure on the left shows an image with a fairly accurate vessel (centerline) segmentation. The image on the right shows in detail the boxed region from the image on the left. Note the inaccuracies in the vessel boundary points caused by poor contrast or noise. Also note how for each trace point, the corresponding boundaries are often not perpendicular to the orientation of the vessel and as such are not accurate for use in measuring vessel width. **(See color insert.)**

direction from a point on a central axis). However, the definition of the edge location and thus the width measurements vary from method to method.

One such method is to determine vessel boundaries at the locations on a cross section where the intensity is halfway between the maximum and minimum intensities of the cross-sectional profile [2; 41]. This method for determining the boundary is referred to as half-height intensity change. This method was used in manual microdensitometry, which used film exposure profiles, film density profiles, or film transmission profiles to determine the boundaries. A semi-automated procedure in which a user estimates the vessel central axis and the computer determines the half heights is used in [42–45]. Another semi-automated algorithm [35] uses computer measured widths based on user input to initialize computer-determined vessel edges.

A different method to determine the vessel boundaries uses parameters of a parabola fit to a cross-sectional intensity profile to determine the width [46]. Others have fit Gaussian curves to the profile and define the boundaries at some distance from the Gaussian's mean [14; 47]. These Gaussian curves are defined using a single parameter, (σ).

Not all methods require the determination of two points as boundaries in order to determine width. Gregson et al. [48] determine width based on fitting an area-equivalent rectangle to the actual image cross section profile of a vessel. Gang et al.

[29] have proposed a method that does not use the distance between two edges to determine the width (though from their method one can infer the edge locations). They determine a vessel's width from a parameter (σ) in an amplitude modified 2nd order Gaussian equation. They construct a 1D filter using Equation 9.2, which they then use to adaptively find a value for σ that maximizes the filter response of a given vessel cross section.

$$f(x) = \frac{1}{\sqrt{2\pi}\sigma^{3.5}}(x^2 - \sigma^2)e^{-x^2/2\sigma^2}. \tag{9.2}$$

They demonstrate that such a filter will have a peak response for a vessel of a particular diameter when the correct value for σ is used. They empirically determine that there is a linear relation between vessel diameter and σ as described by the following equation:

$$w = 2.03\sigma + 0.99. \tag{9.3}$$

This method, originally used to detect and measure retina vessels, becomes the basis for refinement of boundary locations in an innovative active contour methodology as presented in Section 9.8.4.

9.6   Precise Boundary Detection

Essential for any system to detect vessel width change is the ability to accurately measure width. The previous section presented both manual [41] and automated methods [29; 37; 47; 49] that have been developed to measure vessel width. The commonality between all these methods is that all are based on finding the vessel boundaries and then measuring vessel cross sections. However, as the following discussion explains, these measurements are all error prone.

In the case of the vessel tracing algorithm, the boundaries are simply the edges that are detected. The cross sections from which the widths are measured are defined by a set of boundary points. These boundary points represent the center of a detected locally straight (i.e., typically 5, 9, or 13 pixels in length) edge. These edges are found from a search that uses filters created at a discrete set of angular orientations and are often inaccurate. Additionally, the resulting cross section formed from corresponding boundary points is not truly perpendicular to the local orientation of the blood vessel as demonstrated in Figure 9.3. To eliminate these inaccuracies, the boundaries must be determined or refined so that vessel boundaries are defined at any point along a vessel and widths are determined perpendicular to the vessel.

In developing an alternate method to find vessel boundaries, the goal is to create a different vessel boundary model that utilizes the entire length of the vessels (longitudinally) and has a smooth, continuous representation of the boundary. This will be accomplished by using B-splines combined with active contours as described in the next section. The B-splines will supply the desired continuity longitudinally and the active contours will supply the refinement. Vessel boundary points from the vessel tracing algorithm will be used to initialize the B-spline based models and the boundaries will be refined using active contours or "snakes" [50; 51]. This method will be subject to the constraint that the opposite boundary is near-parallel, which introduces another component to the model, producing what will be known as a "ribbon snake" [52]. In such a snake, two (near)-parallel boundaries are discovered simultaneously. This provides a basis for modeling smoother, more accurate vessel boundaries. This will be discussed in detail in the next section.

9.7 Continuous Vessel Models with Spline-Based Ribbons

B-spline ribbon-like objects can be used to represent blood vessels. For a full understanding, it is necessary to present foundation information about B-splines, ribbons, and active contours (or "snakes"). Multiple varieties of these objects will be discussed, all of which can be used to provide a continuous representation of blood vessels and used in algorithms to find vessel boundaries.

9.7.1 Spline representation of vessels

As discussed in Section 9.6, a vessel representation that is continuous at all points along the vessel length is desired. One way to do this is with splines. A spline is a representation of a curve in which individual segments are each defined differently, often by polynomial equations of the same or varying degree. The places where each segment connects to the adjacent segments are called knots. Splines can be defined to ensure certain properties are met at knots, such as first or second order continuity.

An advantage of splines is that since they are defined by mathematical equations, they are defined continuously over a given interval. This now allows a vessel location to be precisely determined at any point between the vessel's ends. Previous point-based methods, where a vessel is defined by a set of points as in the results generated by the vessel tracing algorithm, required that some form of interpolation be performed to determine the vessel locations at points other than those in the set. This introduced a loss of precision depending on the spacing between points. Splines eliminate this need for interpolation and increase the precision in determining a vessel's location.

9.7.1.1 B-Splines

A B-spline is a representation of a curve in which individual parametric segments are determined based on a combination of "basis" functions, where the basis function can be of any polynomial order that meets the desired knot point characteristics [53]. Thus any spline is uniquely characterized based on its polynomial order, the number and the location of the knots/control points. If the desired spline is to have as little curvature as possible to accurately represent the target curve, a third order, or cubic B-spline is required. This is due to the minimum curvature property of cubic B-splines (described in [54]) and is why cubic B-splines tend to be used in most applications.

Cubic B-splines have the additional property that they are second-order continuous so long as control points are not permitted to be co-located. When two control points are co-located, they allow a (first-order) discontinuity and allow corners to be formed. The vessel boundaries modeled by the B-splines in this research are assumed to be without corners and, as such, co-located control points are not allowed. In the remainder of this research, cubic B-splines are defined using $m + 1$ basis functions (where the minimum value for m is 3). Each basis function is defined as a combination of four individual pieces, each expressed as a function of parameter u as follows:

$$B_i(u) = \begin{cases} \frac{1}{6}u^3 & i \leq u < i+1 \\ \frac{1}{6}(1+3u+3u^2-3u^3) & i+1 \leq u < i+2 \\ \frac{1}{6}(4-6u^2+3u^3) & i+2 \leq u < i+3 \\ \frac{1}{6}(1-3u+3u^2-u^3) & i+3 \leq u < i+4 \\ 0 & \text{otherwise.} \end{cases} \tag{9.4}$$

These spline segments combine to form a single curve or basis function.

To form a curve, multiple (at least four) B-spline basis functions are necessary. These functions differ only in that they are translated versions of the basis function B_i described above and are weighted by different values, the values of the corresponding control points. The complete B-spline is evaluated across all intervals in which four segments from four different basis functions are present. Each piece of the basis function is scaled or weighted based on the value of a control point that has a value for each dimension of the space in which the curve is embedded. For instance, for a curve in two dimensions, each basis function has control points with a value for the x dimension and the y dimension. These control points have a local effect on the curve (i.e., only across the four intervals for which the basis function is defined).

Before proceeding, a further explanation of the parameter u is necessary. For each individual spline segment, where a segment is defined as the combination of four basis functions weighted by the corresponding control points evaluated at u, u is defined from 0 to 1. However when describing the parameter over the $m - 2$ intervals of the spline, the parameter u is defined on the range $[3, m+1]$. Thus, the integer portion of the parameter denotes the spline segment and the decimal portion describes the parameter within the segment. For example, when u is 4.7, the segment is the second (i.e., the interval $[4, 5]$) and the value of u used in the basis function is .7. Having now clarified the different contexts of u, let us now return to the discussion of B-splines.

Given the above definition of the basis function B_i, a simple equation can be used to define a spline. The equation to represent an n-dimensional curve, p, as a function of parameter u, consisting of $m + 1$ basis functions (B_i) with corresponding $m + 1$ n-dimensional control points (c_i), can be defined as:

$$p(u) = \sum_{i=0}^{m} B_i(u)c_i \tag{9.5}$$

9.7.1.2 Fitting a B-spline to a set of points

Two issues arise when considering the problem of fitting a B-spline to a set of points. The most obvious is how to arrive at the proper placement of the control points to best fit the data. The second is how to arrive at the correct number of control points to use. If an interpolation of the data is required, then the number of control points must equal the number of data points. However, if an approximation is satisfactory, then the number of control points can be significantly less. In this study, splines are fit initially with control points at uniform arc length intervals as in [55; 56]. Subsequent refinement of the splines using active contour permits the final splines to have nonuniform arc-length control point intervals. The following sections describe the methods used in this research to arrive at an acceptable number and placement of control points.

9.7.1.3 Least squares fit

One way to fit a B-spline curve to a set of $n+1$ data points, d, is to find the $m+1$ control points that minimize the distance between the B-spline and the data points. This can be done using a least squares fitting approach in which the idea is to minimize the total squared distance, S, as expressed in the following equation:

$$S = \sum_{j=0}^{n} [d_j - \sum_{i=0}^{m} c_i B_i(u_j)]^2. \tag{9.6}$$

The value of the parameter u_j is determined based on an arc-length ratio described as follows. If D is the total length of all the line segments connecting successive data points in d_n and U is the total length of the B-spline curve, then

$$\frac{|d_j - d_0|}{D} = \frac{|u_j - u_0|}{U} \tag{9.7}$$

where $|d_j - d_0|$ and $|u_j - u_0|$ are arc length distances. This allows us to compute the values for u_i using the following recurrence

$$u_0 = 3$$

$$u_{i+1} = u_i + (m-2)\frac{|d_{i+1} - d_i|}{D}$$

To find the optimal set of control points to fit the data, we differentiate Equation 9.6 with respect to the control points and equate to zero. This yields

$$\frac{\partial E}{\partial c_k} = -2\sum_{j}([d_j - \sum_{i=0}^{m} c_i B_i(u_j)]B_k(u_j)) = 0. \tag{9.8}$$

Rearranging gives:

$$\sum_{i=0}^{m} c_i[\sum_{j} B_i(u_j)B_k(u_j)] = \sum_{j} d_j B_k(u_j). \tag{9.9}$$

Setting up as a system of linear equations and expressing in matrix form yields a solution for the control points $\vec{c}$:

$$\sum_{j=0}^{n} \begin{bmatrix} B_0(u_j)B_0(u_j) & B_1(u_j)B_0(u_j) & \ldots & B_n(u_j)B_0(u_j) \\ \vdots & \vdots & \vdots & \vdots \\ B_0(u_j)B_k(u_j) & B_1(u_j)B_k(u_j) & \ldots & B_n(u_j)B_k(u_j) \\ \vdots & \vdots & \vdots & \vdots \\ B_0(u_j)B_n(u_j) & B_1(u_j)B_n(u_j) & \ldots & B_n(u_j)B_n(u_j) \end{bmatrix} \begin{bmatrix} c_0 \\ \vdots \\ c_k \\ \vdots \\ c_n \end{bmatrix} = \sum_{j=0}^{n} d_j \begin{bmatrix} B_0(u_j) \\ \vdots \\ B_n(u_j) \end{bmatrix}$$

$$\sum_{j=0}^{n} \vec{B}(u_j)\vec{B}(u_j)^T \vec{c} = \vec{r}$$

$$\vec{c} = (\sum_{j=0}^{n} \vec{B}(u_j)\vec{B}(u_j)^T)^{-1}\vec{r}$$

where the vector $\vec{B}(u_j)$ is defined as:

$$\begin{bmatrix} B_0(u_j) \\ \vdots \\ B_k(u_j) \\ \vdots \\ B_n(u_j) \end{bmatrix}.$$

9.7.1.4 Weighted least squares

While the last section dealt with determining the set of control points to best fit a given set of data points, it may not be desired to attempt a fit to all data points equally. That is, it may be desired to fit some points more closely than others based on some provided measure. This measure or "weight" may be indicative of the confidence in a given data point and as such indicates how closely the fit curve is desired to fit each data point. These weights can be constant or vary in an iterative procedure such as an iteratively weighted least squares fitting. The method for a weighted least squares fit using the same notation and following the previously derived equations is presented as follows:

$$S = \sum_{j=0}^{n} w_j [d_j - \sum_{i=0}^{m} c_i B_i(u_j)]^2 \tag{9.10}$$

where w_j is used to represent the weight of each data point.

$$\frac{\partial E}{\partial c_k} = -2\sum_{j} w_j([d_j - \sum_{i=0}^{m} c_i B_i(u_j)]B_k(u_j)) = 0. \tag{9.11}$$

$$\sum_{i=0}^{m} c_i [\sum_{j} w_j B_i(u_j)B_k(u_j)] = \sum_{j} w_j d_j B_k(u_j). \tag{9.12}$$

$$\sum_{j=0}^{n} w_j \begin{bmatrix} B_0(u_j)B_0(u_j) & B_1(u_j)B_0(u_j) & \cdots & B_n(u_j)B_0(u_j) \\ \vdots & \vdots & \vdots & \vdots \\ B_0(u_j)B_k(u_j) & B_1(u_j)B_k(u_j) & \cdots & B_n(u_j)B_k(u_j) \\ \vdots & \vdots & \vdots & \vdots \\ B_0(u_j)B_n(u_j) & B_1(u_j)B_n(u_j) & \cdots & B_n(u_j)B_n(u_j) \end{bmatrix} \begin{bmatrix} c_0 \\ \vdots \\ c_k \\ \vdots \\ c_n \end{bmatrix} = \sum_{j=0}^{n} w_j d_j \begin{bmatrix} B_0(u_j) \\ \vdots \\ B_n(u_j) \end{bmatrix}$$

$$\sum_{j=0}^{n} w_j \vec{B}(u_j)\vec{B}(u_j)^T \vec{c} = \vec{r}$$

$$\vec{c} = (\sum_{j=0}^{n} w_j \vec{B}(u_j)\vec{B}(u_j)^T)^{-1} \vec{r}$$

9.7.1.5 Determining the number of control points

The number and placement of control points determine the flexibility of the spline. As discussed in Section 9.7.1.2, this study initially places the control points uniformly based on the total arc length of the curve. In determining the number of control points necessary to approximate the set of data points, an acceptable error tolerance needs to be determined. One such measure is that the mean of the residual vector be below a certain tolerance value, where the mean of the residuals, μ_r, is computed as:

$$\mu_r = \frac{\sum_{j=0}^{n} |d_j - \sum_{i=0}^{m} c_i B_i(u_j)|}{n} \tag{9.13}$$

where u_j is the arc-length parameter corresponding to data point j. This tolerance μ_r is equivalent to the "normalized distance" measure used by Saint-Marc and Medioni in [57]. As part of determining the correct number of control points, an acceptable minimum and maximum should be determined. The absolute minimum number of control points is four. The absolute maximum is equal to the number of data points and will result in an exact interpolation. To arrive at a suitable number of control points, it is possible to start at the minimum and iteratively add control points until μ_r is below the acceptable threshold. Since a sub-pixel boundary is desired, this threshold was set to 0.5.

An alternative method for adding control points is to weight the residuals based on how closely the spline is expected to fit the points. These weights could be the same used for the weighted least squares fitting or could be based on some other weighting criteria. For instance, there may be a confidence score associated with each data point indicating that some points are more accurate or relevant than others based on such factors as local contrast or edge strength of local curvature. This score would indicate that the fit spline should better model the points with higher confidence and put less emphasis on those of low confidence. These confidence levels can be assembled into a weight vector, w, which is then used to scale the residuals, and changes Equation 9.13 to

$$\mu_r = \frac{\sum_{j=0}^{n} |(d_j - \sum_{i=0}^{m} c_i B_i(u_j))w_j|}{n}. \tag{9.14}$$

Once the residuals are weighted, there is no longer any relation between μ_r and the desired accuracy of the fit unless care is taken in selecting the weights. To accomplish this, all weights need to be between zero and one, where a one indicates a point with highest confidence and hence the desire to be best fit. These weights can be scaled by normalizing or by using a robust estimator [58]. If the threshold for μ_r is set below 1 then intuitively the relationship between the fit curve and the desired sub-pixel accuracy can again be realized but only for the points of highest confidence. The lower confidence points will not have a guarantee of a close (i.e., sub-pixel) fit.

In this study, the mean weighted residual threshold is set to 0.25 pixels. The number of control points is initially set to one-tenth the number of data points or four, whichever is greater. The number of control points is then increased until the mean weighted residual threshold is met or until the number of control points is more than one-third the number of data points the spline is expected to fit. In practice this upper limit is rarely met. The weights used are the strengths associated with each trace point, which is a measure of the image contrast at the vessel boundary (i.e., it is equal to the template response found during tracing). A final consideration is to normalize the weights so that each weight is between 0 and 1. This is done to maintain the desired sub-pixel fit accuracy for points with the highest strength. The weights are normalized using the infinity norm as shown in the following equation:

$$\mu_r = \frac{\sum_{j=0}^{n}[(d_j - \sum_{i=0}^{m} c_i B_i(u_j)) \frac{w_j}{\|w\|_\infty}]}{n}. \tag{9.15}$$

9.7.2   B-spline ribbons

A variety of different models referred to as "ribbons" are used to describe a two-dimensional region/object that is symmetric about a central axis. These objects can be described from both the perspective of generation (given the axis, create the shape) and recovery (given the shape, find the axis) [59]. A ribbon object is usually generated by using a geometric "generator" such as a disc [60] or a line segment where the line segment is required to have a fixed angle with the axis [61] or a fixed angle with both sides of the shape [62]. These generators can be constant in size and orientation or vary along the length of the axis. Amongst other things, ribbons have been used to find skewed symmetries [63]; to segment wires, plant roots, and bacteria [64]; and to find roads in satellite images [52]. Ribbon-like objects were selected to model retina vessels as most (nonpathological) vessels exhibit a symmetry about a central axis. These models were then used as the basis for active contour methods to more precisely identify the vessel boundaries as described in Section 9.8.3.

Initially, a form of a ribbon commonly referred to as Brooks ribbon [61] was used to model a given vessel based on the data supplied from the modified vessel tracing algorithm described in Section 9.4 (i.e., center point and width in normal direction). These ribbons are formed by line segments making a constant angle with the central axis (in this case they are orthogonal). To continuously and smoothly model the

Ribbon

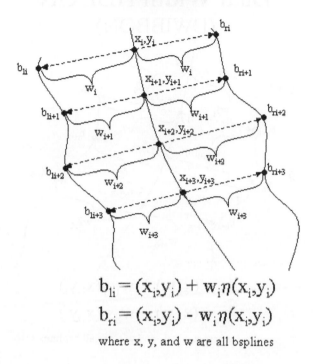

$$b_{li} = (x_i, y_i) + w_i \eta(x_i, y_i)$$

$$b_{ri} = (x_i, y_i) - w_i \eta(x_i, y_i)$$

where x, y, and w are all bsplines

FIGURE 9.4

Ribbon object definition. (x_i, y_i) is the axis center at point i, $\eta(x_i, y_i)$ is the normal at center point i, and w_i is the width. b_l and b_r are the left and right boundary points, respectively.

vessels, each dimension (x, y, and width) is fit with a B-spline, each B-spline using the same parameterization as described in Section 9.7.1.1. The ribbons represented as a set of B-splines will be referred to interchangeably as "ribbon" or "B-spline ribbon" in the remainder of this chapter. This definition of a ribbon can be seen in Figure 9.4. The B-spline representation provides (a) an implicit smoothness for modeling the vessel boundaries and (b) an implicit flexibility in the active contour models based on the number and location of the knots (or the parameterization of the data points).

Since ribbons have only a single width they are most true to the idea that vessels have near-parallel boundaries. However, vessels do not always have near-parallel boundaries, particularly in pathological cases. In these cases, vessels are not symmetric around a central axis, or even if symmetry does exist, allowing only a single degree of freedom in the width parameter may not be sufficient to represent the vessel. This may be because the central axis is not truly centered or because the

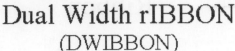

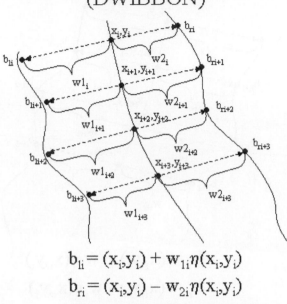

$$b_{li} = (x_i, y_i) + w_{1i}\eta(x_i, y_i)$$

$$b_{ri} = (x_i, y_i) - w_{2i}\eta(x_i, y_i)$$

where x, y w1, and w2 are all bsplines

FIGURE 9.5

Dual Width Ribbon (DWibbon) object definition. (x_i, y_i) is the axis center at point i, $\eta(x_i, y_i)$ is the normal at center point i, and $w1_i$ and $w2_i$ are both widths. b_l and b_r are the left and right boundary points, respectively.

spline is not flexible enough to handle a specific region with varying widths. To address this issue, two other ribbon-like objects were examined, the dual-width ribbon (DWibbon) and the normal-offset ribbon (NORibbon) as described in the following paragraphs. In both cases, a similar ribbon can created from each by identifying the corresponding boundary points for any point on the central axis and estimating a new centered axis point and width. These new axis points and widths can then be converted into a B-spline ribbon.

In attempting to allow more variability in the width along the central axis, the idea of having two widths ("dual widths") one for each side of the central axis was examined. This resulting "DWibbon" object is actually no longer guaranteed to be symmetric about the axis and can be argued is technically not a ribbon. As mentioned above, however, it can be easily transformed into a ribbon. This representation has the advantage that when used as the basis for an active contour, the central axis can be fixed and then each width still has the ability to find the correct boundary, even

Normal Offset RIBBON
(NORIBBON)

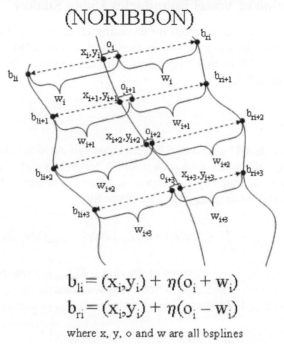

$$b_{li} = (x_i, y_i) + \eta(o_i + w_i)$$
$$b_{ri} = (x_i, y_i) + \eta(o_i - w_i)$$

where x, y, o and w are all bsplines

FIGURE 9.6
Normal Offset Ribbon (NORibbon) object definition. (x_i, y_i) is the axis center at point i, $\eta(x_i, y_i)$ is the normal at center point i, w_i is the width, and o_i is the offset. b_l and b_r are the left and right boundary points, respectively.

when the axis is not in the center of the vessel. This is not possible for ribbons when the ribbon axis is not located in the center of the vessel. The definition of the DWibbon is shown in Figure 9.5.

The final ribbon-like object studied is one that has a single width but rather than applying that width on the central axis, the width is applied at a point that is located at some offset in the normal direction. This is illustrated in Figure 9.6. Again, both the width and the offset can be modeled with splines. This implies that like the DWibbon, the normal-offset ribbon is not truly a ribbon because it is not symmetric about the central axis. But like the DWibbon, this allows the central axis to be fixed when used in an active contour method. It is also capable of being converted to a ribbon. However, the real utility of a NORibbon lies in its ability to be used with an active contour that uses a matched filter as its basis for determining the ribbon width. This will be described in Section 9.8.4.

9.8 Estimation of Vessel Boundaries Using Snakes

Previous sections discussed methods for modeling retina vessels. In this section we present a method for locating the vessels using active contour techniques based on the ribbon models of Section 9.7 initialized with the results of the modified Can's algorithm of Section 9.4.1.

9.8.1 Snakes

As originally introduced by Kass et al. [50], a snake is a curve or contour represented by a set of parametric points, with each position denoted as $v(s) = (x(s), y(s))$. The idea is to position the snake by "attracting" it to certain image features. A snake's motion is controlled by an energy function given by

$$E_{snake} = \int_0^1 E_{int}(v(s)) + E_{image}(v(s)) + E_{con}(v(s))ds, \qquad (9.16)$$

where E_{int} denotes the internal energy of the snake; E_{image} represents external image forces for such features in an image as lines, edges, and terminations of line segments and corners; and E_{con} is an external constraint force. E_{int} is commonly represented as

$$E_{int} = \frac{\alpha(s)|v_s(s)|^2 + \beta(s)|v_{ss}(s)|^2}{2} \qquad (9.17)$$

where the first term controls the elasticity of the snake and the second term controls the rigidity. In the context of vessel boundary detection, E_{image} should be attracted to edges. It is represented as $E_{image} = -|\nabla I(x,y)|^2$ and $E_{con} = 0$.

Using the set of detected boundary points for a single vessel boundary as the initial points, a snake can be used to solve for the final set of boundary points by minimizing the energy in Equation 9.17. This can be done by expressing and solving Equation 9.17 as the following set of Euler-Lagrange differential equations:

$$\frac{\partial x}{\partial t} = \frac{\partial E_{image}}{\partial x} - \frac{\partial}{\partial s}\left(\alpha(s)\frac{\partial x}{\partial s}\right) + \frac{\partial^2}{\partial s^2}\left(\beta(s)\frac{\partial^2 x}{\partial s^2}\right) \qquad (9.18)$$

$$\frac{\partial y}{\partial t} = \frac{\partial E_{image}}{\partial y} - \frac{\partial}{\partial s}\left(\alpha(s)\frac{\partial y}{\partial s}\right) + \frac{\partial^2}{\partial s^2}\left(\beta(s)\frac{\partial^2 y}{\partial s^2}\right) \qquad (9.19)$$

This method will yield a curve that is attracted to the boundary (as defined by the gradient). It is a better representation of the vessel boundary than the current vessel tracing code boundary points because the curve generated is smooth and is known to have converged on the best local boundary. This methodology can be applied to find both boundaries of a single vessel separately. However, a more appropriate application of snakes to vessel boundary location is described in the next section.

9.8.2 Ribbon snakes

Ribbon snakes extend the basic idea of a snake to the detection of linear features that have width. The idea is to attract the two boundaries of the ribbon to the boundaries of the linear feature. Ribbon snakes have been used to extract roads [52; 65; 66] in aerial images and are appropriate for vessel boundary detection because they can be used to model the road-like properties of a vessel. These properties can be described as a locally linear feature with width, symmetric about a central axis, bounded by two edges of relatively high contrast.

Ribbon snakes are defined similarly to snakes by introducing a third parametric component, namely a width component [67]. Where snakes are defined only in terms of x and y, in a ribbon snake each position is now represented as $v(s) = (x(s), y(s), w(s))$ where $x(s), y(s)$ represents the blood vessel center and $w(s)$ determines the vessel boundaries. Since we are trying to find two boundaries, E_{image} needs to be "attracted" to the two edges that have the locally greatest gradient. Thus E_{image} becomes

$$E_{image}(v(s)) = |(\nabla I(v_l(s))|^2 + |\nabla I(v_r(s)))|^2 \qquad (9.20)$$

This energy term should be further modified to favor points of maximal gradient where the gradient is strongest in the direction perpendicular to the detected edge. This is equivalent to requiring that the direction of the gradient be (closely) aligned with the normal. Taking a dot product of the normal and the gradient increases the contribution to the final energy when the gradient and normal directions are closely aligned while minimizing contributions from locations where the gradient and normal are not so aligned. Thus E_{image} can be modified as follows:

$$E_{image}(v(s)) = (\nabla I(v_r(s)) \cdot n(s))^2 + (\nabla I(v_l(s))) \cdot n(s))^2 \qquad (9.21)$$

where $n(s)$ is the unit normal at $x(s), y(s)$ and $v_r(s)$ and $v_l(s)$ are the vessel right and left boundaries, which can be expressed as

$$v_r(s) = w(s)n(s), \qquad v_l(s) = -w(s)n(s). \qquad (9.22)$$

By supplying the centerline positions and widths for a vessel obtained from the modified Can's algorithm, the ribbon snake can be initialized and solved in much the same manner as normal snakes. The major difference is that the results can be used to generate two contours representing both boundaries of the vessel. Additionally, ribbon snakes intrinsically maintain the "almost parallel" boundaries while allowing some degree of variability in width.

9.8.3 B-spline ribbon snake

The idea of combining splines with snakes is not new. Klein et al. used B-spline snakes for vessel single-boundary detection in [68] and Leitner and Cinquin to find contours in computed tomography (CT) and magnetic resonance imaging slices of images of the vertebra [69]. In this application, a B-spline ribbon snake is created to find retina vessels and is a unique combination of B-splines, snakes, and ribbons. A

B-spline ribbon snake behaves similar to snakes described in Section 9.8.1. However, the internal energy is no longer explicitly a part of the snake energy. Instead the smoothness of the snake is controlled implicitly by the parameters used to define the B-spline. Thus in a B-spline framework, the general equation for a snake described in Equation 9.16 becomes:

$$E_{snake} = \int_0^1 E_{image}(v(s))ds \qquad (9.23)$$

Similarly, the image energy E_{image} for a B-spline ribbon snake is affected. Instead of maximizing the energy equation to fit a single contour to the desired image feature, the idea is to fit the two sides of a ribbon B-spline to the desired image features, which in this study are the opposite boundaries of a blood vessel. This is done by simultaneously fitting the two (near)-symmetric contours to the vessel boundaries or edges, where an edge is defined as local areas of maximum gradient. Given an initial estimate of the B-spline ribbon in which the control points are assumed to be evenly spaced along the length of the curve, where the spacing is determined by arc-length, the energy equation for the ribbon B-spline is very similar to Equation 9.21 but is modified based on the B-spline ribbon parameters. This is explained in the following paragraphs. By maximizing the energy equation, an optimal solution representing the best local boundaries is found.

Let E_{snake} be the energy function for the B-spline ribbon snake expressed as a function of the $m+1$ control points, $\vec{c}_0, \ldots, \vec{c}_m$, and recall that each $\vec{c}_i$ has three components, namely x, y, and w (where w controls the width of the ribbon snake, and x and y control the x and y coordinates respectively). Recall that the B-spline ribbon is defined as a parametric function of u where at each u, $r(u) = (v(u), w(u))$ and $v(u) = (x(u), y(u))$ is the coordinate of the ribbon's central axis which is also the axis of symmetry, and $w(u)$ is the corresponding width in the normal direction. The B-spline's $m+1$ control points make $m-2$ spline segments, numbered from 3 to m, with u defined on the interval $(3..m+1)$.

$$E_{snake}(\vec{c}_0, \ldots, \vec{c}_m) = \int_3^{m+1} 1/2[\nabla I(\vec{p}_l(u)) \cdot \hat{\eta}(u)]^2 + 1/2[\nabla I(\vec{p}_r(u)) \cdot \hat{\eta}(u)]^2 du \qquad (9.24)$$

where $\hat{\eta}(u)$ is the unit normal, $\vec{p}_l$ is the left boundary curve defined by $\vec{p}_l(u) = \vec{v}(u) + w(u)\hat{\eta}(u)$, and $\vec{p}_r$ is the right boundary curve defined by $\vec{p}_r(u) = \vec{v}(u) - w(u)\hat{\eta}(u)$. The dot products with the unit normal in Equation 9.24 serve to emphasize the edges where the gradient is more closely aligned with the normal. Having now defined the energy function, all that needs to be done is to determine the control points that maximize the energy. Having now defined the energy equation for a ribbon, similar equations can be defined for both the DWibbon and NORibbon. The only difference is in how $\vec{p}_l(u)$ and $\vec{p}_r(u)$ are calculated.

However, Equation 9.24 fails to take advantage of the direction of the gradient when computing the energy. The objective function is defined to give more "energy" to the gradient that is more closely perpendicular to the orientation of the vessel (i.e., more closely aligned with the normal as shown in Figure 9.7). We do this by taking

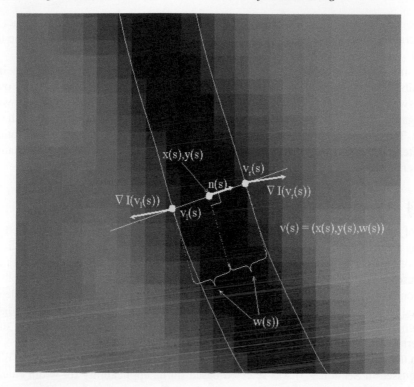

FIGURE 9.7
Illustration showing the parameters of a ribbon snake. Note the projection of the gradient on the unit norm $(n(s))$ used to further improve the boundary extraction. **(See color insert.)**

the dot product of the normal and the gradient. When they are more closely aligned, the value of the dot product will be close to the value of $|\nabla I|$ or $-|\nabla I|$ and thus contribute more to the energy.

However, we can leverage one additional piece of knowledge: the vessel is darker than the surrounding area. Thus on one side of the ribbon snake, the left, the intensity goes from light background to dark vessel, and on the other side of the ribbon, the right, from dark to light. This information can be utilized to modify the energy equation. The idea is to use the same dot products to require the projection of the gradient vector onto the ribbon's unit normal vector to be positive on the ribbon's left boundary and negative on its right. Thus Equation 9.24 is modified by dropping the square term and changing the addition to a subtraction. Thus E_{image} as used for all ribbon snake objects is defined as:

$$E_{snake}(\vec{c}_0,\ldots,\vec{c}_m) = \int_3^{m+1} \nabla I(\vec{p}_l(u)) \cdot \hat{\eta}(u) - \nabla I(\vec{p}_r(u)) \cdot \hat{\eta}(u)du \qquad (9.25)$$

For an image in which the vessels are lighter than the background (e.g., fluorescein angiograms) the sign of dot products would be switched so that the dot product of the gradient and normal would be negative on the left boundary and positive on the right.

Using this equation offers two advantages over the previous. First, it is now impossible during the active contour process for the sides of the ribbons to cross over and switch to the opposite side. Doing so would result in less energy as the side with a negative dot product would subtract a positive dot product, reducing the overall energy. The second advantage involves vessels that are in close proximity to each other. It often happens that two vessels appear side by side in an image and this equation prevents the boundary from moving to the nearest boundary of a nearby vessel.

9.8.4 Cross section-based B-spline snakes

All of the ribbon snakes discussed thus far are based on aligning ribbon object edges along areas of maximum intensity gradient, with an additional criteria that the direction of the gradient is close to perpendicular to the ribbon edge. These properties are represented in the objective function that we wish to maximize. For these reasons, a ribbon snake can be thought of as "edge-based" where a good fit to a vessel is determined by the magnitude and direction of the image gradient along the ribbon edges. Another approach is to determine a good fit based on an alternate criteria. One such criterion developed is the use of matched filters in conjunction with snakes.

In this research, the Amplitude Modified Second Order Gaussian (AMSOG) filter (discussed in Section 9.5) was selected based on its applicability for width change detection. This filter has been demonstrated as effective at locating and measuring vessel widths [29]. It also provides a precise definition of a vessel width based on the parameter σ given in Equation 9.3.

Given Equation 9.2 for the filter shape, an object that could utilize this filter in an active contour method was created by using both the Ribbon and the NORibbon as discussed in Section 9.7.2. These objects will be referred to as an AMSOG Ribbons and AMSOG NORibbons respectively and in more general terms are referred to as "cross section" snakes. Instead of fitting ribbon edges to the contours of maximum gradient, the idea is to position a ribbon-like object based on how closely its cross-sectional shape fits the image cross section.

The AMSOG Ribbon object is initialized by solving for the parameter σ using Equation 9.3 based on the original vessel tracing width. This is done by calculating the value for σ based on a sampled cross section centered at the appropriate location. For the ribbon, this point is on the central axis. For the NORibbon, it is at the offset point. The response of this cross section and filter is calculated with the filter center and the cross section center aligned. This response contributes to the new objective function, that is the new energy equation of the AMSOG NORibbon as shown by the following equation:

$$E = \sum_i I(p_i(x,y)) \otimes f(\sigma_i) \tag{9.26}$$

where $f(\sigma_i)$ denotes the filter (i.e., Equation 9.2), σ_i is the value of the parameter sigma at point i, $I(p_i(x,y))$ is the cross section in the normal direction centered at p_i

Table 9.1: Summary of the Parameters of each B-Spline Ribbon Method (showing which parameters are fixed and which are allowed to vary in determining the final position of the ribbon.)

Method	Fixed	Free
Ribbon		x,y,w
DWibbon	x,y	w_1, w_2
NORibbon	x,y	o,w
AMSOG Ribbon		x,y,σ
AMSOG NORibbon	x,y	o,σ

and $\otimes$ represents the operation of calculating the filter response. For a ribbon,

$$p_i = (x_i, y_i) \tag{9.27}$$

and for a NORibbon,

$$p_i = (x_i, y_i) + \eta_i \cdot o_i \tag{9.28}$$

where η_i and o_i are the normal and offset at point i.

Maximizing the energy in Equation 9.26 yields an optimal solution of either $\vec{\sigma}$ for AMSOG Ribbons or $\vec{\sigma}_i$ and $\vec{o}_i$ for AMSOG NORibbons.

9.8.5 B-spline ribbon snakes comparison

Several ribbon models have been discussed in an effort to produce vessel boundaries that are smooth and continuous and from which a vessel width can be determined. Ribbon snakes are initialized with the results from the tracing algorithm but all then use the original image intensity structure to refine the final boundary locations. Each snake differs based on the ribbon it uses and its energy equation. Three-edge-based ribbon snakes, namely ribbon, DWibbon, and NORibbon were presented. Additionally, a new, novel methodology referred to as cross section-based ribbon snakes was presented. Two cross section based snakes, the AMSOG Ribbon and the AMSOG NORibbon, were presented. Each ribbon method differed based on the parameters that define it and each snake differs in the ribbons parameters that are held constant or allowed to vary within the "snake" framework. These differences are summarized in Table 9.1.

All these methods address the identified shortcomings of the tracing algorithm, particularly in the areas of continuity and smoothness. Empirical evidence not reported in this chapter has suggested that the boundaries generated by the AMSOG NORibbon are more applicable for change detection.

9.9   Vessel Width Change Detection

A prerequisite in the task of detecting change is the ability to account for projective geometry differences between two images by aligning the images through a process known as registration. By registering two images, transformations are created that can be used to convert images to a common scale space. These transformations ensure that the distance and direction between any two corresponding points in transformed images are equal. Without this ability to register and transform images, it would not be possible to compare distances and hence detect changes in width. The DBICP Registration algorithm provides this needed capability to reliably and accurately register almost any set of fundus images that contain detectable features [70].

Once registered, differences in measurements between two images may be attributed to the variation in the method of estimation of vessel width from image to image. This stochastic variation is influenced by multiple factors such as variable focus, variable illumination, and physiological changes from pathologies or even the pulsation of vessels caused by the beating of the heart. These variations result in vessel boundary estimation that is erroneous. This section presents a method that addresses these stochastic challenges by presenting decision criteria designed to account for this uncertainty.

9.9.1   Methodology

Any approach at width change detection would need to follow three basic steps. The first step is to find the vessels in each image with the boundaries being identified to sub-pixel accuracy. Second is the step of transforming all vessels into the same coordinate system and identifying corresponding vessel pieces. Last is the ability to measure to sub-pixel accuracy the vessel widths and to identify changes in width over time. These requirements will be discussed in the following sections. A final step not mentioned is displaying the detected differences. The object of detecting the differences is to draw the attention of the physician to the regions that appeared to have changed. A method to call out the regions of change that does not obstruct the observer's view of the region of change in the original image is needed. To accomplish this, a box is drawn around vessel segments that are determined to have changed as can be seen in sample change detection results in Figure 9.9.

9.9.1.1   Vessel detection

The first requirement in the detection of vessel width change is to be able to accurately and consistently identify vessels in retinal images. This includes the accurate location and continuous definition of the vessel boundaries. The AMSOG NORibbon discussed in Section 9.8.4 is used because it was empirically determined to identify more repeatable continuous vessel boundaries than other methods.

9.9.1.2 Image registration and determining corresponding vessels

The second requirement in the detection of vessel change is the ability to accurately register images. By using the DBICP registration algorithm, it is possible to determine transformations that can be used to accurately align both images as well as results generated from these images. Once aligned it is then possible to determine corresponding vessel cross sections and directly compare their widths. However, finding corresponding vessels is a challenge, particularly in the cases where a vessel has disappeared or has failed detection in one image but is detected in another. Thus this possibility must be considered when determining corresponding vessel sections.

When a vessel detected in one image coincides with a vessel in another image, then the vessels in both images are accepted as being the same. If a vessel is within some distance δ of another vessel, such as one vessel width, then an additional constraint needs to be applied to ensure they are the same vessel. This additional constraint is a check to see if both vessels are generally progressing in the same direction. If this condition is not met, then it is assumed that the vessels are different. If no other vessel is found, then it can be concluded that the corresponding vessel has either escaped detection or does not exist. In this case, the image that is missing the vessel is once again consulted to determine if the vessel is truly not there or if it was a failed detection. Only after this second attempt to test for the presence of the vessel is the vessel considered as being not present.

9.9.1.3 Width change detection

Once vessels are detected, the boundaries identified, and the images registered, it is then possible to identify corresponding vessel points and compare widths to identify width change.

9.9.1.4 Comparison of widths

All widths for a given vessel segment are measured from two points on opposite sides of a vessel. These two points are determined from the B-spline ribbons representing the detected vessel boundaries. The measured width between them is along a line that is guaranteed to be perpendicular to the vessel orientation. A separate algorithm determines corresponding cross sections between images. Once corresponding points on corresponding vessels are discovered, widths can be compared directly to identify differences. By following these steps, there are no problems caused by differences in scale, discontinuities or discretization of the boundaries or cross section angle; and there are no issues with how a cross section's end points are defined.

In determining vessel width change, it becomes necessary to define what constitutes change. What difference between corresponding vessel regions should be construed as change? Other research has shown that the "normal" expected difference between vessels over time caused by the cardiac cycle is approximately 5% (4.8% in [71], 5.4% in [45]). Thus this serves as the basis for comparison of two vessels — any vessel portions that exhibit more than this change should be flagged as sites where differences exist.

However, comparing widths using this value as an absolute threshold does not take into account the uncertainty in the vessel segmentation, the uncertainty in identified boundaries, and the variability caused by inter-image inconsistencies. This uncertainty and variability can be caused by a variety of factors such as the presence of pathologies or differences in contrast caused by varying illumination and/or varying focus. The method presented in this chapter takes into account this 5% cardiac change and was designed mindful of these considerations.

9.9.2 Change detection via hypothesis test

A method for testing for width change is based on the generation of statistics for each width measurement and conducting a hypothesis test [72; 73]. This is done as an attempt to consider in a stochastic framework the uncertainty and variability of the images and the detected vessel boundaries from those images. A hypothesis test is a standard statistical inference that uses probability distributions to determine if there is sufficient support for a statement or "hypothesis." In this case, we want to determine if there is sufficient evidence to believe that the two measured widths are the same (within 5%) or different.

In order to determine statistics that could be used in a hypothesis test, the width measurements are modeled in a manner that can be interpreted as a probability distribution. To do this, the image is sampled across a blood vessel cross section from which the width measurement is determined. This sampling is a 1D signal and the derivative of this signal is computed. The resulting signal is treated as two probability density functions (PDF) of two random variables, with the center of the density function being located at the vessel end points and the limits of the pdf defined at the zero crossing or at the first relative minima. From these functions, values for the standard deviation, σ, can be determined. This idea is illustrated in Figure 9.8. The average values for the standard deviation of each width's end points can be used to provide a value that can be used in a hypothesis test.

In hypothesis testing, we are trying to determine if the probability distribution of two separate measurements are the same. This is done based on the measurement's mean and standard deviation. The first step of the hypothesis test is to identify the hypothesis — that is to identify what exactly it is we are trying to prove. If the hypothesis test is successful, it means that there is substantive support for the hypothesis at a specific significance level. The significance level is a parameter that is used to help control Type 1 errors. (A Type 1 error is defined as rejecting the hypothesis when it is true, i.e., false negatives). As the significance level increases, the number of rejections decreases, decreasing the number of false negatives. The effect of this is an increase in the number of positives, both true and false.

In setting up a hypothesis test, the negation of the hypothesis is termed the null hypothesis (H_0) and the hypothesis itself is termed the alternative (H_a). Mathematically, a hypothesis test is set up as shown below in Equation 9.29. The values of μ_1 and μ_2 are the mean values of the measurements with Δ_0 indicating the amount of difference in the measurement allowed by the hypothesis test. If the difference in the measurement is greater than this value, the null hypothesis is rejected. A value

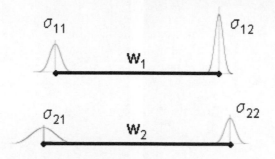

FIGURE 9.8

Two measured widths, w_1 and w_2 are illustrated. For each width measurement, the derivatives of the image intensity along the cross section on which the width is measured result in two probability density functions centered at the end points. From these, values for the standard deviation of the width measurement can be estimated.

of $\Delta = 0$ indicates that there is no tolerance for a difference in the measurements — both measurements are expected to be the same.

$$H_0 : \mu_1 - \mu_2 = \Delta_0 \tag{9.29}$$
$$H_a : \mu_1 - \mu_2 \neq \Delta_0 \tag{9.30}$$

To conduct the hypothesis test, a test statistic, z, is computed as follows. Note that:

$$z = \frac{\mu_1 - \mu_2 - \Delta_0}{\sqrt{\sigma_1^2 + \sigma_2^2}}. \tag{9.31}$$

This statistic is compared against a value, z_α, that would be expected from a normal distribution at a certain significance level, α.

The goal of this method is to determine if vessels have changed (where we have defined change as a difference of more than 5%). However we only want to arrive at this conclusion when there is strong evidence to support it. Thus the hypothesis is that changed vessels are those that show more than a 5% change. In Equation 9.29 the values of μ_1 and μ_2 are the two widths that are to be compared. Replacing this with δ_w, the amount of measured change, (i.e., the difference between w_i and w_2), then the hypothesis is that there is change when $\delta_w > 0.05w_{max}$ where w_{max} is the maximum of the two widths and Δ_0 in Equation 9.29 is replaced with $0.05w_{max}$.

So, Equation 9.29 becomes

$$H_0 : \delta_w \leq .05w_{max}(\text{there is no change}) \tag{9.32}$$
$$H_a : \delta_w > .05w_{max}(\text{there is change}) \tag{9.33}$$

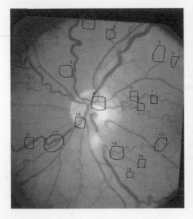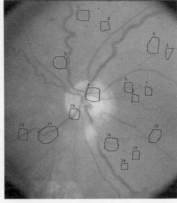

FIGURE 9.9
Illustrating the results of change detection. Boxes are drawn around vessels with suspected width change. The image on the left has been transformed into the same coordinate system as the image on the right. (**See color insert.**)

and Equation 9.31 becomes

$$z = \frac{\delta_w - .05 w_{max}}{\sqrt{\sigma_1^2 + \sigma_2^2}}. \tag{9.34}$$

Since we are interested in accepting the hypothesis when the change is greater than 5%, H_0 is rejected if $z \geq z_\alpha$. A value of $\alpha = 0.95$ was used to generate the sample results shown in Figure 9.9.

9.9.3 Summary

This section presented a method for detection of vessel width change. This method judged change based on a 5% threshold of acceptable width variance due to the changes in vessel widths caused by the cardiac cycle. The method judged change based on descriptive statistics at each vessel end point. The end points of a cross section are treated as random variables and the variance is computed based on the derivative of the intensities at the end point. These variances then are used in a hypothesis test.

9.10 Conclusion

This chapter presented a method by which to compare fundus images for indications of blood vessel width change. It started by presenting several blood vessel models and an improved algorithm for extracting blood vessels. Then several longitudinally continuous ribbon-like blood vessel models using B-splines were described, whose purpose was to continuously define a blood vessel and allow the identification of an orthogonal cross section for accurate vessel width determination. These ribbons then utilized a snake algorithm that allowed for further refinement of the vessel boundary locations. Once final blood vessel boundary locations are determined, it is then possible to transform images into common coordinate systems through the process of registration. Once registered, widths can be compared utilizing the described hypothesis test framework, attributing any change of 5% or less to normal vessel changes caused by the cardiac rhythm.

References

[1] Gao, X., Bharath, A., Stanton, A., et al., A method of vessel tracking for vessel diameter measurement on retinal images, in *Proceedings IEEE International Conference on Image Processing*, 2001, 881–884.

[2] Heier, H. and Brinchmann-Hansen, O., Theoretical relations between light streak characteristics and optical properties of retinal vessels, *Acta Ophthalmologica*, 64, 33, 1986.

[3] Brinchmann-Hansen, O., Heier, H., and Myhre, K., Fundus photography of width and intensity profile of the blood column and the light reflex in retinal vessels, *Acta Ophthalmologica*, 64, 20, 1986.

[4] Brinchmann-Hansen, O. and Sandvik, L., The intensity of the light reflex on retinal arteries and veins, *Acta Ophthalmologica*, 547–552, 1986.

[5] Roberts, D., Analysis of vessel absorption profiles in retinal oximetry, *Medical Physics*, 14, 124, 1987.

[6] Pinz, A., Bernogger, S., Datlinger, P., et al., Mapping the human retina, *IEEE Transactions on Medical Imaging*, 17, 606, 1998.

[7] Tascini, G., Passerini, G., Puliti, P., et al., Retina vascular network recognition, in *SPIE Conference on Image Processing*, 1993, vol. 1898 of *Proc. SPIE*, 322–329.

[8] Can, A., Shen, H., Turner, J.N., et al., Rapid automated tracing and feature extraction from live high-resolution retinal fundus images using direct exploratory algorithms, *IEEE Transactions on Information Technology in Biomedicine*, 3, 125, 1999.

[9] Wang, Y. and Lee, S., A fast method for automated detection of blood vessels in retinal images, in *Conference Record of the 32nd Asilomar Conference on Signals, Systems & Computers*, 1997, vol. 2, 1700–1704.

[10] Solouma, N., Youssef, A., Badr, Y., et al., Real-time retinal tracking for laser treatment planning and administration, in *Medical Imaging 2001: Image Processing*, 2001, vol. 4322 of *Proc. SPIE*, 1311–1321.

[11] Li, H. and Chutatape, O., Fundus image features extraction, in *Proceedings of the IEEE International Conference Engineering in Medicine and Biology*, Chicago, IL, 2000, vol. 4, 3071–3073.

[12] Kochner, B., Schuhmann, D., Michaelis, M., et al., Course tracking and contour extraction of retinal vessels from color fundus photographs: Most efficient use of steerable filters for model-based image analysis, in *SPIE Conference on Image Processing*, 1998, vol. 3338 of *Proc. SPIE*, 755–761.

[13] Jasiobedzki, P., Taylor, C., and Brunt, J., Automated analysis of retinal images, *Image and Vision Computing*, 3, 139, 1993.

[14] Zhou, L., Rzeszotarski, M., Singerman, L., et al., The detection and quantification of retinopathy using digital angiograms, *IEEE Transactions on Medical Imaging*, 619–626, 1994.

[15] Chaudhuri, S., Chatterjee, S., Katz, N., et al., Detection of blood vessels in retinal images using two-dimensional matched filters, *IEEE Transactions on Medical Imaging*, 8, 263, 1989.

[16] Hoover, A., Kouznetsova, V., and Goldbaum, M., Locating blood vessels in retinal images by piecewise threshold probing of a matched filter response, *IEEE Transactions on Medical Imaging*, 19, 203, 2000.

[17] Chutatape, O., Zheng, L., and Krishman, S., Retinal blood vessel detection and tracking by matched Gaussian and Kalman filters, in *Proceedings of the 20th IEEE International Conference Engineering in Medicine and Biology*, 1998, vol. 20, 3144–3149.

[18] Frame, A., Undrill, P., Olson, J., et al., Structural analysis of retinal vessels, in *6th International Conference on Image Processing and its Applications (IPA 97)*, 1997, 824–827.

[19] Ballerini, L., An automatic system for the analysis of vascular lesions in retinal images, in *Proc. 1999 IEEE Nuclear Science Symposium*, 1999, vol. 3, 1598–1602.

[20] Hammer, M., Leistritz, S., Leistritz, L., et al., Monte-Carlo simulation of retinal vessel profiles for the interpretation of *in vivo* oxymetric measurements by imaging fundus reflectometry, in *Medical Applications of Lasers in Dermatology and Ophthalmology, Dentistry, and Endoscopy*, 1997, vol. 3192 of *Proc. SPIE*, 211–218.

[21] Jagoe, J., Blauth, C., Smith, P., et al., Quantification of retinal damage done during cardiopulmonary bypass: Comparison of computer and human assessment, *IEE Proceedings Communications, Speech and Vision*, 137, 170, 1990.

[22] Jiang, X. and Mojon, D., Adaptive local thresholding by verification-based multithreshold probing with application to vessel detection in retinal images, *IEEE Transactions on Pattern Analysis and Machine Intelligence*, 25, 131, 2003.

[23] Akita, K. and Kuga, H., A computer method of understanding ocular fundus images, *Pattern Recognition*, 15, 431, 1982.

[24] Jasiobedzki, P., McLeod, D., and Taylor, C., Detection of non-perfused zones in retinal images, in *Proceedings of the 4th IEEE Symposium on Computer-Based Medical Systems*, 1991, 162–169.

[25] Zana, F. and Klein, J.C., Robust segmentation of vessels from retinal angiography, in *Proceeding International Conference Digital Signal Processing*, 1997, 1087–1090.

[26] Zana, F. and Klein, J.C., Segmentation of vessel-like patterns using mathematical morphology and curvature evaluation, *IEEE Transactions on Image Processing*, 10, 1010, 2001.

[27] Staal, J., Kalitzin, S., Abramoff, M., et al., Classifying convex sets for vessel detection in retinal images, in *IEEE International Symposium on Biomedical Imaging*, Washington, DC, 2002, 269–272.

[28] Heneghan, C., Flynn, J., O'Keefe, M., et al., Characterization of changes in blood vessel width and tortuosity in retinopathy of prematurity using image analysis, *Medical Image Analysis*, 6, 407, 2002.

[29] Gang, L., Chutatape, O., and Krishnan, S., Detection and measurement of retinal vessels in fundus images using amplitude modified second-order Gaussian filter, *IEEE Transactions on Biomedical Engineering*, 49, 168, 2002.

[30] Luo, G., Chutatape, O., and Krishman, S., Performance of amplitude modified second order Gaussian filter for the detection of retinal blood vessel, in *SPIE Conference Ophthalmic Technologies XI*, 2001, vol. 4245 of *Proc. SPIE*, 164–169.

[31] Jasiobedzki, P., Williams, C., and Lu, F., Detecting and reconstructing vascular trees in retinal images, in *SPIE Conference on Image Processing*, 1994, vol. 2167 of *Proc. SPIE*, 815–825.

[32] Sinthanayothin, C., Boyce, J., Cook, H., et al., Automated localisation of the optic disc, fovea, and retinal blood vessels from digital colour fundus images, *British Journal of Ophthalmology*, 83, 902, 1999.

[33] Truitt, P., Soliz, P., Farnath, D., et al., Utility of color information for segmentation of digital retinal images: Neural network-based approach, in *SPIE Conference on Image Processing*, 1998, vol. 3338 of *Proc. SPIE*, 1470–1481.

[34] Tan, W., Wang, Y., and Lee, S., Retinal blood vessel detection using frequency analysis and local-mean-interpolation filters, in *Medical Imaging 2001: Image*

Processing, 2001, vol. 4322 of *Proc. SPIE*, 1373–1384.

[35] Schwartz, B., Takamoto, T., and Lavin, P., Increase of retinal vessel width in ocular hypertensives with timolol therapy, *Acta Ophthalmologica*, 215, 41, 1995.

[36] Lalonde, M., Gagnon, L., and Boucher, M.C., Non-recursive paired tracking for vessel extraction from retinal images, in *Vision Interface 2000*, Montreal, Quebec, 2000.

[37] Pedersen, L., Grunkin, M., Ersbøll, B., et al., Quantitative measurement of changes in retinal vessel diameter in ocular fundus images, *Pattern Recognition*, 21, 1215, 2000.

[38] Kurokawa, T., Kondoh, M., Lee, S., et al., Maze-tracing algorithm applied to eye-fundus blood vessels, *Electronics Letters*, 34, 976, 1998.

[39] Gagnon, L., Lalonde, M., Beaulieu, M., et al., Procedure to detect anatomical structures in optical fundus images, in *Medical Imaging 2001: Image Processing*, 2001, vol. 4322 of *Proc. SPIE*, 1218–1225.

[40] TargetJr Consortium, The VXL book, 2000, http://public.kitware.com/vxl/doc/release/books/core/book.html.

[41] Delori, F., Fitch, K., Feke, G., et al., Evaluation of micrometric and microdensitometric methods for measuring the width of retinal vessel images on fundus photographs, *Graefes Archive for Clinical and Experimental Ophthalmology*, 226, 393, 1988.

[42] Wong, T., Klein, R., Sharrett, A., et al., Retinal arteriolar narrowing and risk of diabetes mellitus in middle-aged persons, *JAMA*, 287, 2528, 2002.

[43] Wong, T., Klein, R., Sharrett, A., et al., Retinal arteriolar narrowing and risk of diabetes mellitus in middle-aged persons, *JAMA*, 287, 1153, 2002.

[44] Newsom, R., Sullivan, P., Rassam, S., et al., Retinal vessel measurement: comparison between observer and computer driven methods, *Graefes Archive for Clinical and Experimental Ophthalmology*, 230, 221, 1992.

[45] Dumskyj, M., Aldington, S., Dore, C., et al., The accurate assessment of changes in retinal vessel diameter using multiple frame electrocardiograph synchronized fundus photography, *Current Eye Research*, 15, 625, 1996.

[46] Miles, F. and Nutall, A., Matched filter estimation of serial blood vessel diameters from video images, *IEEE Transactions on Medical Imaging*, 12, 147, 1993.

[47] Gao, X., Bharath, A., Stanton, A., et al., Measurement of vessel diameters on retinal images for cardiovascular studies, in *Proceedings of Medical Image Understanding and Analysis*, 2001.

[48] Gregson, P., Shen, Z., Scott, R., et al., Automated grading of venous beading, *Computers and Biomedical Research*, 28, 291, 1995.

[49] Chapman, N., Witt, N., Gao, X., et al., Computer algorithms for the automated measurement of retinal arteriolar diameters, *British Journal of Ophthalmology*, 85, 74, 2001.

[50] Kass, M., Witkin, A.P., and Terzopoulos, D., Snakes: Active contour models, *International Journal of Computer Vision*, 1, 321, 1988.

[51] Neuenschwander, W.M., Fua, P., Iverson, L., et al., Ziplock snakes, *International Journal of Computer Vision*, 25, 191, 1997.

[52] Mayer, H., Laptev, I., Baumgartner, A., et al., Automatic road extraction based on multiscale modeling, *International Archives of Photogrammetry and Remote Sensing*, 32, 47, 1997.

[53] Bartels, R.H., Beatty, J.C., and Barsky, B.A., *An introduction to splines for use in computer graphics and geometric modeling*, Morgan Kaufmann, San Mateo, CA, 1987.

[54] Unser, M., Splines a perfect fit for signal and image processing, *IEEE Transactions on Signal Processing*, 16, 22, 1999.

[55] Figueiredo, M., Leitao, J., and Jain, A., Unsupervised contour representation and estimation using B-splines and a minimum description length criterion, *IEEE Transactions on Image Processing*, 9, 1075, 2000.

[56] Menet, S., Saint-Marc, P., and Medioni, G., B-snakes: Implementation and application to stereo, in *Proceedings of the DARPA Image Undertanding Workshop*, Pittsburgh, PA, 1990, 720–726.

[57] Saint-Marc, P. and Medioni, G., B-spline contour representation and symmetry detection, in *Proceedings of the First European Conference on Computer Vision*, 1990, 604–606.

[58] Stewart, C.V., Robust parameter estimation in computer vision, *SIAM Reviews*, 41, 513, 1999.

[59] Rosenfeld, A., Axial representations of shape, *Computer Vision, Graphics and Image Processing*, 33, 156, 1986.

[60] Blum, H. and Nagel, R., Shape description using weighted symmetric axis features, *Pattern Recognition*, 10, 167, 1978.

[61] Brooks, A., Symbolic reasoning among 3-D models and 2-D images, *Artificial Intelligence*, 17, 285, 1981.

[62] Brady, M. and Asada, H., Smoothed local symmetries and their implementation, MIT Artifical Intelligence Laboratory Memo 757, 1984.

[63] Ponce, J., On characterizing ribbons and finding skewed symmetries, *Computer Vision, Graphics and Image Processing*, 52, 328, 1990.

[64] Huang, Q. and Stockman, G., Generalized tube model: Recognizing 3D elon-

gated objects from 2D intensity images, in *Proceedings of the IEEE Conference on Computer Vision and Pattern Recognition*, 1993, 104–109.

[65] Laptev, I., *Road extraction based on snakes and sophisticated line extraction*, Master's thesis, Royal Institute of Technology, Stockholm, Sweden, 1997.

[66] Laptev, I., Mayer, H., Lindeberg, T., et al., Automatic extraction of roads from aerial images based on scale space and snakes, *Machine Vision and Applications*, 12, 23, 2000.

[67] Fua, P. and Leclerc, Y.G., Model driven edge detection, *Machine Vision Applications*, 3, 45, 1990.

[68] Klein, A., Egglin, T., Pollak, J., et al., Identifying vascular features with orientation specific filters and B-spline snakes, in *Proceedings of Computers in Cardiology*, 1994, 113–116.

[69] Leitner, F. and Cinquin, P., From splines and snakes to snake splines, *Geometric Reasoning: From Perception to Action, Lecture Notes in Computer Science*, 708, 477, 1990.

[70] Stewart, C., Tsai, C.L., and Roysam, B., The dual-bootstrap iterative closest point algorithm with application to retinal image registration, *IEEE Transactions on Medical Imaging*, 22, 1379, 2003.

[71] Chen, H., Patel, V., Wiek, J., et al., Vessel diameter changes during the cardiac cycle, *Eye*, 8, 97, 1994.

[72] Bhattacharyya, G.K. and Johnson, R.A., *Statistical Concepts and Methods*, John Wiley and Sons, Chichester, West Sussex, United Kingdom, 1977.

[73] Devore, J.L., *Probability and Statisitics for Engineering and the Sciences*, Duxbury, Belmont, CA, 2000.

10

Geometrical and Topological Analysis of Vascular Branches from Fundus Retinal Images

Nicholas W. Witt, M. Elena Martínez-Pérez, Kim H. Parker, Simon A. McG. Thom, and Alun D. Hughes

CONTENTS

10.1 Introduction 305
10.2 Geometry of Vessel Segments and Bifurcations 306
10.3 Vessel Diameter Measurements from Retinal Images 312
10.4 Clinical Findings from Retinal Vascular Geometry 315
10.5 Topology of the Vascular Tree 318
10.6 Automated Segmentation and Analysis of Retinal Fundus Images 323
10.7 Clinical Findings from Retinal Vascular Topology 328
10.8 Conclusion 329
      References 330

10.1   Introduction

The retinal fundus is a site where the microcirculation (arteries and veins between 20–200 μm) can readily be viewed and imaged. Evidence that the retinal microcirculation is affected by diabetes [1], renal disease, and hypertension [2] followed rapidly once the ophthalmoscope was invented by Helmholtz in 1851 [1]. In the context of hypertension, Keith, Wagener, and Barker showed that mortality increased with increasing severity of retinopathy [3] and their work led to the most widely known eponymous classification system of hypertensive retinopathy. Subsequently, a number of alternative classification schemes have been proposed [4; 5].

Fundoscopy is a routine part of the assessment of the hypertensive patient [6–8]. However with better levels of control of blood pressure the frequency of severe retinopathy such as that seen by Keith, Wagener, and Barker has declined markedly. Current estimates suggest that retinopathy occurs in only around 2% to 15% of the nondiabetic adult population aged 40 years and older [9–16]. Consequently the value of routine fundoscopy in hypertension has been increasingly questioned on the grounds of poor reproducibility and indifferent predictive value [17; 18]. In contrast, diabetic retinopathy remains an immense health problem and is one of the commonest causes of blindness in adults [19].

Hypertension is a major cause of mortality and morbidity, currently affecting nearly a billion individuals worldwide [20], and it accounts for approximately one in eight of all deaths [21]. Moreover, blood pressure shows a continuous relationship with cardiovascular disease risk [22] and the majority of cardiovascular disease that is attributable to increased blood pressure occurs in individuals that are not categorized as hypertensive. Therefore, identification of individuals at risk of cardiovascular events within the range of "normal" blood pressure would be of considerable value.

10.2   Geometry of Vessel Segments and Bifurcations

Interest in quantifiable geometrical parameters of vessel segments and bifurcations has been driven by the hypothesis that alterations in such parameters can provide an indication of cardiovascular risk independent of blood pressure and other known risk factors.

An important consideration in the measurement of retinal vascular geometry is that an unknown refraction is introduced by the lens, cornea, and aqueous humour in the optical path of the eye through which a retinal image is captured, rendering absolute measurements of physical distances uncertain [23]. It has been estimated that the effects of refraction may give rise to variability of up to 20% in absolute vascular diameter measurements from retinal fundus photographs [24]. Accordingly, the greatest attention has been given to nondimensional geometrical parameters, typically involving a ratio of distances, which are more robust to confounding effects of variations in the optical path. Examples of geometrical parameters not influenced by ocular refraction include:

- Arterial to venous diameter ratio (AVR)

- Bifurcation geometry, including diameter relationships and angles

- Vessel length to diameter ratio (LDR)

- Vessel tortuosity.

Further definitions of these parameters are given in the following sections.

10.2.1   Arterial to venous diameter ratio

One of the first parameters describing vascular geometry to receive attention was the ratio of arterial to venous vascular diameters, commonly known as the AVR, which can be found in the literature as early as 1879 [25]. The principal objective of this parameter is to provide sensitivity to general arterial narrowing, while reducing the impact of refractive variation through normalization by the venous diameter. Confirmation of the insensitivity of AVR to refraction has been reported by Wong et al. [24].

Stokoe and Turner [25] drew attention to the importance of calculating the AVR from measurements of arterial and venous diameters at comparable orders of division in their respective vascular trees, and also highlighted the practical difficulty of achieving this, not least because the more peripheral retinal arteries and veins tend to be dissociated. In order to overcome some of these problems, the AVR for a single eye has commonly been calculated by a technique based on work originated by Parr and Spears [26; 27], and subsequently modified by Hubbard [28], in which diameter measurements of a series of arteries or veins are combined into an equivalent diameter of the central retinal artery or vein, respectively. The ratio of these equivalent central vessel diameters can then be calculated to yield the AVR.

Parr and Spears derived an empirical formula relating vessel diameters at an arterial bifurcation, based on measurements from a sample of red-free monochrome retinal photographs of normotensive adults [26]. Their approach was guided by the observation that the ratio of areas of the daughter vessels to that of the parent generally decreased with increasing asymmetry of the bifurcation, suggesting a general form of an expression relating the diameters. A computer search algorithm was used to determine the parameters based on a least-squares criterion, yielding a relationship giving the parent arterial diameter

$$d_{a_0} = \sqrt{0.87d_{a_2}^2 + 1.01d_{a_1}^2 - 0.22d_{a_1}d_{a_2} - 10.76} \qquad (10.1)$$

where d_{a_1} and d_{a_2} are the diameters of the larger and smaller daughter vessels respectively, all measured in μm. An equivalent formula for the veins was later derived by Hubbard by a similar approach, giving the parent venous diameter as

$$d_{v_0} = \sqrt{0.72d_{v_2}^2 + 0.91d_{v_1}^2 + 450.05} \qquad (10.2)$$

where d_{v_1} and d_{v_2} are defined in the same way as for the arteries, also measured in μm.

In order to yield the central vessel equivalent diameter from a series of arterial diameter measurements, Hubbard [28] proposed a simplified pairing of vessels, compared to the original Parr and Spears technique that involved reconstructing the actual arterial tree [27]. In the simplified scheme, the largest vessel is paired with the smallest, the next largest with the next smallest and so on, irrespective of the bifurcations actually observed. The parent vessel diameters are calculated by the appropriate formula, and are carried together with any odd remaining vessel to the next order of division where the pairing procedure is repeated. The process is continued until a diameter estimate for the single central vessel has been achieved. This process is illustrated in Figure 10.1(a), where measured arterial vessels [27] are shown in the left-hand column, and the diameters of subsequent orders of vessels are calculated by the Parr and Spears empirical formula, eventually yielding the equivalent diameter of the central retinal artery, d_{cra}.

The process is repeated separately for the venous tree, yielding the equivalent diameter of the central retinal vein, d_{crv}. Hence the arterial to venous ratio is given by

$$\text{AVR} = \frac{d_{\text{cra}}}{d_{\text{crv}}}. \tag{10.3}$$

In a previously unpublished analysis, we have compared the diameter relationships predicted at an arterial bifurcation by the empirical Parr and Spears formula with those suggested theoretically in an optimum bifurcation by Murray's Law [29], as discussed in the following section. In perfectly symmetrical bifurcations, the Parr and Spears formula consistently gives rise to a parent diameter in the region of 2.2% greater than that indicated by Murray's Law, but more importantly, this relationship appears to be maintained within a tolerance of better than $\pm 0.5\%$ of parent diameter over a wide range of bifurcations, the only exceptions being cases of extreme asymmetry. This consistency between the empirical Parr and Spears approach and the theoretical treatment by Murray should not be unexpected, bearing in mind that the Parr and Spears formula was derived from images of healthy normotensive subjects. It suggests that the AVR calculated by the Parr, Spears and Hubbard technique might be sensitive not only to general arterial narrowing, but also to deviations from the optimal bifurcation geometry predicted by Murray's Law.

The Parr and Spears technique depends on measurement of all vessel diameters being undertaken at a consistent location in the vascular tree. One approach to achieve this involves an annular grid, consisting of concentric rings centered on the optic disc, superimposed on a retinal image [28]. Diameter measurements are taken from all vessels traversing a measurement zone between the concentric rings, as illustrated in Figure 10.1(b), before being combined by the method described earlier to yield their central vessel equivalent diameters, from which the AVR can be calculated.

10.2.2   Bifurcation geometry

The geometry of bifurcating vessels may have a significant impact on the hemodynamics of the vascular network. Important parameters characterizing the geometry of an arterial bifurcation are the bifurcation angle ψ, defined as the internal angle between the daughter vessels, and the junction exponent x, defined by the relationship

$$d_0^x = d_1^x + d_2^x \tag{10.4}$$

where d_0 and d_1, d_2 are the diameters of the parent and daughter vessels respectively. Early work by Murray [29; 30] predicted that optimum values of both the junction exponent and bifurcation angle should exist, minimizing the power required to maintain circulation through the bifurcation (including losses due to viscous drag, and the metabolic energy to maintain the blood and tissue volume). Murray indicated that the optimum value of the junction exponent is 3, generally referred to as Murray's Law. Sherman [31] and LaBarbera [32], based on data from a variety of other workers, have shown that with the exception of the very largest vessels, healthy arteries

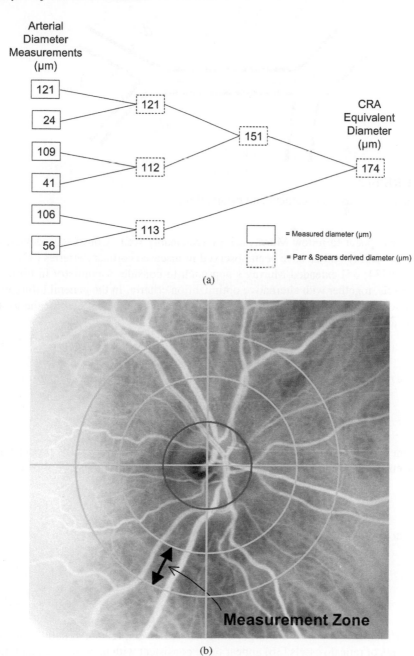

Arterial
Diameter
Measurements
(µm)

121

24

121

109

41

112

151

CRA
Equivalent
Diameter
(µm)

174

106

56

113

□ = Measured diameter (µm)

⬚ = Parr & Spears derived diameter (µm)

(a)

Measurement Zone

(b)

FIGURE 10.1

Measurement of AVR by Parr, Spears, and Hubbard technique: (a) derivation of central retinal arterial (CRA) equivalent diameter, and (b) measurement of vessels in zone defined by a predetermined annular grid.

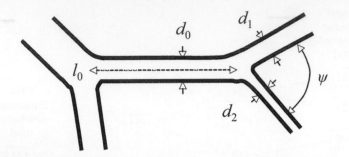

FIGURE 10.2

A generalized vascular segment and bifurcation.

and veins appear to follow Murray's Law reasonably well. Conversely, deviations from the Murray optima have been observed in diseased coronary arteries [33].

Zamir [34; 35] extended Murray's approach to consider asymmetry in bifurcating vessels, together with alternative optimization criteria. In the general bifurcation illustrated in Figure 10.2, nondimensional parameters can be defined for the asymmetry ratio

$$\alpha = \frac{d_2^2}{d_1^2} \tag{10.5}$$

and the ratio of vessel cross-sectional areas, sometimes referred to as expansion ratio

$$\beta = \frac{d_1^2 + d_2^2}{d_0^2}. \tag{10.6}$$

From Murray's principal hypothesis that the diameter of a vessel is proportional to the cube root of the flow that the vessel is intended to carry, it can be shown that

$$\beta = (1+\alpha)\left(1+\alpha^{3/2}\right)^{-2/3} \tag{10.7}$$

and that

$$\frac{d_1}{d_o} = \left(1+\alpha^{3/2}\right)^{-1/3} \tag{10.8}$$

$$\frac{d_2}{d_0} = \alpha^{1/2}\left(1+\alpha^{3/2}\right)^{-1/3}, \tag{10.9}$$

where d_1 is the diameter of the larger daughter vessel. Experimental data from measurements of retinal vessels [36] appear to be consistent with these theoretical ratios, albeit with some scatter of observed data around the theoretical values.

From the above ratios, theoretical optimum branching angles can be predicted given the asymmetry ratio and taking into account specific optimization criteria. Four such criteria have been considered [34–37]: lumen surface, lumen volume, pumping power, and endothelial drag. The spread observed in data from retinal bifurcations suggests that more than one optimality criterion may be involved, although some bias in favor of the principles of minimum lumen volume and pumping power has been observed [36]. In general, for a given optimality criterion, the optimum bifurcation angle ψ depends on both the junction exponent x and also the asymmetry ratio α [37], but for reasonably symmetrical bifurcations (say $\alpha > 0.4$) obeying Murray's Law, the optimum angle ψ for a bifurcation is approximately constant at 75 degrees.

It is generally believed that the endothelium plays an important role in the maintenance of optimal geometry at bifurcations. Inhibition of endothelial nitric oxide *in vitro* has been shown to cause deviations in the junction exponent from optimum values [38], and observations in the retina from young normal subjects have shown acute alteration of bifurcation geometry when synthesis of endothelial nitric oxide was suppressed by infusion of N^G-mono-methyl-L-arginine (L-NMMA) [39]. Accordingly, it has been hypothesised that deviations from optimal bifurcation geometry are associated with endothelial dysfunction. Given that impairment of endothelial function has been found in the early stages of atherosclerosis [40], speculation has arisen that altered bifurcation geometry may even precede clinical presentation of cardiovascular disease.

It has been noted that the junction exponent is not an ideal parameter to characterize the optimality of diameter relationships at a bifurcation, since it is poorly behaved in the presence of measurement noise [41]. For this reason, an alternative parameter based on mean nondimensional daughter diameter, corrected for the effects of asymmetry, was used in a recent study [41] as a more robust surrogate for junction exponent.

10.2.3 Vessel length to diameter ratios

The length to diameter ratio (LDR) of a vessel segment is typically measured between consecutive bifurcations, represented by l_0/d_0 in Figure 10.2. The LDR will tend to increase in value in the presence of general arterial narrowing, as well as rarefaction, both of which are associated with increased peripheral vascular resistance and hypertension [42]. Furthermore, the LDR, like the AVR, is robust to variability in refraction by virtue of its nondimensionality.

A practical issue arises in the measurement of LDR from typical retinal images. Since the length of a vessel segment is measured between consecutive bifurcations, a risk exists that a measurement of LDR may vary, depending on the ability to detect a bifurcation involving a very small daughter vessel branching from a larger parent. This, in turn, is likely to be affected by image quality, increasing scatter in L/D measurements, and reducing reproducibility. In order to minimize any association between L/D measurements and image quality, it is necessary to establish criteria to reject small daughter vessels close to the threshold of imaging or visualization, so that these are not regarded as terminating vessel segments undergoing LDR measurement.

10.2.4 Tortuosity

Vascular tortuosity in the retina has been qualitatively assessed by physicians since the invention of the ophthalmoscope, but quantitative measurement of tortuosity of retinal vessels has been a more recent development. A large number of computational techniques are available for the measurement of vascular tortuosity, and Hart et al. [43] have compared the characteristics of seven different measures, without conclusively recommending a particular approach.

A simple and widely used technique is based on the ratio of arc length l_a to chord length l_c in the form

$$\tau_{\text{simple}} = \frac{l_a}{l_c} - 1. \tag{10.10}$$

This measure is sensitive to the increase in arc length in a tortuous vessel, but does not necessarily reflect the extent to which a vessel changes direction. An alternative measure of tortuosity also offering sensitivity to the latter characteristic can be derived from the curvature of the vessel κ, normalized by the arc length as follows

$$\tau_{\text{curve}} = \frac{1}{l_a} \int_{\xi_{\text{start}}}^{\xi_{\text{end}}} [\kappa(\xi)]^2 \, d\xi, \tag{10.11}$$

where ξ is the distance along the vessel path. This measure benefits from a property referred to as "compositionality," meaning that if a vessel is composed of two smoothly connected segments, then the tortuosity of the entire vessel must lie between those of the constituent segments [43]. Measures having such a property have been considered *a priori* to correspond most closely to the tortuosity judged qualitatively by ophthalmologists [43]. However it should be noted that the curvature-based measure (τ_{curve}) is not dimensionless.

The distinction between these alternative measures may be appreciated by reference to Figure 10.3 illustrating three vessels of equal arc and chord length, but with zero, one, and two inflection points. All three vessels are constructed from concatenated semi-circles, allowing both measures of tortuosity to be calculated analytically. Bearing in mind that curvature-based tortuosity is not dimensionless, this measure has been computed assuming a typical vessel length of 353 pixels from a retinal field of approximately 2800 pixels in diameter corresponding to a 30 degree view. Simple tortuosity is equal in all three cases since the arc or chord lengths remain unchanged, whereas curvature tortuosity progressively increases with the number of inflection points.

10.3 Vessel Diameter Measurements from Retinal Images

Several of the parameters discussed above, such as AVR, bifurcation diameter optimality, and LDR, involve measurement of vessel diameter for their computation. The most accurate source from which to determine the diameter of retinal vessels

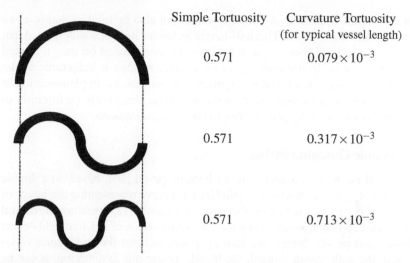

	Simple Tortuosity	Curvature Tortuosity (for typical vessel length)
	0.571	0.079×10^{-3}
	0.571	0.317×10^{-3}
	0.571	0.713×10^{-3}

FIGURE 10.3

Comparison of alternative tortuosity measures. (Adapted from Witt, N.W., Wong, T.Y., Chaturvedi, N., et al., *Hypertension,* 47, 975, 2006. With permission.)

would generally be considered to be fluorescein angiography, but such an invasive procedure is unsuitable for routine clinical imaging, and the preferred technique is to measure vascular geometry from red-free monochrome images, or else from color images, usually by selection of the green layer. Measurement of vessel diameter from images acquired without fluorescein is more challenging since the contrast between vessel and background is much lower, and the edges of vessels are poorly defined. The presence of a pronounced central light reflex may also cause problems. Three techniques are described here, which have been proposed to tackle the challenge of measuring the diameter of a retinal vessel from red-free images. All these techniques are based upon measurement of diameter from a single intensity cross section normal to the direction of flow in the vessel and, typically, an overall estimate of diameter would be made from a sequence of such cross sections a few pixels apart.

10.3.1 The half-height method

Brinchmann-Hansen and Engvold [44] proposed a method of measuring the width of a retinal vessel from a single intensity cross section of a fundus photograph, based upon measurement of distance between the points of half intensity. The principle is illustrated in Figure 10.4(a), where the vessel gives rise to increasing intensity, as would arise from a red-free image on monochrome negative film. In summary, the points of maximum and minimum intensity are identified on each side of the vessel center line, and overall extreme intensities are taken to be the means of the values from opposite sides of the profile. The vessel diameter is measured between the points on the profile intercepting the half intensity value, taken to be the midpoint between the overall extremes. A similar process can also be used to measure the width of the central light reflex. This half-height technique has been widely used, but it has been criticized [45] because it makes measurements based on only a limited amount of information in the intensity cross section, making it vulnerable to the effects of image intensity noise and other imaging imperfections. Implementation of a practical measurement system based on this technique would rely on filtration of the image and/or the intensity profile prior to taking measurements.

10.3.2　Double Gaussian fitting

A more general model-based approach has been proposed [46], based on a double Gaussian intensity profile, in which a main Gaussian curve representing the image of the vessel itself is summed with a smaller inverted Gaussian representing the central light reflex. This approach assumes that increased attenuation of red-free light occurs in the lumen as it passes through the blood column, and that the attenuation varies linearly with the path length through the blood. Under this assumption, it can be shown that a Gaussian function is a reasonable approximation of the intensity profile across the vessel [46]. The central light reflex can be modeled as an optical scattering from a rough column of blood, and under the assumption of elliptical scattering functions, gives rise to the narrow inverted Gaussian [47–49]. The double Gaussian curve can be characterized by up to seven parameters, a_1 to a_7, such that the intensity I varies as a function of the distance along the cross section x

$$I(x) = a_1 e^{-((x-a_2)/a_3)^2} + a_4 - a_5 e^{-((x-a_6)/a_7)^2} \tag{10.12}$$

as illustrated in Figure 10.4(b). Given an intensity cross section from a retinal photograph, the seven parameters characterizing the double Gaussian profile can be determined from a nonlinear fitting technique, such as the Levenberg-Marquardt method [50], although robustness to noise can be improved by fixing some of the parameters, such as a_2 and/or a_7 to reduce the degrees of freedom. It should be noted that the parameter a_3 characterizing the width of the main Gaussian curve does not correspond directly to the diameter of the vessel, and must be multiplied by a scaling factor to allow direct comparison with the results from other measurement methods. In a comparison of vessel measurement techniques, including the double Gaussian model, Chapman et al. [45] took the vessel diameter to be $2.33a_3$.

10.3.3　The sliding linear regression filter (SLRF)

The SLRF method [45] is based upon the fitting of a line by linear regression, relating image intensity against distance along the cross section, within a window of W points centered on the nth point. The window is progressively moved by a single point at a time across the entire cross section of interest, and the slope of the best least-squares line attributed to the nth point as m_n. Hence

$$m_n = \frac{W \sum_i x_i z_i - \sum_i x_i \sum_i z_i}{W \sum_i x_i^2 - \left(\sum_i x_i \right)^2} \tag{10.13}$$

for all i such that $-W/2 \leq (i-n) \leq W/2$, x_i and z_i being the position and intensity respectively at the ith point. This principle is illustrated in Figure 10.4(c).

To determine the positions of the maximum positive going and negative going slope, the resulting values of m are subject to a threshold test, and those points falling beyond a specified range are used to compute the actual position of the edge. The diameter is taken as the distance between the opposite edges.

An important consideration in the SLRF method is the choice of window size W. Generally, a smaller window size gives better resolution of edges of small vessels, but at the expense of less noise rejection, whereas a larger window gives better consistency in measurements from larger vessels. It can be concluded that the window size should be adapted to reflect the size of the vessel under examination, which has also been found to improve the linearity of the measurement technique. A suitable value of W can be derived from an initial estimate of the vessel under measurement, either from a moment-based calculation or else application of the half-height technique.

In a comparison of automated vessel measurement techniques [45], including the double Gaussian and SLRF techniques, it was found that the SLRF method yielded the most consistent and most repeatable automated measurements.

10.4 Clinical Findings from Retinal Vascular Geometry

Early clinical studies have pointed to associations between altered retinal vascular geometry and cardiovascular risk. Increased LDR was found to be associated with hypertension in a small study comparing men with normal blood pressure and hypertension [51]. This is consistent with previous findings of increased vessel length and reduced caliber [42] in hypertension. Furthermore, a significant association has been found between increasing age and decreasing junction exponent in retinal arterial bifurcations, both in normotensive and hypertensive individuals [52]. This study was performed in a group of 25 subjects undergoing fluorescein angiography, and is consistent with other reports of abnormal endothelial function with aging [53]. The same study found that bifurcation angles also reduced with age, and were smaller for people with hypertension than those with normal blood pressure.

A later study found significantly narrower bifurcation angles in a group of men with low birth weight [54] (although no difference in junction exponent) compared to a similar group having high birth weight, independent of blood pressure. Bearing in mind that interesting associations have been reported between low birth weight and increased cardiovascular mortality [55] as well as increased prevalence of hypertension [56–58], these findings in the retina may point to a mechanistic link between low birth weight and subsequently increased cardiovascular risk, and add support to the suggestion that abnormalities in retinal vascular geometry can precede other manifestations of disease.

Significant deviations in junction exponents of retinal arterial bifurcations have also been found in normotensive men with peripheral vascular disease [59], whereas

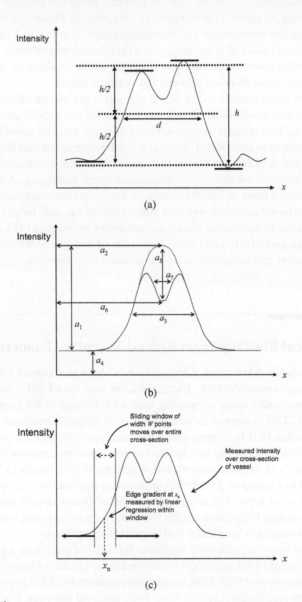

FIGURE 10.4
Techniques for vessel diameter measurement: (a) the half-height method, (b) the double Gaussian method, and (c) the SLRF method. (Part (c) from Chapman, N., Witt, N.W., Gao, X., Bharath, A.A., et al., *Br. J. Ophthalmol.,* 85, 74, 2001. With permission.)

healthy controls, matched for age and blood pressure, exhibited optimal junction exponents as predicted by Murray's Law.

Important evidence of the power of AVR and other geometrical characteristics of the retinal vasculature to predict vascular disease have come from prospective population-based studies, most notably the Atherosclerosis Risk in Communities (ARIC) study [60] and the Beaver Dam Eye Study [61]. Reduced AVR measured by the Parr, Spears, and Hubbard method has been shown to predict independently incident hypertension over a 3-year period in the ARIC study [62], and in the Beaver Dam Eye Study [63] over a 10-year period. These findings are consistent with the hypothesis that arterial narrowing is associated with the occurrence and development of hypertension, although neither study distinguishes between functional or structural narrowing of arteries. Furthermore, in the ARIC study reduced AVR has been shown to predict stroke independently of other risk factors [64], coronary heart disease (CHD) in women (but not men) [65], and type 2 diabetes mellitus [66]. In the Beaver Dam Eye Study, AVR was found to predict cardiovascular death in a cohort of 879 younger persons (age 43–74 years) although not in older individuals [67]. However, in a larger analysis of 4926 individuals from the same population, a U-shaped association was found in which very large or very small values of AVR were associated with increased mortality over 10 years, both from all causes and vascular disease [68]. This latter finding contrasts with those from earlier studies, suggesting that further investigation is needed to understand fully the association between AVR and systemic disease.

An extensive analysis of retinal vascular geometry has been undertaken in a cohort of 528 subjects participating in the Beaver Dam Eye Study [41]. This nested case-control study found that sub-optimal diameter relationships at retinal arterial bifurcations were associated with risk of death within 10 years from ischemic heart disease (IHD), independently of other known risk factors including age, gender, and history of cardiovascular disease. This study provides the most compelling evidence to date of the power of abnormal bifurcation geometry to predict incident cardiovascular disease. In the same study LDR was found again to be significantly associated with resting blood pressure, and furthermore was found to predict death from stroke, although not independently of blood pressure. Reduced simple tortuosity (τ_{simple}) was found to be significantly associated with risk of death from IHD, independently of other risk factors. The association between reduced tortuosity and death from IHD was unexpected and is not consistent with earlier qualitative assessments of retinal vascular tortuosity from fundoscopy of subjects with coronary artery disease [69]. However, tortuosity assessed by fundoscopy may be less reliable than that measured quantitatively from retinal photographs and, in addition, confounding factors such as age, hypertension, and diabetes were not taken into account in the earlier study. Given that the endothelium plays a major role in the regulation of microvascular flow and angiogenesis, the finding from the Beaver Dam cohort has given rise to speculation that lowered retinal arterial tortuosity may be linked to endothelial dysfunction, and to widespread impairment of perfusion or oxygenation in the microvasculature.

In the Beaver Dam cohort discussed above, the trend observed in both simple and curvature tortuosity was very similar, although increased scatter was observed in the curvature-based parameter, most likely due to noise associated with the measurement of vector derivatives. However, in a study of plus disease in retinopathy of prematurity (ROP) [70], it was found that measurements of tortuosity based on curvature gave a more significant association with disease than simple tortuosity. Hence further work may be warranted to establish the clinical value of alternative quantitative measures of microvascular tortuosity.

10.5   Topology of the Vascular Tree

The foregoing discussion has focused on geometrical characteristics of individual vascular segments and bifurcations, but an association has also been found between more global topological characteristics of the retinal vascular arcades and cardiovascular health [71].

Branching structures are common in nature, occurring in both geographical and biological phenomena. Some of the earliest work on topology of branching structures was performed by geographers, and subsequently applied to other branching structures, particularly in biology, such as in the study of dendrites, bronchial airways, and arterial trees. Studies of biological branching trees, particularly from image processing techniques, can be found widely in the literature, such as coronary artery trees from X-ray angiograms [72; 73], pulmonary vascular trees from X-ray computer tomography [74], and airway trees from computer tomography [75]. However, the topology of retinal vascular trees has been less widely studied.

Vascular trees are branching structures that are typically treated as binary rooted trees, a special type of graph. A graph is a set of points (or vertices) connected by edges. A tree is a graph with no cycles. A rooted tree is one in which a single vertex is distinguished as the root and a binary tree is one in which at most three edges are contiguous to any vertex [76]. Figure 10.5(a) shows a retinal vessel tree and Figure 10.5(b) shows its schematic representation as a rooted binary tree graph.

In order to study the global properties of branching structures, it has been usual to group bifurcations into schemes based on their order, or generation. The order is a number assigned to an edge, the value of this number depending on the ordering scheme in use, whereas the generation represents the hierarchical level at which a particular bifurcation belongs, as in a family tree. The generational representation is found mainly in symmetrical models. Ordering schemes can be either centrifugal, ordering from the root of the tree toward the periphery, or else centripetal, commencing at the periphery and progressing toward the root. Some schemes assume all branches are symmetrical, incorporating diameters and length but not branching angles, whereas others assume all branches with the same order have the same diameter, the same length, and bifurcate with the same asymmetry. This means that some schemes are strictly topological whereas others combine geometry with topology in their representations.

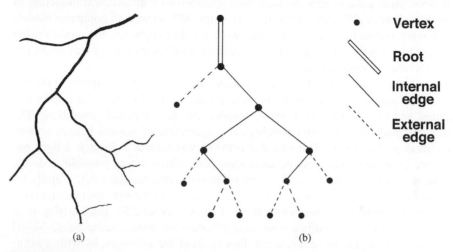

FIGURE 10.5

(a) Segmented retinal vessel tree and (b) its schematic representation as a rooted binary tree graph.

The different methods give different assessments of the number of orders. The more asymmetrical the branching structure, the more critical becomes the choice of an appropriate ordering scheme. The consensus among geographers has led to the choice of the Strahler method (1952) by the majority of biologists. Horsfield and coworkers [77], who have worked extensively on bronchial trees, have adopted Strahler ordering in their studies, which facilitates comparison of their results with those of other authors.

Strahler ordering is a centripetal scheme that assigns all external edges (excluding the root) an order of $m = 1$. Where two edges of order m come together, the third edge is assigned order $m + 1$. Where an edge of order m meets an edge of order n, the third edge is assigned order $\max(m,n)$. This ordering scheme is purely topological, and an example can be found in Figure 10.6(c).

A large amount of work has been done in relating geometrical features such as lengths, diameters, and cross-sectional areas as a function of order or generation in biological branching trees, most commonly those from lungs. A widely adopted model has been the symmetrical model developed by Weibel in 1963, who carried out detailed measurements of dimensions in casts of both arteries and airways in human lungs. An alternative classification method, more suited to describe asymmetrical trees, was developed by Horsfield and Cumming in 1968. They produced a series of models based on their own ordering technique and on the Strahler system [76–78]. Further interesting work was performed by Huang et al. [79], in which casts of arterial and venous trees from human lungs were prepared and measured. This model modified Horsfield's Strahler ordering scheme, introducing a rule to adjust the order based on relative vessel diameters at junctions. Based on experimental and theoretical work, other authors have focused their attention on mathematical modeling of bronchial airways [78] and arterial trees in lungs [80], as well as computer models of coronary arterial trees [81]. The latter work sought to optimize the models using different functional seeds as parameters, and statistical morphometry was employed to characterize anatomical variations.

In the human retina, Schroder [82] developed an interesting description of the microvascular network, including the branching pattern, the number of arterioles and venules, and the distribution of vessel lengths and diameters per generation. The study was made *in vitro* from histological preparations of normal human retinas, three days post mortem. The vascular network was recorded through a light microscope onto photomicrographic montages, from which it was possible to divide the network into dichotomous, asymmetric arteriolar and venular trees. Capillaries were considered as order 1 using the Strahler method, but the precapillary and postcapillary vessels were not taken into account so as to avoid difficulties arising from capillary loops and to facilitate separation of arteriolar from venular trees. Vessel diameters and lengths were measured directly from the micrographs with a semiautomatic calibrated morphometric analyzer. Vessel length in the microcirculation typically shows a log-normal distribution, and so median lengths of different orders were compared. On the other hand, microvascular diameters typically show an almost symmetrical distribution within each vessel order, and so mean diameter values were used. Both arterial and venous trees contained 6 Strahler orders, incorporating 1173 and 507 vessel segments respectively in the largest trees. Their results showed a tendency of vessel segments above the third order to increase progressively in length, which was approximated by a second degree polynomial curve. Diameters rose sharply with increasing orders both in arteriolar and venous trees, which was approximated by an exponential curve.

The studies mentioned above have generally involved analysis of geometrical features as a function of the order, across six or more generations. However, retinal trees from fundus images often show fewer orders than this (sometimes only three), insufficient to allow effective analysis of diameters and lengths as a function of order. For this reason we confine our description here to purely topological indices that can characterize retinal vascular trees extracted from clinical fundus images and that may give us insight into possible changes in the topology associated with cardiovascular disease.

Some important topological features of a biological branching tree are those describing whether it is unbalanced or elongated, in other words the extent to which deviates from a purely dichotomous tree, i.e., one that is perfectly balanced [76]. Figures 10.6(a) and (b) show examples of two extreme branching topologies.

The topological indices we list here are the most commonly used indices within biological applications [83]:

- Strahler branching ratio (R)

- Maximum tree exterior path length or altitude (A)

- Total exterior path length (P_e)

- Number of external-internal edges (N_{EI}) and the total number of external (or terminal) edges (N_T)

- Tree asymmetry index (A_s).

Further definitions are provided in the following sections.

10.5.1 Strahler branching ratio

The Strahler branching ratio is calculated by ordering all the edges within a given tree using the Strahler ordering scheme. At a given order m, the branching ratio is defined as

$$R_m = \frac{N_m}{N_{m+1}} \tag{10.14}$$

where N is the number of edges, as shown in Figure 10.6(c).

The significance of R_m is that it indicates a degree of topological self-similarity in the branching structure. This idea has been applied by other authors to investigate regularities corresponding to other geometrical self-similarity, such as

$$R_d = \frac{\bar{d}_m}{\bar{d}_{m+1}} \quad ; \quad R_L = \frac{\bar{L}_m}{\bar{L}_{m+1}} \tag{10.15}$$

where $\bar{d}$ is the mean diameter, $\bar{L}$ the mean length and m the order.

The branching ratio R for the whole tree is typically calculated by taking the antilog of the absolute value of the slope of $\log N_m$ against m.

10.5.2 Path length

The altitude, A, is defined as the largest external path length, where an external path length is the number of edges between the root and the terminal edge. The total path length, P_e, is the sum of all the external path lengths. Figure 10.6(d) shows an example where $A = 5$ and $P_e = 30$.

10.5.3 Number of edges

The count of external-internal edges is designated N_{EI}, where an external-internal edge is terminal while its sister is nonterminal. The total count of terminal edges is designated N_T. In Figure 10.6(e), $N_{EI} = 3$ and the total number of terminal edges is $N_T = 7$. The number of external-external edges $N_{EE} = N_T - N_{EI}$. It should be noted that the number of edges is very dependent on the field of view of the image under consideration.

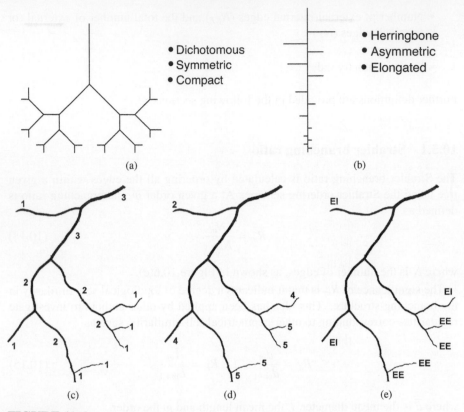

(a)   (b)

(c)   (d)   (e)

FIGURE 10.6
(a) and (b) two extreme branching topologies, (c) Strahler ordering gives $N_1 = 7$, $N_2 = 4$, and $N_3 = 2$, (d) altitude $A = 5$ and total path length $P_e = 30$, and (e) number of external-internal edges $N_{EI} = 3$ and total number of terminal edges $N_T = 7$.

10.5.4 Tree asymmetry index

The final index we consider is the tree asymmetry index, A_s. In order to render it magnitude independent, it is defined in terms of the total number of segments, $N = 2N_T - 1$ and the altitude, A as:

$$A_s = \frac{N + 1 - 2A}{2^A - 2A}. \tag{10.16}$$

Its value ranges from 0 for a herringbone tree to 1 in a perfectly symmetric case.

10.6 Automated Segmentation and Analysis of Retinal Fundus Images

Algorithms have been described earlier that concentrate on measurement of vessel diameters from a sequence of vessel intensity profiles, but to facilitate topological analysis of the retinal vasculature, an automated approach to segmentation and analysis of the whole vascular network from retinal fundus images is desirable.

Most of the work on segmentation of retinal blood vessels can be categorized into three approaches; those based on line or edge detectors with boundary tracing [84; 85], those based on matched filters, either 1-D profile matching with vessel tracking and local thresholding [86–89] or 2-D matched filters [90–92], and those supervised methods that require manually labeled images for training [93; 94]. However, due to the large regional variations in intensity inherent in retinal images and the very low contrast between vessels and the background, particularly in red-free photographs, these techniques have several shortcomings. Techniques based on line or edge detectors lack robustness in defining blood vessels without fragmentation and techniques based on matched filters are difficult to adapt to the variations of widths and orientation of blood vessels. Furthermore, most of these segmentation methods have been developed to work either on red-free or fluorescein images, but not on both.

During the last few decades the computer vision and image processing communities have been studying and developing tools to describe image structures at different scales. Koenderink [95] advocated deriving a set of images at multiple scales by a process of diffusion, equivalent to convolution by a family of Gaussian kernels, and describing image properties in terms of differential geometric descriptors possessing invariance properties under certain transformations. Detection of tube-like structure features using multiscale analysis has been carried out by many researchers [96–101]. The main principle underlying all of these works was to develop a line-enhancement filter based on eigenvalue analysis of the Hessian matrix. Analysis of this kind has also been applied previously to optical images and particularly to retinal images [94; 102; 103], to extract the center lines and perform measurements of diameter using a medialness function.

We present an approach for segmenting blood vessels from fundus images, rather than enhancing them, based upon the principles of multiscale differential geometry in combination with gradient information and a region growing algorithm. This algorithm was originally presented at MICCAII'99 [104], where the segmentation method was tested on a small sample of images without validation. As far as we are aware, this was the first reported analysis of this kind applied to retinal images. An extension of this work [105] reports testing on two local databases and two public databases of complete manually labeled images [92; 94] that have also been used by other authors for the same validation purposes [89; 92; 94]. In addition, validation of diameters and branching angles measured from segmented vessels has also been presented [106]. This approach works equally well with both red-free fundus images

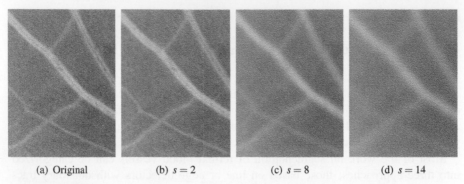

(a) Original   (b) $s = 2$ (c) $s = 8$ (d) $s = 14$

FIGURE 10.7

Multiscale convolution outputs for $s = 0, 2, 8$ and 14 pixels of a portion (720×580 pixels) of a negative of a red-free retinal image (2800×2400 pixels).

and fluorescein angiograms.

Under the multiscale framework, representation of information at different scales is achieved by convolving the original image $I(x, y)$ with a Gaussian kernel $G(x, y; s)$ of variance s^2:

$$I_s(x, y; s) = I(x, y) \otimes G(x, y; s) \tag{10.17}$$

where G is:

$$G(x, y; s) = \frac{1}{2\pi s^2} e^{-\frac{x^2 + y^2}{2s^2}} \tag{10.18}$$

and s is a length scale factor. The effect of convolving an image with a Gaussian kernel is to suppress most of the structures in the image with a characteristic length less than s. Figure 10.7 shows different convolution outputs of a portion of a negative red-free retinal image, for $s = 0, 2, 8$, and 14 pixels, showing the progressive blurring of the image as the length scale factor increases.

The use of Gaussian kernels to generate multiscale information ensures that the image analysis is invariant with respect to translation, rotation, and size [95; 107]. To extract geometrical features from an image, a framework based on differentiation is used. Derivatives of an image can be numerically approximated by a linear convolution of the image with scale-normalized derivatives of the Gaussian kernel:

$$\delta^n I_s(x, y; s) = I(x, y) \otimes s^n \delta^n G(x, y; s) \tag{10.19}$$

where n indicates the order of the derivative.

10.6.1 Feature extraction

The first directional derivatives describe the variation of image intensity in the neighborhood of a point. Under a multiscale framework, the magnitude of the gradient

$$|\nabla I_s(s)| = \sqrt{(\delta_x I_s)^2 + (\delta_y I_s)^2} \tag{10.20}$$

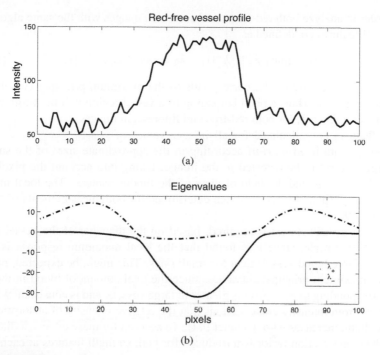

FIGURE 10.8

(a) Intensity profile across a blood vessel from a negative red-free image and (b) Eigenvalues, λ_+ (dash-dot line) and λ_- (solid line). Ridges are regions where $\lambda_+ \approx 0$ and $\lambda_- \ll 0$.

represents the slope of the image intensity for a particular value of the scale parameter s.

The second directional derivatives describe the variation in the gradient of intensity in the neighborhood of a point. Since vessels appear as ridge-like structures in the images, we look for pixels where the intensity image has a local maximum in the direction for which the gradient of the image undergoes the largest change (largest concavity) [108]. The second derivative information is derived from the Hessian of the intensity image $I(x, y)$:

$$H = \begin{pmatrix} \delta_{xx}I_s & \delta_{xy}I_s \\ \delta_{yx}I_s & \delta_{yy}I_s \end{pmatrix}. \tag{10.21}$$

Since $\delta_{xy}I_s = \delta_{yx}I_s$, the Hessian matrix is symmetrical with real eigenvalues and orthogonal eigenvectors that are rotation invariant. The eigenvalues λ_+ and λ_-, where we take $\lambda_+ \geq \lambda_-$, measure convexity and concavity in the corresponding eigendirections. Figure 10.8 shows the profile across a negative red-free vessel and the corresponding eigenvalues of the Hessian matrix, where $\lambda_+ \approx 0$ and $\lambda_- \ll 0$ for pixels in the vessel. For a negative fluorescein vessel profile, where vessels are darker than the background, the eigenvalues are $\lambda_- \approx 0$ and $\lambda_+ \gg 0$ for vessel pixels.

In order to analyze both red-free and fluorescein images with the same algorithm, additional features are defined as

$$\lambda_1 = \min\left(|\lambda_+|, |\lambda_-|\right); \quad \lambda_2 = \max\left(|\lambda_+|, |\lambda_-|\right). \tag{10.22}$$

The maximum eigenvalue λ_2, corresponds to the maximum principal curvature of the Hessian tensor. Thus, a pixel belonging to a vessel region will be weighted as a vessel pixel if $\lambda_2 \gg 1$, for both red-free and fluorescein images.

The features are calculated for all integer values of s, $s_{\min} \leq s \leq s_{\max}$, where s_{min} and s_{max} are fixed *a priori* according to the approximate sizes of the smallest and largest vessel to be detected in the image, taking into account the pixel resolution of the image and the field of view of the fundus camera. The local maxima over the scales (pixel by pixel) is then determined for both measurements of feature strength [109].

However, an adjustment is required, based on the diameter of the vessel that is sought at each scale, since it is found that the local maximum response is much higher for large blood vessels than for small ones. This might be expected, particularly for maximum principal curvature, since the total amount of blood in the light path corresponding to each pixel is greater in large vessels, and is consistent with observations from intensity cross sections that the relative intensity of absorption in a blood column increases with diameter [44]. To account for these effects, a diameter-dependent equalization factor is introduced for both strength features at each scale. Since vessels with diameter $d \approx 2s$ are most strongly detected when the scale factor is s, each feature is normalized along scales by d and the local maxima are sought over the scales as follows:

$$\gamma = \max_s \left[\frac{|\nabla I_s(s)|}{d}\right]; \quad \kappa = \max_s \left[\frac{\lambda_2(s)}{d}\right]. \tag{10.23}$$

Figures 10.9(a) and (b) show the local maxima over the scales after applying the diameter-dependent equalization factor, d, to each scale.

10.6.2 Region growing

The features γ and κ are used to classify pixels in the image into two region classes, either background or vessel, using a multiple pass region growing procedure based on an iterative relaxation technique. All the parameters used in the region growing are automatically calculated for each image from the histograms of the extracted features.

The algorithm begins by planting seeds for each class based primarily upon the maximum principal curvature, using thresholds determined from the histogram of κ. This gives rise to each pixel being classified initially as either vessel, background, or unknown. After the seeds are planted, growth proceeds iteratively in two stages, based on classification of the 8-neighboring pixels. In the first stage growth is constrained to regions of low gradient magnitude allowing a relatively broad and fast classification while suppressing classification in the edge regions where the gradients are large. In the second stage, the classification constraint is relaxed and classes

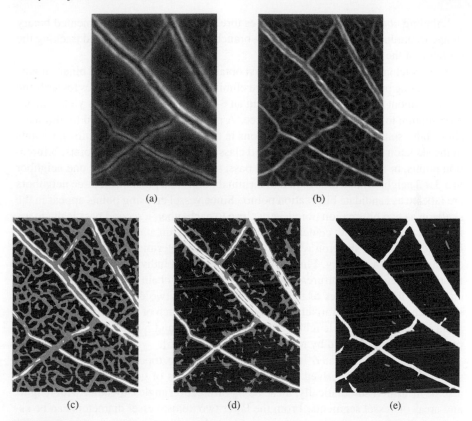

(a)   (b)

(c)   (d)   (e)

FIGURE 10.9

Local maxima responses over the scales for (a) diameter-dependent equalized gradient magnitude γ, and (b) diameter-dependent equalized maximum principal curvature κ. Region growing algorithm consists of (c) planting seeds (white = vessel seeds, black = background seeds, and gray = unknown pixels) followed by (d) growth restricted to regions with low gradients, and, finally, (e) growth without the gradient restriction to define borders between classes.

grow based solely upon κ to allow the definition of borders between regions. Figure 10.9(c) through Figure 10.9(e) illustrate the successive stages of the region growing algorithm. The overall result is an adaptive thresholding that depends on both spectral and spatial local information.

10.6.3   Analysis of binary images

Following completion of the segmentation process, a semi-automatic labeling of the skeleton trees is performed, followed by an automatic procedure to extract and measure the basic topological and geometrical properties.

Labeling of each vascular tree involves three steps; thinning the segmented binary image to produce its skeleton, detecting branch and crossing points, and tracking the skeleton of the tree.

The skeleton of the vascular tree is first obtained from the segmented binary image by a thinning process in which pixels are eliminated from the boundaries towards the center without destroying connectivity in an 8-connected scheme. This yields an approximation to the medial axis of the tree. A pruning process is applied to eliminate short, false spurs, due to small undulations in the vessel boundary. Significant points in the skeleton must then be detected and classified as either terminal points, bifurcation points, or crossing points. In a first pass, skeleton pixels with only one neighbor in a 3×3 neighborhood are labeled as terminal points and pixels with three neighbors are labeled as candidate bifurcation points. Since vessel crossing points appear in the skeleton as two bifurcation points very close to each other, a second pass is made using a fixed size window centered on the candidate bifurcations, and the number of intersections of the skeleton with the window frame determines whether the point is a bifurcation or a crossing. Finally, each tree is tracked individually, commencing at the root. When the first bifurcation point is reached the chain of the current branch is ended and the coordinates of the starting points of the two daughters are found and saved. The process is iteratively repeated for every branch of the tree until a terminal point is reached and all daughters have been detected and numbered. The complete process has been reported by Martinez-Perez et al. [106].

Using the data generated in the labeling stage, the topological parameters described earlier can be derived. In addition, three types of geometrical features can also be measured automatically, these being bifurcation angles, together with lengths and areas of vessel segments. From the latter two items, vessel diameters can be estimated allowing nondimensional geometrical characteristics described earlier to be calculated, such as bifurcation optimality and length to diameter ratios.

10.7   Clinical Findings from Retinal Vascular Topology

A recent investigation compared the topology and architecture of the retinal microvasculature in 20 normotensive subjects, 20 patients with uncomplicated essential hypertension (EHT), and 20 patients with malignant phase hypertension (MHT) [71]. Digitized red-free monochrome retinal photographs, reduced to 1400x1200 pixels, were analyzed to quantify geometrical and topological properties of arteriolar and venular trees.

Mean arteriolar LDR was significantly increased in essential hypertensives ($p = 0.002$) and malignant hypertensives ($p < 0.001$), as shown in Figure 10.10(a), consistent with other studies reported earlier. LDR in venules did not differ significantly between groups.

Both EHT and MHT were associated with significant changes in arteriolar topology. EHT and MHT were associated with reductions in N_T; this was most marked in

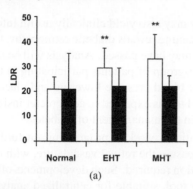
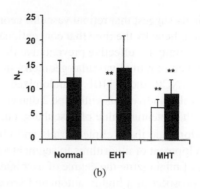

(a)   (b)

FIGURE 10.10

(a) Length diameter ratio (LDR) and (b) number of terminal branches (N_T) of arterioles (open bars) and venules (filled bars) in normal subjects (Normal), essential hypertensives (EHT) and malignant hypertensives (MHT). Data are means $\pm$SD, $**p < 0.01$ by ANOVA and Dunnett's multiple comparison test. (From Hughes, A.D., Martinez-Perez, M., Jabbar, A.-S., Hassan, A., Witt, N.W., Mistry, P.D., et al., *J. Hypertens.* 24, 889, 2006. With permission.)

MHT, as in Figure 10.10(b). Similarly, the total path length was reduced in EHT and significantly so in MHT, even after adjustment for N_T. Neither EHT nor MHT were associated with significant changes in any measure of venular topology after adjustment for N_T. The symmetry of the arteriolar and venous trees was also unaffected by either EHT or MHT.

These changes in the arteriolar network topology are indicative of rarefaction and were exaggerated in MHT. Furthermore, there was also increased venular tortuosity and venular rarefaction in MHT compared with normotensive subjects. This study demonstrated that hypertension is associated with marked topological alterations in the retinal vasculature. The use of automated or semi-automated retinal vascular analyzes should facilitate future investigation of these questions in large populations.

10.8 Conclusion

In this chapter we have presented a growing collection of evidence indicating that alteration of retinal vascular geometry and topology is not only associated with current cardiovascular disease, but in fact arises in advance of other clinical indications, and offers predictive power independent of other recognized risk factors. It may also be of benefit in the clinical assessment of target organ damage in hypertensive patients.

Much of the clinical investigation related to retinal vascular geometry has focused on hypertension and cardiovascular disease, but less attention so far has been given to other systemic diseases such as diabetes. Early unpublished findings in diabetic patients suggest that retinal vascular geometry may also yield clinically useful information here; by the time that conventional screening reveals diabetic retinopathy, the opportunity for effective preventative therapy may have passed. Analysis will be undertaken of retinal vascular geometry in a sub-group of patients participating in the ADVANCE study [110], a randomized trial of blood pressure lowering and glucose control in individuals with type 2 diabetes, and this is expected to add greater insight into the potential value of vascular geometry in the management of diabetes.

Alongside these clinical trials and observations, work is progressing on further development of algorithms to segment and measure the retinal vasculature, with the aim of minimizing the degree of user intervention required. Such developments offer the prospect of a highly automated screening tool, suitable for centralized analysis of retinal photographs captured locally using existing digital fundus cameras, for example during routine examinations by optometrists. Such an arrangement might offer a highly cost effective opportunity to screen large populations for risk factors in a range of systemic diseases.

References

[1] Wolfensberger, T.J. and Hamilton, A.M., Diabetic retinopathy — an historical review, *Semin Ophthalmol*, 16(1), 2, 2001.

[2] Liebreich, R., Ophthalmoskopischer Befund bei Morbus Brightii, *Graefes Arch Clin Exp Ophthalmol*, 5, 265, 1859.

[3] Keith, N.M., Wagener, H.P., and Barker, N.W., Some different types of essential hypertension: their cause and prognosis, *Am J Med Sci*, 197, 332, 1939.

[4] Dodson, P.M., Lip, G.Y., Eames, S.M., et al., Hypertensive retinopathy: a review of existing classification systems and a suggestion for a simplified grading system, *J Hum Hypertens*, 10(2), 93, 1996.

[5] Wong, T.Y. and Mitchell, P., Hypertensive retinopathy, *N Engl J Med*, 351(22), 2310, 2004.

[6] Chobanian, A.V., Bakris, G.L., lack, H.R., et al., Seventh report of the joint national committee on prevention, detection, evaluation and treatment of high blood pressure, *Hypertens*, 42, 1206, 2003.

[7] Williams, B., Poulter, N.R., Brown, M.J., et al., Guidelines for management of hypertension: report of the fourth working party of the British Hypertension Society, 2004-BHS IV, *J Hum Hypertens*, 18(3), 139, 2004.

[8] Lip, G.Y., Beevers, M., and Beevers, D.G., Complications and survival of 315 patients with malignant-phase hypertension, *J Hypertens*, 13(8), 915, 1995.

[9] Wong, T.Y., Klein, R., Klein, B.E.K., et al., Retinal microvascular abnormalities and their relationship with hypertension, cardiovascular disease, and mortality, *Surv Ophthalmol*, 46(1), 59, 2001.

[10] Klein, R., Klein, B.E.K., and Moss, S.E., The relation of systemic hypertension to changes in the retinal vasculature: the Beaver Dam Eye Study, *Trans Am Ophthalmol Soc*, 95, 329, 1997.

[11] Wang, J.J., Mitchell, P., Leung, H., et al., Hypertensive retinal vessel wall signs in a general older population: the Blue Mountains Eye Study, *Hypertens*, 42(4), 534, 2003.

[12] Wong, T.Y., Klein, R., Klein, B.E.K., et al., Retinal vessel diameters and their associations with age and blood pressure, *Invest Ophthalmol Vis Sci*, 44(11), 4644, 2003.

[13] Wong, T.Y., Hubbard, L.D., Klein, R., et al., Retinal microvascular abnormalities and blood pressure in older people: the Cardiovascular Health Study, *Br J Ophthalmol*, 86(9), 1007, 2002.

[14] Klein, R., Sharrett, A.R., Klein, B.E., et al., Are retinal arteriolar abnormalities related to atherosclerosis?: The Atherosclerosis Risk in Communities Study, *Arterioscler Thromb Vasc Biol*, 20(6), 1644, 2000.

[15] Couper, D.J., Klein, R., Hubbard, L.D., et al., Reliability of retinal photography in the assessment of retinal microvascular characteristics: the Atherosclerosis Risk in Communities Study, *Am J Ophthalmol*, 133(1), 78, 2002.

[16] Cuspidi, C., Meani, S., Valerio, C., et al., Prevalence and correlates of advanced retinopathy in a large selected hypertensive population. The evaluation of target organ damage in hypertension (ETODH) study, *Blood Press*, 14(1), 25, 2005.

[17] Dimmitt, S.B., West, J.N., Eames, S.M., et al., Usefulness of ophthalmoscopy in mild to moderate hypertension, *Lancet*, 1(8647), 1103, 1989.

[18] van den Born, B.J., Hulsman, C.A., Hoekstra, J.B., et al., Value of routine funduscopy in patients with hypertension: systematic review, *Br Med J*, 331(7508), 73, 2005.

[19] Fong, D.S., Aiello, L., Gardner, T.W., et al., Retinopathy in diabetes, *Diabetes Care*, 27(Suppl 1), S84, 2004.

[20] Kearney, P.M., Whelton, M., Reynolds, K., et al., Global burden of hypertension: analysis of worldwide data, *Lancet*, 365(9455), 217, 2005.

[21] World Health Organisation, The world health report 2002: reducing risks, promoting healthy life, 2002.

[22] Lewington, S., Clarke, R., Qizilbash, N., et al., Age-specific relevance of usual blood pressure to vascular mortality: a meta-analysis of individual data for one

million adults in 61 prospective studies, *Lancet*, 360(9349), 1903, 2002.

[23] Arnold, J.V., Gates, J.W.C., and Taylor, K.M., Possible errors in the measurement of retinal lesions, *Invest Ophthalmol Vis Sci*, 34, 2576, 1993.

[24] Wong, T.Y., Wang, J.J., Rochtchina, E., et al., Does refractive error influence the association of blood pressure and retinal vessel diameters? The Blue Mountains Eye Study, *Am J Ophthalmol*, 137, 1050, 2004.

[25] Stokoe, N.L. and Turner, R.W.D., Normal retinal vascular pattern. Arteriovenous ratio as a measure of arterial calibre, *Br J Ophthalmol*, 50, 21, 1966.

[26] Parr, J.C. and Spears, G.F.S., Mathematic relationships between the width of a retinal artery and the widths of its branches, *Am J Ophthalmol*, 77, 478, 1974.

[27] Parr, J.C. and Spears, G.F.S., General calibre of the retinal arteries expressed as the equivalent width of the central retinal artery, *Am J Ophthalmol*, 77, 472, 1974.

[28] Hubbard, L.D., Brothers, R.J., King, W.N., et al., Methods for evaluation of retinal microvascular abnormalities associated with hypertension/sclerosis in the Atherosclerosis Risk in Communities Study, *Ophthalmology*, 106, 2269, 1999.

[29] Murray, C.D., The physiological principle of minimum work: the vascular system and the cost of blood volume, *Proc Natl Acad Sci USA*, 12, 207, 1926.

[30] Murray, C.D., The physiological principle of minimum work applied to the angle of branching of arteries, *J Gen Physiol*, 9, 835, 1926.

[31] Sherman, T.F., On connecting large vessels to small. The meaning of Murray's law, *J Gen Physiol*, 78, 431, 1981.

[32] LaBarbera, M., Principles of design of fluid transport systems in zoology, *Science*, 249(4972), 992, 1990.

[33] Hutchins, G.M., Miner, M.M., and Boitnott, J.K., Vessel caliber and branch angle of human coronary artery branch points, *Circ Res*, 38, 572, 1976.

[34] Zamir, M., Optimality principles in arterial branching, *J Theor Biol*, 62, 227, 1976.

[35] Zamir, M., Nonsymmetrical bifurcations in arterial branching, *J Gen Physiol*, 72, 837, 1978.

[36] Zamir, M., Medeiros, J.A., and Cunningham, T.K., Arterial bifurcations in the human retina, *J Gen Physiol*, 74, 537, 1979.

[37] Woldenberg, M.J. and Horsfield, K., Relation of branching angles to optimality for four cost principles, *J Theor Biol*, 122, 187, 1986.

[38] Griffith, T.M., Edwards, D.H., Davies, R.L., et al., EDRF coordinates the behaviour of vascular resistance vessels, *Nature*, 329, 442, 1987.

[39] Chapman, N., Baharudin, S., King, L., et al., Acute effects of L-NMMA on the retinal arteriolar circulation in man, *J Hum Hypertens*, 14, 841, 2000.

[40] McLenachan, J.M., Williams, J.K., Fish, R.D., et al., Loss of flow-mediated endothelium-dependent dilation occurs early in the development of atherosclerosis, *Circ*, 84, 1273, 1991.

[41] Witt, N., Wong, T.Y., Hughes, A.D., et al., Abnormalities of retinal microvascular structure and risk of mortality from ischemic heart disease and stroke, *Hypertension*, 47, 975, 2006.

[42] Struijker-Boudier, H.A.J., le Noble, J.L.M.L., Messing, M.W.J., et al., The microcirculation and hypertension, *J Hypertens*, 10(Suppl 7), S147, 1992.

[43] Hart, W.E., Goldbaum, M., Côté, B., et al., Measurement and classification of retinal vascular tortuosity, *Int J Med Inform*, 53, 239, 1999.

[44] Brinchmann-Hansen, O. and Engvold, O., Microphotometry of the blood column and the light streak on retinal vessels in fundus photographs, *Acta Opthalmologica*, Suppl 179, 9, 1986.

[45] Chapman, N., Witt, N., Gao, X., et al., Computer algorithms for the automated measurement of retinal arteriolar diameters, *Br J Ophthalmol*, 85, 74, 2001.

[46] Gao, X., Bharath, A.A., Hughes, A.J., et al., Towards retinal vessel parameterization, *Proc SPIE*, 3034, 734, 1997.

[47] Brinchmann-Hansen, O. and Heier, H., Theoretical relations between light streak characteristics and optical properties of retinal vessels, *Acta Opthalmologica*, Suppl 179, 33, 1986.

[48] Brinchmann-Hansen, O. and Engvold, O., The light streak on retinal vessels. I. A theoretical modelling of the reflex width, *Acta Opthalmologica*, Suppl 179, 38, 1986.

[49] Brinchmann-Hansen, O. and Engvold, O., The light streak on retinal vessels. II. A theoretical modelling of the reflex intensity, *Acta Opthalmologica*, Suppl 179, 46, 1986.

[50] Press, W.H., Teukolsky, S.A., Vetterling, W.T., et al., *Numerical Recipes in C — The art of scientific computing*, Cambridge University Press, Cambridge, 2nd ed., 1997.

[51] King, L.A., Stanton, A.V., Sever, P.S., et al., Arteriolar length-diameter (L:D) ratio: a geometric parameter of the retinal vasculature diagnostic of hypertension, *J Human Hypertens*, 10, 417, 1996.

[52] Stanton, A.V., Wasan, B., Cerutti, A., et al., Vascular network changes in the retina with age and hypertension, *J Hypertens*, 13(12 Pt2), 1724, 1995.

[53] Egashira, K., Inou, T., Hirooka, Y., et al., Effects of age on endothelium-dependent vasodilation of resistance coronary artery by acetylcholine in hu-

mans, *Circ*, 88, 77, 1993.

[54] Chapman, N., Mohamudally, A., Cerutti, A., et al., Retinal vascular network architecture in low-birth-weight men, *J Hypertens*, 15(12 Pt1), 1449, 1997.

[55] Barker, D.J.P., Osmond, C., Golding, J., et al., Growth in utero, blood pressure in childhood and adult life, and mortality from cardiovascular disease, *Br Med J*, 298, 564, 1989.

[56] Law, C.M. and Shiell, A.W., Is blood pressure inversely related to birth-weight? The strength of evidence from a systematic review of the literature, *J Hypertens*, 14, 935, 1996.

[57] Curhan, G.C., Willet, W., Rimm, E.B., et al., Birth weight and adult hypertension and diabetes mellitus in U.S. men, *Am J Hypertens*, 9(4 Suppl 1), 11A, 1996.

[58] Poulter, N., Chang, C.L., McGregor, A., et al., Differences in birth weight between twins and subsequent differences in blood pressure levels, *J Human Hypertens*, 12(11), 792, 1998.

[59] Chapman, N., Dell'omo, G., Sartini, M.S., et al., Peripheral vascular disease is associated with abnormal diameter relationships at bifurcations in the human retina, *Clinical Science*, 103, 111, 2002.

[60] The ARIC Investigators, The Atherosclerosis Risk in Communities (ARIC) study: design and objectives, *Am J Epidemiol*, 129, 687, 1989.

[61] Klein, R., Klein, B.E.K., Linton, K.L.P., et al., The Beaver Dam Eye Study: visual acuity, *Ophthalmology*, 98, 1310, 1991.

[62] Wong, T.Y., Klein, R., Sharrett, A.R., et al., Retinal arteriolar diameter and risk for hypertension, *Ann Intern Med*, 140, 248, 2004.

[63] Wong, T.Y., Shankar, A., Klein, R., et al., Prospective cohort study of retinal vessel diameters and risk of hypertension, *Br Med J*, 329, 79, 2004.

[64] Wong, T.Y., Klein, R., Couper, D.J., et al., Retinal microvascular abnormalities and incident stroke: the Atherosclerosis Risk in Communities Study, *Lancet*, 358(9288), 1134, 2001.

[65] Wong, T.Y., Klein, R., Sharrett, A.R., et al., Retinal arteriolar narrowing and risk of coronary heart diseases in men and women: the Atherosclerosis Risk in Communities Study, *JAMA*, 287, 1153, 2002.

[66] Wong, T.Y., Klein, R., Sharrett, A.R., et al., Retinal arteriolar narrowing and risk of diabetes mellitus in middle-aged persons, *JAMA*, 287, 2528, 2002.

[67] Wong, T.Y., Klein, R., Nieto, F.J., et al., Retinal microvascular abnormalities and 10-year cardiovascular mortality: a population based case-control study, *Ophthalmology*, 110, 933, 2003.

[68] Wong, T.Y., Knudtson, M.D., Klein, R., et al., A prospective cohort study of retinal arteriolar narrowing and mortality, *Am J Epidemiol*, 159, 819, 2004.

[69] Michelson, E.L., Morganroth, J., Nichols, C.W., et al., Retinal arteriolar changes as an indicator of coronary artery disease, *Arch Intern Med*, 139, 1139, 1979.

[70] Gelman, R., Martinez-Perez, M.E., Vanderveen, D.K., et al., Diagnosis of Plus disease in retinopathy of prematurity using retinal image multi-scale analysis, *Invest Ophthalmol Vis Sci*, 46, 4734, 2005.

[71] Hughes, A.D., Martinez-Perez, M.E., Jabbar, A.S., et al., Quantification of topological changes in retinal vascular architecture in essential and malignant hypertension, *J Hypertens*, 24(5), 889, 2006.

[72] Ezquerra, N., Capell, S., Klein, L., et al., Model-guided labeling of coronary structure, *IEEE Trans Med Imag*, 17, 429, 1998.

[73] Harris, K., Efstratiadis, S.N., Maglaveras, N., et al., Model-based morphological segmentation and labeling of coronary angiograms, *IEEE Trans Med Imag*, 18, 1003, 1999.

[74] Williams, J. and Wolff, L., Analysis of the pulmonary vascular tree using differential geometry-based vector fields, *Comp Vis Image Und*, 65, 226, 1997.

[75] Sauret, V., Goatman, K.A., Fleming, J.S., et al., Semi-automatic tabulation of the 3D topology and morphology of branching networks using CT: application to the airway tree, *Phys Med Biol*, 44, 1625, 1999.

[76] MacDonald, N., *Trees and Networks in Biological Models*, John Wiley & Sons, New York, 1983.

[77] Horsfield, K., Relea, F.G., and Cumming, G., Diameter, length and branching ratios in the bronchial tree, *Resp Physiol*, 26, 351, 1976.

[78] Phillips, C.G., Kaye, S.R., and Schroter, R.C., Diameter-based reconstruction of the branching pattern of the human bronchial tree. Part I. Description and application, *Resp Physiol*, 98, 193, 1994.

[79] Huang, W., Yen, R.T., McLaurine, M., et al., Morphometry of the human pulmonary vasculature, *J Appl Physiol*, 81(5), 2123, 1996.

[80] Dawson, C.A., Krenz, G.S., Karau, K.L., et al., Structure-function relationships in the pulmonary arterial tree, *J Appl Physiol*, 86(2), 569, 1999.

[81] Schreiner, W., Neumann, F., Neumann, M., et al., Anatomical variability and funtional ability of vascular trees modeled by constrained constructive optimization, *J Theor Biol*, 187, 147, 1997.

[82] Schröder, S., Brab, M., Schmid-Schönbein, G.W., et al., Microvascular network topology of the human retinal vessels, *Fortschr Ophthalmol*, 87, 52, 1990.

[83] Berntson, G.M., The characterization of topology: a comparison of four topological indices for rooted binary trees, *J Theor Biol*, 177, 271, 1995.

[84] Akita, K. and Kuga, H., A computer method of understanding ocular fundus images, *Pattern Recogn*, 15, 431, 1982.

[85] Wu, D.C., Schwartz, B., Schwoerer, J., et al., Retinal blood vessel width measured on color fundus photographs by image analysis, *Acta Ophthalmol Scand*, Suppl 215, 33, 1995.

[86] Zhou, L., Rzeszotarski, M.S., Singerman, L.J., et al., The detection and quantification of retinopathy using digital angiograms, *IEEE Trans Med Imag*, 13, 619, 1994.

[87] Tolias, Y.A. and Panas, S.M., A fuzzy vessel tracking algorithm for retinal images based on fuzzy clustering, *IEEE Trans Med Imag*, 17, 263, 1998.

[88] Gao, X., Bharath, A., Stanton, A., et al., Quantification and characterisation of arteries in retinal images, *Comput Meth Prog Biomed*, 63(2), 133, 2000.

[89] Jiang, X. and Mojon, D., Adaptive local thresholding by verification-based multithreshold probing with application to vessel detection in retinal images, *IEEE Trans Pattern Anal Mach Intell*, 25, 131, 2003.

[90] Chaudhuri, S., Chatterjee, S., Katz, N., et al., Detection of blood vessels in retinal images using two-dimensional matched filters, *IEEE Trans Med Imag*, 8, 263, 1989.

[91] Zana, F. and Klein, J.C., Robust segmentation of vessels from retinal angiography, in *Proc 13th Int Conf Digital Signal Processing*, Santorini, Greece, 1997, vol. 2, 1087–90.

[92] Hoover, A., Kouznetsova, V., and Goldbaum, M., Locating blood vessels in retinal images by piecewise threshold probing of a matched filter response, *IEEE Trans Med Imag*, 19, 203, 2000.

[93] Sinthanayothin, C., Boyce, J.F., Cook, H.L., et al., Automated localisation of the optic disc, fovea and retinal blood vessels from digital colour fundus images, *Br J Ophthalmol*, 83, 902, 1999.

[94] Staal, J., Abràmoff, M.D., Niemeijer, M., et al., Ridge-based vessel segmentation in color images of the retina, *IEEE Trans Med Imag*, 23, 501, 2004.

[95] Koenderink, J.J., The structure of images, *Biol Cybern*, 50, 363, 1984.

[96] Koller, T.M., Gerig, G., Székely, G., et al., Multiscale detection of curvilinear structures in 2D and 3D image data, in *Fifth International Conference on Computer Vision*, 1995, 864–69.

[97] Lorenz, C., Carlsen, I.C., Buzug, T.M., et al., Multi-scale line segmentation with automatic estimation of width, contrast and tangential direction in 2D and 3D medical images, in *Proc CVRMed-MRCAS'97*, J. Troccaz, E. Grimson,

and R. Mösges, eds., 1997, vol. 1205 of *Lecture Notes in Computer Science*, 233–242.

[98] Sato, Y., Nakajima, S., Atsumi, H., et al., 3D multi-scale line filter for segmentation and visualization of curvilinear structures in medical images, in *CVRMed-MRCAS'97*, J. Troccaz, E. Grimson, and R. Mösges, eds., 1997, vol. 1205 of *Lecture Notes in Computer Science*, 213–222.

[99] Frangi, A.F., Niessen, J.W., Vincken, K.L., et al., Multiscale vessel enhancement filtering., in *Medical Image Computing and Computer-Assisted Intervention MICCAI'98*, W.M. Wells, A. Colchester, and D. S., eds., Springer, 1998, vol. 1496 of *Lecture Notes in Computer Science*, 130–7.

[100] Krissian, K., Malandain, G., Ayache, N., et al., Model-based detection of tubular structures in 3D images, *Computer Vision and Image Understanding*, 80(2), 130, 2000.

[101] Aylward, S.R. and Bullitt, E., Initialization, noise, singularities, and scale in height ridge traversal for tubular objects centerline extraction, *IEEE Trans Med Imag*, 21(2), 61, 2002.

[102] Jomier, J., Wallace, D.K., and Aylward, S.R., Quantification of retinopathy of prematurity via vessel segmentation, in *Medical Image Computing and Computer-Assisted Intervention (MICCAI'03)*, 2003, vol. 2879 of *Lecture Notes in Computer Science*, 620–626.

[103] Sofka, M. and Stewart, C.V., Retinal vessel centerline extraction using multiscale matched filters, confidence and edge measures, *IEEE Trans Med Imag*, 25(12), 1531, 2006.

[104] Martinez-Perez, M.E., Hughes, A.D., Stanton, A.V., et al., Retinal blood vessel segmentation by means of scale-space analysis and region growing, in *Medical Image Computing and Computer-Assisted Intervention (MICCAI'99)*, 1999, vol. 1679 of *Lecture Notes in Computer Science*, 90–97.

[105] Martinez-Perez, M.E., Hughes, A.D., Thom, S.A., et al., Segmentation of blood vessels from red-free and fluorescein retinal images, *Med Image Anal*, 11(1), 47, 2007.

[106] Martinez-Perez, M.E., Hughes, A.D., Stanton, A.V., et al., Retinal vascular tree morphology: a semi-automatic quantification, *IEEE Trans Biomed Eng*, 49(8), 912, 2002.

[107] Witkin, A.P., Scale-space filtering: a new apporach to multi-scale description, in *Image Understanding*, S. Ullman and W. Richards, eds., Ablex Publishing Co., Norwood, NJ, 79–95, 1984.

[108] Eberly, D., *Ridges in Image and Data Analysis, Computational Imaging and Vision*, Kluwer Academic, Netherlands, 1996.

[109] Lindeberg, T., On scale selection for differential operators, in *Proc 8th Scan-*

dinavian Conference on Image Analysis, K. Heia, K.A. Hogdra, and B. B., eds., Tromso, Norway, 1993, vol. 2, 857–866.

[110] Stolk, R.P., Vingerling, J.R., Cruickshank, J.K., et al., Rationale and design of the AdRem study: evaluating the effects of blood pressure lowering and intensive glucose control on vascular retinal disorders in patients with type 2 diabetes mellitus, *Contemp Clin Trials*, 28, 6, 2007.

11

Tele-Diabetic Retinopathy Screening and Image-Based Clinical Decision Support

Kanagasingam Yogesan, Fred Reinholz, and Ian J. Constable

CONTENTS

11.1 Introduction 339
11.2 Telemedicine 339
11.3 Telemedicine Screening for Diabetic Retinopathy 344
11.4 Image-Based Clinical Decision Support Systems 346
11.5 Conclusion 347
     References 348

11.1 Introduction

Telemedicine services such as specialist referral services, patient consultation, remote patient monitoring, medical education, and consumer medical and health information use provide major benefits to health systems. Telemedicine services reduce health care costs and enables early detection of blinding eye conditions, e.g., diabetic retinopathy. Several feasibility studies of telemedicine screening for diabetic retinopathy have been reported. These studies demonstrate the enormous usefulness of the technology for the communities living in rural and remote areas. In combination with automated image analysis tools and clinical decision support systems, telemedicine could provide widespread screening with the help of less expensive staff and empower local clinicians in the decision making process for eye conditions.

11.2 Telemedicine

With an increasing population it is a challenge to provide specialist health care to all. The advent of telemedicine has opened new vistas in patient care and disease

339

management. Telemedicine means exchange of clinical data via communication networks to improve patient care. Application of telemedicine in ophthalmology and teleophthalmology has already become a common tool in mainstream eye care delivery in many countries [1]. Telemedicine service delivery offers a number of significant advantages over conventional face-to-face consultations. Major benefits of telemedicine are: (1) service access can be improved considerably in remote areas, (2) telemedicine is cost effective due to reduction in patient or staff transfers [2], (3) patients have the benefit of receiving treatment where they live without travelling, and (4) training of local medical officers and nurses to gain knowledge about eye diseases and diagnosis.

There are two modes of delivery in telemedicine. One is real-time video conferencing, which is widely used for emergency and psychiatry consultations. Real-time consultations require high-bandwidth and scheduling. They need both clinician and patient to be present at the same time. This may be not possible in the case of specialists like ophthalmologists. In ophthalmology, high-resolution color images are required to capture the fine detail in the eye. Image files can be large and transmission of these high-resolution images can be time intense. Therefore, teleophthalmology is normally not suitable for video conferencing.

The second mode is called store-and-forward, where images are captured, compressed, and stored in the computer for transmission at a later stage. This is a cost-effective mode that utilizes low bandwidth (Internet) and can send high resolution images. Ophthalmology is an image-based diagnostic field, and most of the diseases can be identified from retinal and anterior segment images. Therefore, specialist ophthalmic care can be easily delivered using the store-and-forward method.

11.2.1 Image capture

One of the procedures of the store-and-forward method is image capture. It is the most important part of the system. There are three different imaging devices, namely the slitlamp, fundus camera, and ophthalmoscope, to image the anterior segment and retina. Corneal opacification from trachomatous scarring, vitamin A deficiency, injuries, or bacterial and viral keratitis can be readily imaged using a video slitlamp biomicroscope or external macro-photography. Cataract can also be documented by each of these methods, or by the use of more complicated photographic systems. Glaucomatous cupping of the optic disc can be detected by standard ophthalmoscopy, fundus photography, and stereo fundus photographic systems or by scanning laser ophthalmoscopy [3; 4]. Diabetic retinopathy is detected by slitlamp biomicroscopy with a fundus lens (+78 to +90D), fundus photography (large or small pupil instruments), or by conventional ophthalmoscopy. The relative efficacy of these methods has been examined in several field trials [5; 6]. Each examination method has advantages and disadvantages related to portability, cost of equipment, ability to obtain hard copy or digitized records, resolution of images, and ease of use. There are other, more advanced but also very expensive imaging devices such as OCT (Optical Coherent Tomography) and SLO (Scanning Laser Ophthalmoscope) to study the retina. These devices are limited to major eye clinics.

Table 11.1: Camera Pixel Number Required to Resolve Detail of Various Resolutions at the Retina

Resolution (μm)	Pixel number (megapixels)	
	30° FOV	50° FOV
3.5 (Sparrow limit)	12	32
4.5 (Rayleigh criterion)	7	20
10 (Typical photographic fundus camera resolution)	1.5	4.5
20	0.4	1

11.2.2 Image resolution

Image resolution, which impacts on image quality, is very important for the diagnosis of eye conditions. Poor quality images may lead to poor diagnosis. The resolution of any optical instrument is defined as the shortest distance between two points on a specimen that can still be distinguished as separate entities, first by the optical camera system and second by the observer. The pixelated camera sensor samples the continuous optical images of the retina that the human ocular system and optical components form on the surface of the sensor. For both, the optical image formation and the periodic sampling at discrete points in time and space, there are well established theories that describe the dependence of the achievable resolution on myriads of imaging conditions and parameters (such as wavelength, illumination or imaging cone, spatial or temporal cut-off frequencies, signal-to-noise ratio, and signal strengths).

It is an important design consideration for ophthalmoscopic instruments to match the optical and the digital resolutions. If the digital resolution is too small, then information may be lost. On the other hand, an increase in digital resolution above the optimum value will not improve the definition of the image. However, the disadvantages are: (1) a sensor with a larger pixel number is more expensive; (2) the light sensed per pixel is less, which gives rise to more noise in the image; and (3) the image file size increases, making it more time consuming to process and transmit the file.

Due to considerations for eye safety (maximum permissible exposure) and patient comfort the power of the illuminating light is restricted to certain upper limits, depending on wavelengths and exposure time. As a consequence, the information being reflected off the retina containing light is very weak. Or in other words, the number of signal photons arriving at the sensor for detection is small. This, together with the inherent shot noise (Poisson statistics) of light bursts, limits the number of distinguishable grey levels in digital ophthalmic instruments. A dynamic range of 8-bit in each color band is therefore more than sufficient for the presentation of such images to ophthalmologists or for quantitative data analyses.

In Table 11.1, the required digital image resolution (pixel number) of the camera is given in terms of the desired retinal feature size to be resolved (the smallest value of 3.5 μm results from the maximum obtainable optical resolution with normal human eyes) and the field of view (FOV). As can be seen, a 7 megapixel camera allows a diagnostic resolution similar to that of a photographic-based fundus camera with a 50° field of view. The smallest lesions are microaneurysms with the size varying from 10 to 25 μm in diameter [7]. If a camera achieves this resolution or better then it can be suitable for diabetic retinopathy screenings.

11.2.3   Image transmission

Digital high resolution images require substantial storage space (> 3 MB) and the transmission of these images over the Internet can be time consuming. The conventional telephone line with a maximum speed of 56 000 bits per second takes 140 seconds to send a 1 megabyte image. But a high speed Internet connection such as DSL (digital subscriber line) needs only 1 second to send a 1 megabyte image. Presently, high speed broadband connections are widely used at homes. The most common broadband connection is called ADSL (asymmetric digital subscriber line). ADSL operates over the existing telephone line without interfering with the normal telephone line. There are two speeds involved with broadband. One is download speed — this is the speed at which information is received. The other is called the upload speed — this is the speed at which information is sent from your computer. The standard ADSL connection provides speeds from 256 to 8000 kbps. Therefore, the time to send images is becoming less significant. However, this can still be an issue if large numbers of images or videos are to be transmitted for telemedicine purposes.

A feasibility study of teleophthalmology by Chen et al. [8] indicated that image transmission via ADSL communication was not stable and required resending of digital images in 88% of the cases (required five or fewer attempts at transmission). The authors indicated that they used JPEG compression ratio of 20:1 for fundus photographs with an average transmission time of around 60 to 90 seconds per patient.

In another study [9] of Web-based real-time telemedicine consultation over cable connection, ADSL and VDSL (very high speed digital subscriber line), concluded that ADSL may be not sufficient for use as a real-time transmission line of telemedicine data. The study recommended a VDSL line for both transmitting and receiving units.

11.2.4   Image compression

Image compression techniques are commonly used in telemedicine systems to increase the transmission speed and also to reduce the storage space. Image compression can be lossy or lossless. The lossless techniques allow perfect reconstruction of the original images but yield modest compression rates. However, lossy compression provides higher compression rates at the expense of some information loss from the original image when it is reconstructed. Loss of information may lead to wrong interpretation of the images. This is critical in the case of retinal images where small pathologies (microaneurysms) provide significant information about disease.

In one of our previous studies [10] we have compared the effect of two commonly used compression algorithms, JPEG (Joint Photographic Experts Group) and Wavelet, on the quality of the retinal images. We investigated the effect of digital compression and the level of compression tolerable. The quality of the retinal images was assessed by both objective (root mean square error) and subjective methods (by four ophthalmologists). Our results indicated that both JPEG and Wavelet compression techniques are suitable for compression of retinal images. Wavelet compression of a 1.5 MB image to 15 kB (compression ratio of 100:1) was recommended when transmission time and costs are considered. The computational time for Wavelet was comparably longer than for JPEG. JPEG compression of a 1.5 MB image to 29 kB (compression ratio of 71:1) was a good choice when compatibility and/or computational time were issues.

In another study, Basu et al. [11] evaluated the JPEG compression technique on images obtained from diabetic retinopathy screenings. An objective assessment was carried out by counting the lesions in compressed and original images (compressed at four different compression levels). They concluded that compression ratios of 20:1 to 12:1 with file sizes of 66–107 kB (original image size 1.3 MB) are acceptable for diabetic retinopathy screenings.

Baker et al. [12] studied the effect of JPEG compression of stereoscopic images on the diagnosis of diabetic retinopathy. The retinal images (original image size 6 MB) from 20 patients with type 2 diabetes mellitus were compressed at two different compression ratios, 55:1 and 113:1 (file size of less than 110 kB). The outcome of their study showed that JPEG compression at ratios as high as 113:1 did not significantly influence the identification of specific diabetic retinal pathology, diagnosis of level of retinopathy, or recommended follow-up. This study demonstrated that JPEG compression could be successfully utilized in a teleophthalmology system for the diagnosis of diabetic retinopathy.

Lee et al. [13] have studied the effects of image compression for drusen identification and quantification. They concluded that JPEG compression ratio of 30:1 may be suitable for archiving and telemedicine application. A group from the Netherlands [14] studied the influence of JPEG compression on diagnosis of diabetic retinopathy using two-field digital images. Using JPEG compression ratio of 30:1, they obtained a sensitivity of 0.72 to 0.74 and specificity of 0.93 to 0.98 for the detection of vision threatening diabetic retinopathy. The original TIFF (tagged image file format) images gave a sensitivity of 0.86 to 0.92 and specificity of 0.93. The group concluded that the compression of digital images could influence the detection of diabetic retinopathy.

It is evident from these studies that the JPEG compression algorithm may be suitable for use in teleophthalmology systems for the diagnosis of diabetic retinopathy. The JPEG compression ratios in the order of 50:1 can reduce the image file size from 6 MB to around 100 kB in order to obtain real-time transmission of images over a standard modem.

11.3   Telemedicine Screening for Diabetic Retinopathy

Diabetic eye disease is the most common cause of new cases of blindness in the Western world [15]. About one-third of diabetics have diabetic retinopathy at any given time point and nearly all will develop it within 20 years after diagnosis. The earliest clinical indication (nonproliferative stage) can be microaneurysms (MA), hemorrhages, hard exudates, cotton wool spots, intraretinal microvascular abnormalities, and venous beading. It is important to note that early stages of diabetic retinopathy are asymptomatic but they are the prelude to the sight-threatening complications. The outcome of treatment for diabetic retinopathy depends on the timing of laser treatment. If the disease is identified early then appropriate laser treatment can be delivered to prevent loss of vision. Regular eye screening for diabetic retinopathy can optimize the timing for laser treatment. It is reported that the incidence and prevalence of blindness can be much lower in communities where diabetic retinopathy screening is well established compared to populations without proper screening for the disease [16]. People living in rural and remote areas have limited access to specialist care and therefore tele-diabetic retinopathy screening by trained staff can be an excellent alternative. The imaging devices such as nonmydriatic fundus cameras should ideally be easy to operate and low cost such that allied health professionals and laypeople can operate the devices and software to obtain high quality images and videos. The patient data, images, medical history, and family history could be sent to a centralized disease control center for reading and diagnostic advice [17; 18].

Cavallerano et al. [19; 20] have successfully implemented and are using telemedicine for diabetic retinopathy screening in the Veterans Affairs Medical Centre. They have been using the Joslin Vision Network (JVN) eye health care model, which is based on a centralized image reading center. With the help of a health worker (imager) certified by the Joslin Diabetes Center, digital fundus images are obtained. Together with patient data images are transmitted via the Internet to the JVN Reading and Evaluation Center at the Joslin Diabetes Center in Boston. There the images are evaluated by an expert team of ophthalmologists, optometrists, and clinical staff. They provide appropriate treatment guidance based on the data received for each patient. This model demonstrates the possibility of using telemedicine based diabetic retinopathy screening in a nonophthalmic setting.

The teleophthalmology program in Western Australia [2] is one of the ongoing and successful programs in the world. The Gascoyne region lies 900 km north of the Perth metropolitan area with a population of approximately 11 000. No permanent eye specialist services exist in the Gascoyne region. The current practice is for an ophthalmologist and a registrar to make a week-long visit to Carnarvon Regional Hospital four times a year for consultations. Community-based screenings for early onset of eye-related disease including glaucoma, diabetic retinopathy, active trachoma, corneal scarring, trichiasis, pterygium, and cataract were conducted. A nurse is trained to use the fundus camera (Canon CR4-45NM), the portable slit-lamp (developed by the Lions Eye Institute; see Figure 11.1) and a puff tonometer.

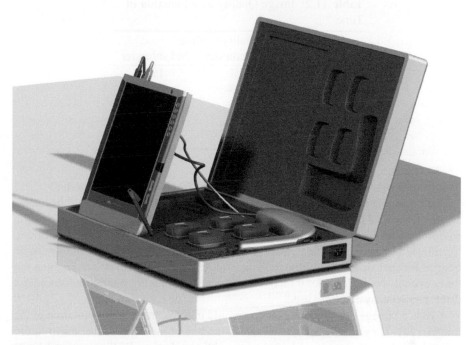

FIGURE 11.1

Low-cost, easy-to-operate, and portable imaging device for both anterior segment and retinal imaging. This device is ideal for telemedicine consultations. (Developed by the Lions Eye Institute in Perth, Australia.)

The nurse also obtains visual acuity and other relevant patient data (medical and family history, medications, and other complications). These data are then sent via a Web-based secure telemedicine system to a centralized telemedicine server. The nurse can choose the referring ophthalmologist and an automatic e-mail alert will be sent to that ophthalmologist about the referral. On average 10 patients per week are referred via this telemedicine service. About 37% of the referrals are related to diabetic retinopathy and 3% of the patients have been referred to ophthalmologists in Perth. If this service were not available all the patients would have been sent to Perth.

During the trial period (one year), 352 people in the Gascoyne region presented for a face-to-face ophthalmic consultation at a cost of $91 760 or $260 per consultation. The Teleophthalmology Project Trial indicated that equivalent funding of teleophthalmology services would benefit 850 patients, costing $107 per consultation.

We have also analyzed the image quality (for diagnosis) during the trial period (Table 11.2). Analysis of the images showed that over time and with experience the images taken by the newly recruited and trained nurse improved significantly. For example, 58% of images were assessed as either "good" or "excellent" in the first six

Table 11.2: Image Quality as a Function of Time

	Image Quality Coding	
Codes	1st semester	2nd semester
1 = Very Poor	2%	1%
2 = Poor	40%	19%
3 = Good	53%	68%
4 = Excellent	5%	12%
All images	100%	100%

months of the program. This figure increased to 80% in the second semester.

The Lions Eye Institute provides regular training to upgrade the skills of the nurses and local medical officers (twice a year). The training is provided for the use of the equipment and software. We also educate the participants about the eye disease, treatment, and disease grading. The imager should know the region of interest to be imaged for each disease, e.g., for glaucoma optic disc is the focal point. Training the trainees could be made easier if image-based decision support systems and automatic disease grading systems are used.

Advanced image processing techniques could improve human interpretation of the images [21]. They could improve our understanding of the findings that may require referral for more thorough analysis by an ophthalmologist. Williamson and Keating [22] have suggested that automated acquisition of images and analysis of digital images without intervention by technical staff either at the site or after transmission to a centralized reading center will indicate to patients whether they have abnormal fundi. Advanced digital image analysis tools could provide objective and more accurate measurements from retinal images. It could be automatic counting and area measurement of microaneurysm for diabetic retinopathy and cup:disc ratio and volume of optic disc for glaucoma. These automatic measurements could be performed on images taken over a period of time to objectively compare them for pathological changes over time. In other words, computer-aided diagnosis could provide objective measurements to monitor disease progression. In teleophthalmology systems, image compression, especially lossy compression techniques, could influence the digital image analysis tools. However, more advanced image compression techniques are still evolving and could have less influence on the outcomes of advanced digital imaging techniques.

11.4   Image-Based Clinical Decision Support Systems

Clinical (or diagnostic) decision support systems (CDSS) are interactive software, which directly assist clinicians and other health professionals with decision-making tasks using clinical observations and health knowledge. Advanced image analysis tools could further support the decision-making process. These tools could automatically identify abnormal pathologies. Presence or absence of various pathologies together with other parameters such as family history could lead to automatic disease grading. A medical decision support system for diabetic retinopathy will further enhance the management of the disease and empower the rural and remote health professionals and patients. Image-based automatic grading systems could provide faster and more efficient screening with the help of trained health care personnel [23; 24]. Telemedicine and widespread screening combined with image-based clinical decision support will enable early detection of disease and therefore prevent blindness.

In fundus photography, exposure setting and focus are the important and difficult skills. Stumpf et al. [25] have demonstrated that an online continuous quality improvement protocol could support and reinforce fundus imaging skills in diabetic retinopathy screenings over a significant period of time even when considerable turnover was experienced.

The TOSCA-Imaging project established by European countries [26; 27] is one of the advanced projects that utilizes advanced image analysis techniques for telemedicine-based diabetic retinopathy screenings. An Internet-based image processing software for screening and diagnosis of diabetic retinopathy was tested in the field. A preliminary validation of this software showed a sensitivity and specificity of 80% for the detection of normality based on precise detection of individual lesions. Decisions that depend on the detection of lesion patterns such as clinically significant macular edema showed a sensitivity and specificity of more than 95%. Validation by two expert graders suggested a sensitivity and specificity of below 90% for any lesion and of more than 95% for predicting overall retinopathy grade.

Another group from Spain, Hornero et. al [28], has evaluated an automated retinal image analysis in a telemedicine screening program for diabetic retinopathy. Automatic image analysis technique was utilized to visually discriminate between hard exudates, cotton wool spots, and hemorrhages. The main focus of this program was to detect all hard exudates. 35 out of 52 digital fundus photographs presented hard exudates. A sensitivity of 75% and a specificity of 99% were obtained. The long-term goal of this project is to automate the telemedicine screening for diabetic retinopathy.

11.5 Conclusion

Major barriers for the introduction of teleophthalmology are fees for service and indemnity, but we can see major changes happening around the world in recent times. In the United States, teleophthalmology consultations can be reimbursed in California. The other states and other countries may follow the path in the very near future.

Telemedicine screening by nurses and primary care providers is a feasible solution for early detection and follow-up of diabetic retinopathy in rural, remote, and underserved areas. Teleophthalmology technology combined with image-based CDSS will improve and upgrade skills of local clinicians. It will save many remote patients from unnecessary visits to specialist centers on one hand, and allows more effective diagnosis and intervention on the other.

References

[1] Yogesan, K., Kumar, S., Goldschmidt, L., et al., *Teleophthalmology*, Springer-Verlag, Germany, 2006.

[2] Kumar, S., Tay-Kearney, M.L., Chaves, F., et al., Remote ophthalmology services: cost comparison of telemedicine and alternative service delivery options, *Journal of Telemedicine and Telecare*, 12, 19, 2006.

[3] Wormald, R.P. and Rauf, A., Glaucoma screening, *Journal of Medical Screening*, 2(2), 109, 1995.

[4] Komulainen, R., Tuulonen, A., and Airaksinen, P.J., The follow-up of patients screened for glaucoma with non-mydriatic fundus photography, *Inter. Ophthalmol*, 16(6), 465, 1993.

[5] Buxton, M.J., Sculpher, M.J., Ferguson, B.A., et al., Screening for treatable diabetic retinopathy: A comparison of different methods, *Diabetic Medicine*, 8(4), 371, 1991.

[6] Higgs, E.R., Harney, B.A., Kelleher, A., et al., Detection of diabetic retinopathy in the community using a non-mydriatic camera, *Diabetic Medicine*, 8(6), 551, 1991.

[7] Kohner, E. and Hamilton, A.M.P., Vascular retinopathies — The management of diabetic retinopathy, in *Clinical Ophthalmology*, S. Miller, ed., IOP Publishing Ltd, Bristol, 238, 1987.

[8] Chen, L.S., Tsai, C.Y., Lu, T.Y., et al., Feasibility of tele-ophthalmology for screening for eye disease in remote communities, *Journal of Telemedicine and Telecare*, 10, 337, 2004.

[9] Yoo, S.K., Kim, D.K., Jung, S.M., et al., Performance of a web-based, real-time, tele-ultrasound consultation system over high-speed commercial telecommunication lines, *Journal of Telemedicine and Telecare*, 10, 175, 2004.

[10] Eikelboom, R.H., Yogesan, K., Barry, C.J., et al., Methods and limits of digital image compression of retinal images for telemedicine, *Invest. Ophthalmol. Vis. Sci.*, 41(7), 1916, 2000.

[11] Basu, A., Kamal, A.D., Illahi, W., et al., Is digital image compression acceptable within diabetic retinopathy screening? *Diabet Med*, 20(9), 766, 2003.

[12] Baker, C.F., Rudnisky, C.J., Tennant, M.T., et al., JPEG compression of stereo-scopic digital images for the diagnosis of diabetic retinopathy via teleophthal-mology, *Can J Opththalmol*, 39(7), 746, 2004.

[13] Lee, M.S., Shin, D.S., and Berger, J.W., Grading, image analysis, and stereopsis of digitally compressed fundus images, *Retina*, 20(3), 275, 2000.

[14] Stellingwerf, C., Hardus, P.L.L.J., and Hooymans, J.M.M., Assessing diabetic retinopathy using two-field digital photography and the influence of JPEG-compression, *Documenta Ophthalmologica*, 108, 203, 2004.

[15] American Diabetes Association, Complications of diabetes in the United States, 2008, http://www.diabetes.org/diabetes-statistics/complications.jsp, ac-cessed 17th June 2008.

[16] Stefansson, E., Bek, T., Prota, M., et al., Screening and prevention of diabetic blindness, *Acta Ophthalmologica Scandinavica*, 78, 374, 2000.

[17] Boucher, M.C., Nguyen, Q.T., and Angioi, K., Mass community screening for diabetic retinopathy using a nonmydriatic camera with telemedicine, *Canadian Journal of Ophthalmology*, 40(6), 734, 2005.

[18] Yogesan, K., Constable, I.J., and Chan, I., Telemedicine screening for diabetic retinopathy: Improving patient access to care, *Disease Management and Health Outcomes*, 10(11), 673, 2002.

[19] Cavallerano, A.A., Cavallerano, J.D., Katalinic, P., et al., A telemedicine pro-gram for diabetic retinopathy in a veterans affairs medical center — The Joslin Vision Network eye health care model, *American Journal of Ophthalmology*, 139(4), 597, 2005.

[20] Aiello, L.M., Cavallerano, A.A., Bursell, S.E., et al., The Joslin Vision Network innovative telemedicine care for diabetes: Preserving human vision, *Ophthal-mology Clinics of North America*, 13(2), 213, 2000.

[21] Patton, N., Aslam, T.M., Macgillivray, T., et al., Retinal image analysis: Con-cepts, applications and potential, *Prog Retin Eye Res*, 25(1), 99, 2006.

[22] Williamson, T.H. and Keating, D., Telemedicine and computers in diabetic retinopathy screening, *BJO*, 82, 5, 1998.

[23] Jelinek, H.F., Cree, M.J., Worsely, D., et al., An automated microaneurysm detector as a tool for identification of diabetic retinopathy in a rural optometry practice, *Clinical and Experimental Optometry*, 89(5), 299, 2006.

[24] Cree, M.J., Olson, J.A., McHardy, K., et al., A fully automated comparative microaneurysm digital detection system, *Eye*, 11, 622, 1997.

[25] Stumpf, S.H., Verma, D., Zalunardo, R., et al., Online continuous quality im-provement for diabetic retinopathy tele-screening, *Telemedicine Journal and e-Health*, 10(2), S35, 2004.

[26] Hejlesen, O., Ege, B., Englmeier, K.H., et al., TOSCA-Imaging — developing Internet based image processing software for screening and diagnosis of diabetic retinopathy, in *Medinfo 2004*, 2004, vol. 11, 222–226.

[27] Luzio, S., Hatcher, S., Zahlmann, G., et al., Feasibility of using the TOSCA telescreening procedures for diabetic retinopathy, *Diabetic Medicine*, 21(10), 1121, 2004.

[28] Hornero, R., Sanchez, C., and Lopez, M., Automated retinal image analysis in a teleophthalmology diabetic retinopathy screening program, *Telemedicine Journal and e-Health*, 10(1), S101, 2004.

Index

abnormality, 131
access to care, 54
accuracy, 242–244, 257
active contour, 278, 279, 284–286, 288, 292
age-related macular degeneration, 2, 5, 72
altitude, 320–322
analyzing wavelet, 225, 226, 229
anisotropy, 228, 229, *see also* elongation
area closing, 164
area under curve, 89–90, 243–244, 249, 254, 257
ARIC, *see* Atherosclerosis Risk in Communities Study
arterial venous diameter ratio, 187–190, 192, 193, 196, 198, 205, 306–308, 311, 312, 317
arteriolar narrowing, 11, 12, 185–187, 190–193, 196, 200
arteriovenous nicking, 11, 185, 187, 191, 197, 198
asymmetric digital subscriber line, 342
asymmetry index, 321–322
asymmetry ratio, 310, 311
atherosclerosis, 198
Atherosclerosis Risk in Communities Study, 190–194, 196–198, 200, 317
AUC, *see* area under curve
AVR, *see* arterial venous diameter ratio
A_z, *see* area under curve

B-spline, 278–284
Bayes's formula, 231
Bayesian decision theory, 169, 231
Beaver Dam Eye Study, 189–192, 196, 198, 200, 317

bias, 107–108
bifurcation, *see* vessel
Biometric identification and verification, 223
blindness, 2, 29, 54, 79, 93–95, 306, 344
blood glucose control, 42
blood pressure, 42, 306, 315–317, 330
blood vessel, *see* vessel
Blue Mountains Eye Study, 29, 191–193, 196, 197
boundary detection, 278–279, 288, 289
bounding box closing, 164
branching vessel points, 222, 223, 259

cardiac cycle, 295, 298
cardiovascular disease, 6, 43, 186–191, 201, 306
Cardiovascular Health Study, 197, 198
categorical scale, 104
central retinal arteriolar equivalent diameter, 187, 205
central retinal venular equivalent diameter, 187, 205
cerebrovascular disease, 6, 191–193
change detection, 221, 222, 259
Chaudhuri et al. filter, 235, 242, 244, 254, 258
CHD, *see* coronary heart disease
Chennai Urban Rural Epidemiology Study, 198
chord length, 312
class-conditional probability density function, *see* likelihood
classifier, 158, 159
    Gaussian quadratic, 121, 127
    GMM, 122, 127, 224, 231–233, 235, 242, 244, 245, 249, 254, 256–258

*k*NN, 121, 127, 161, 171, 233, 235,
    242, 244, 245, 249, 254, 256–
    258
LMSE, 234–235, 244, 245, 249,
    256, 258
naïve Bayes, 169, 171
rule based, 159
clinical decision suppport system, 346
Cochrane Collaboration, 101
Cohen's kappa, 108
cohort, 104, 106
color normalization, 133, 166
color retinal photography, 221, 222,
    235, 240, 247, 249
color space
    HLS, 142, 144, 148, 150
    L*ab*, 132, 142, 144, 147, 150, 171
    L*Ch*, 144, 147, 148, 150
    L*uv*, 134
confidence interval, 85, 86, 89, 95, 106
confusion matrix, 242
contingency table, *see* confusion matrix
continuous scale, 87, 90, 104
contrast enhancement, 133, 134, 162
coronary heart disease, 189, 193–194,
    200, 317
correction term, wavelet, 225, 229, 259
correlation coefficients, 141
correlation filter, 223, 227, 256, *see also*
    Chaudhuri et al. filter
correlation matrix, 234
cotton wool spots, 9–10, 35, 36, 38, 70,
    71, 100, 124, 129, 166, 191–
    193, 197, 344, 347
covariate, 90, 108
coverage, 81–82, 90
cross section, 270, 276–278, 292, 293,
    295, 296, 299, 313, 314
crossing vessel points, 222, 223, 259
CRT monitor, 92, 96
curvature, 312, 317, 318, 326
CWS, *see* cotton wool spots

diabetes, 2, 27–29, 35, 40, 42–46, 54,
    55, 79, 80, 122, 186, 187,

    194, 196–198
    prevalence, 28, 80
Diabetes Control and Complications
    Trial, 42, 68
diabetic maculopathy, 128
diabetic macular edema, 11, 29, 35, 37,
    39, 40, 46, 49, 53, 99, 104,
    105
diabetic maculopathy, 98, 122, 124
diabetic retinopathy, 2–5, 27, 29–55,
    69, 90–93, 97–100, 104, 105,
    121, 122, 130, 155, 172, 174,
    176–178, 196, 221, 222, 240,
    260, 306, 339, 340, 343–346
    classification, 40, 53
    definition, 35
    nonproliferative, 35, 36, 38, 40,
        80, 100, 123–124
    pathogenesis, 43–45
    prevalence, 29
    proliferative, 29, 35, 36, 39, 40, 80,
        90, 94, 100, 123, 124, 150,
        222
    screening, 3–5, 48–50, 54, 68, 71,
        156, 160, 165, 172, 175, 176,
        178, 342, 344, 347
    sight threatening, 80, 98
    systemic associations, 42–43
    treatment, 45–47
diagnosis
    early, 79–81
diagnostic performance criterion, 130
digital camera, 49, 92, 172–173, 176
digital subscriber line, 342
directional wavelets, 226, 228–229
distance
    Euclidean, 233
    Mahalanobis, 233
distance measures, 233, 238
DME, *see* diabetic macular edema
DRIVE database, 12, 68, 176, 240–242,
    257
drusen, 9–10, 99, 129
dual width ribbon, 286, 287, 290, 293
DWibbon, *see* dual width ribbon

early diagnosis, *see* diagnosis, early
Early Treatment Diabetic Retinopathy
        Study, 40, 68, 69, 102
    final scale, 104
EBM, *see* evidence-based medicine
edge, 313, 315, 318, 319, 321, 323
edge detection, 12, 163, 226, 227
EHT, *see* essential hypertension
elongation, 228, 229, 237, 247
EM, *see* expectation-maximization
energy, 288–293
essential hypertension, 328, 329
estimation, 85, 86, 95, 108
ETDRS, *see* Early Treatment Diabetic
        Retinopathy Study
ethnicity, 28, 29
Euclidean distance, 233
Euclidean group, 226, 227
evaluation of vessel segmentation, 241–
        245, 259–260
evidence-based medicine, 68, 101
Exeter Standard, 85
expansion ratio, 310
expectation-maximization, 127, 232
external validation, 93
external validity, 101
exudates, 9–10, 35, 36, 38, 43, 70,
        71, 92, 98–99, 121–131, 133,
        135–138, 140, 149, 150, 166,
        344, 347
eye safety, 341

false negative fraction, 85
false negative test, 81
false positive fraction, 84, 87, 89, 109,
        110, 242, 244, 259
false positive test, 81
fast Fourier transform, 99, 227, 256
FDA, 102, 109
feature normalization, 238–239
FFT, *see* fast Fourier transform
fluorescein angiography, 36, 42, 155–
        160, 221, 222, 235, 240, 247,
        249, 313
fluorescence

    choroidal, 157
Fourier analysis, 99, 224
fovea, 11, 71
    automated detection, 11, 129, 159
FPF, *see* false positive fraction
fractal analysis, 12, 222, 225, 226, 259,
        260
fundoscopy, 305, 306, 317
Fundus Photograph Reading Center,
        105

Gabor transform, *see* short-time Fourier
        transform (STFT)
Gabor wavelet, 228–229
Gaussian, 157–159, 167, 222, 225, 228,
        229, 231, 232, 314, 315, 323,
        324
Gaussian cross-sectional profiles, 222
Gaussian mixture model, 122, 127, 224,
        231–233, 254, 256–258
Gaussian quadratic, 121, 127
generalization, 135
glaucoma, 6
global vessel segmentation, 224, 259
GMM, *see* Gaussian mixture model
GMM classifier, 224, 231–233, 235,
        242, 244, 245, 249, 254, 256–
        258
GNU General Public License (GPL),
        245
gold standard, 103–107
GRADE, 110
gradient vector flow, 132, 141, 145
graphical user interface, 245, 247–249
gray-level morphology, 142, 146, 150
ground truth, 125, 132, 141, 147, 148,
        150, 240, 242–244, 260
group, Euclidean, 226, 227
GUI, *see* graphical user interface

hard exudates, *see* exudates
hat wavelet, Mexican, 229
heart disease
    coronary, 317
    ischemic, 28, 317

hemorrhages, 9, 35, 36, 39, 69–71, 92,
97–98, 122, 123, 128, 129,
164–166, 185, 187, 191–193,
197, 344, 347
dot, 9, 35, 36, 38, 39, 155, 156, 164
Hessian, 323, 325, 326
histogram specification, 133, 166
HLS color space, 142, 144, 148, 150
HTML results pages, 245, 246
hue, 147, 148, 150, 161, 166, 171
hypertension, 6, 11, 42, 43, 186, 187,
189–192, 198, 200, 305, 306,
311, 315, 317, 329
essential, 328, 329
malignant phase, 328, 329
hypothesis test, 244, 260, 296–298

IHD, *see* ischemic heart disease
image
capture, 172, 221–222, 340
compression, 92, 173–175, 342–
343, 346
field of view, 49, 50
file format, 50
public databases, 12, 68, 102, 176,
240–241
quality, 72, 91–93, 96–98, 102,
103, 110, 172, 311, 341, 345
red-free, 155, 160, 165, 313
resolution, 50, 92, 98, 157, 159,
161, 163, 173, 174, 176, 341–
342
transmission, 342
variability, 222, 239, 257, 258
image-based, 125, 127, 129, 130, 133,
139, 149
incidence rate, 95
index terms, 101, 103
index test, 105
inner product, *see* scalar product
interaction, user, 224, 239, 240, 258–
260, *see also* graphical user
interface (GUI)
internal validity, 101

International Clinical Diabetic Macular Edema Disease Severity
Scale, 40, 41
International Clinical Diabetic Retinopathy Disease Severity Scale,
40, 41, 69, 104
Internet, 340, 342
intraretinal microvascular abnormalities, 35, 36, 38, 40, 70, 100,
344
IRMA, *see* intraretinal microvascular
abnormalities
ischemic heart disease, 317
IVAN, 201–207

Joslin Vision Network, 344
JPEG compression, 173–175, 343
junction exponent, 308, 311, 315, 317

K nearest neighbor, *see* kNN classifier
kappa, 108
kNN classifier, 121, 127, 161, 171, 233,
235, 242, 244, 245, 249, 254,
256–258

L-NMMA, *see* N^G-mono-methyl-L-
arginine
L*ab* color space, 132, 142, 144, 147,
150, 171
L*ab* components, 132, 150
laser photocoagulation, 45–46
latent decision variable model, 90
LCD monitor, 92
L*Ch* color space, 144, 147, 148, 150
LDR, *see* vessel, length to diameter ratio
lead time, 107
learning dataset, *see* training dataset
least squares fit, 281–284
length to diameter ratio, *see* vessel
length, vessel, 222, 260
lesion-based, 125, 129, 130
lightness, 142, 147, 148
likelihood, 231, 232
linear discriminant analysis (LDA), 159

Lions Eye Institute, 339, 344, 346
Lipid Research Clinic's Coronary Primary Prevention Trial, 193
LMSE classifier, 234–235, 244, 245, 249, 256, 258
localization, 122, 124, 127–132, 140, 141, 144, 145, 147–149
LogMAR, 95, 96
L*uv* color space, 134

machine learning, 102
macula, 10, 35, 122, 123, 130, 131, 140, 158
macular detachment, 39
macular edema, 5–6, *see also* diabetic macular edema
macular involvement, 98
Mahalanobis distance, 233
malignant phase hypertension, 328, 329
manual vessel segmentation, 223, 224, 229, 239–245, 249, 254, 257–260
MAR, 96
masking, 106–107
mass screening, *see* screening
matched filter, 157, 158, 167, 168, 270, 287, 292, *see also* correlation filter
MATLAB, 245–247, 256, 260
McNemar's test, 106
medical subject headings, 103
meta-analysis, 90
metabolic syndrome, 196–197
Mexican hat wavelet, 229
MHT, *see* malignant phase hypertension
micro-infarctions, *see* cotton wool spots
microaneurysms, 8–9, 35, 36, 38, 39, 44, 69–71, 92, 97–99, 102, 108, 122, 123, 128, 129, 155–156, 185, 187, 191–193, 197, 198, 342–344, 346
    appearance, 36, 123, 155
    automated detection, 8–9, 156–175
        standard approach, 157

turnover, 102, 156, 177–178
minimum description length, 137
mlvessel package, 245–249
monochromatic retinal photography, 221, *see also* red-free retinal photography
Morlet wavelet, 225, 228
morphological filtering, 131, 132, 156, 157, 161, 164
morphology, 122, 128, 129, 132, 140–144, 146–148, 150, 158
    color, 143, 144, 148
    gray-level, 132, 142, 150
    reconstruction, 161, 167
morphology of the retinal vasculature, 221–222, 260
mother wavelet, *see* analyzing wavelet
Multi-Ethnic Study of Atherosclerosis, 197, 198, 200
multiresolution, 224
multiscale vessel detection, 223, 229, 235, 238, 241, 258
Murry's Law, 308

National Health Examination Survey, 193
National Screening Committee, 84
negative predictive value, 85
neovascularization, 35–37, 39, 70, 174, 222, 260, *see also* new vessels
neural network, 129, 159, 163
new vessels, 35–37, 39, 70, 71, 100
N^G-mono-methyl-L-arginine (L-NMMA), 311
nonexudate, 121, 134, 135, 137, 138, 149
nonparametric, 135, 149
nonparametric classification, 233
nonproliferative diabetic retinopathy, *see* diabetic retinopathy
nonstationary signals, 224–225
NORibbon, *see* normal offset ribbon
normal offset ribbon, 286, 287, 290, 293
normalization, feature, 238–239
NPV, *see* negative predictive value

NSC, *see* National Screening Committee

OCT, *see* optical coherence tomography
opening operator, 158
ophthalmoscopy, 48, 50, 340
optic disc, 9–11, 37, 53, 71, 122, 124, 126–132, 139–150, 175, 187, 346
optical coherence tomography, 42, 51, 99, 340
ordinal scale, 104
over-fitting, 232, 257
overcalling, 86

Package, mlvessel, 245–249
paired test, 106, 108
parametric classification, 233, 234
parametric density estimation, 135
Parr and Spears, 307, 308
Parr-Hubbard formulae, 187, 188
path length, 314, 320, 321, 329
pathologies, 35, 121, 125, 130–132, 140, 141
pdf, *see* probability density function
PDR, *see* diabetic retinopathy, proliferative
pericytes, 155
peripheral vascular disease, 315
photocoagulation, 98, 100
pipeline architecture, 245
pixel classification, 134, 161
pixel level, 128, 134
pixel resolution, 121, 125, 129, 130, 149, 157
pixel-based, 125, 134, 161
point prevalence, 95
Poisson regression, 95
positive predictive value, 85, 109
posterior probability, 231–233, 242, 244, 249, 259
PPV, *see* positive predictive value
predictive value, 85–87
    negative, 85
    positive, 85, 109

predictivity, 130, 137–139, 149
preprocessing, 125, 131–133, 148, 150
prevalence, 86, 104, 108
    diabetes, 28, 80
principal component analysis, 131, 137
prior probability, 231, 232, 243
probability density function, 135, 296
proliferative diabetic retinopathy, *see* diabetic retinopathy
pseudoinverse, 234
public image databases, 12, 68, 102, 176, 240–241
PubMed, 101, 103
PVD, *see* peripheral vascular disease

QUADAS, 101
quality assurance standards, 84–85

rating scale, 108
receiver operating characteristic, 85, 87–90, 235, 242–244, 259, 260
    free-response, 159
red-free retinal photography, 98, 155, 160, 165, 221, 222, 235, 247, 249, 313
reference test, 103–107
region growing, 158, 161, 162, 165, 326–327
registration, 221–223, 259, 269, 272, 294–295
renal disease, 197–198
retina, 29–35
retinal image, *see* image
retinal pigment epithelium, 29, 97, 98
retinal thickening, 35, 36, 46, 49, 51, 70, 96, 99–100
retinopathy
    diabetic, *see* diabetic retinopathy
    hypertensive, 40, 186, 189–191
Retinopathy Grading Centre, 93, 106
retinopathy of prematurity, 318
Retinopathy Online Challenge, 68, 177
RGC, *see* Retinopathy Grading Centre
ribbon, 279, 284–287, 289–295, 299

dual width, 286, 287, 290, 293
normal offset, 286, 287, 290, 293
ribbon snake, 289–293
risk reduction program, 79, 82, 83, 91, 93, 94, 96, 99
risk score, 101
ROC, *see* receiver operating characteristic, *see also* Retinopathy Online Challenge
ROP, *see* retinopathy of prematurity
Rotterdam Eye Study, 189, 191, 193, 196, 198
RPE, *see* retinal pigment epithelium

saturation, 147, 148
scalar product, 225, 227, 234, 238, 244
scale, wavelet, 223, 225, 229, 235, 238, 241
scale-space skeletonization, 246
scanning laser ophthalmoscope, 340
Scottish Intercollegiate Guidelines Network, 82
screening, 48, 71, 80–84, 339
mass, 68, 83
uptake, 82
screening test, 83–84, 86, 94
SD-OCT, 99
segmentation, 124, 125, 127, 128, 130, 134, 144, 150, 323–327
sensitivity, 48, 84–85, 87, 96, 103, 107, 109, 125, 129–131, 137–139, 149
shade-correction, 157
short-time Fourier transform, 224
sight threatening diabetic retinopathy, *see* diabetic retinopathy
SIGN, *see* Scottish Intercollegiate Guidelines Network
skeletonization, scale-space, 246
skeletonized vasculature, 222, 246, 259
sliding linear regression filter, 314–315
SLRF, *see* sliding linear regression filter
snake, 11, 141, 279
gradient vector flow, 132, 141, 147
soft exudates, *see* cotton wool spots

software, mlvessel, *see* mlvessel package
specificity, 48, 84–85, 87, 96, 107, 109, 125, 129–131, 137, 139, 149
standard photographs, 102, 104, 105
STARD (standards for reporting of diagnostic accuracy), 103
STARE database, 12, 68, 102, 176, 240–242, 257
stationary signals, 224
statistical hypothesis test, 244, 260
STDR, *see* diabetic retinopathy, sight threatening
STFT, *see* short-time Fourier transform
Strahler, 319–321
stroke, 28, 191–193, 317
sum of squared error criterion, 234
supervised pixel classification, 223, 229–231, 235, 239–240, 247, 258
Svensson's method, 106, 108
systematic review, 101

telemedicine, 50, 339–348
store-and-forward, 340
template matching, 127, 129, 131, 132, 140–141, 147
test dataset, 102
threshold, 273–274
time-frequency uncertainty, 224–225, 228
tophat transform, 158, 162, 164, 167
topology, 318–323, 328–329
tortuosity, *see* vessel
TPF, *see* true positive fraction
training dataset, 101, 135
treatment, 45–47
true positive fraction, 84, 87, 242, 244, 259

undercalling, 86
United Kingdom Prospective Diabetes Study, 42
unpaired test, 106
uptake, 82

user interaction, 224, 239, 240, 258–260, *see also* graphical user interface (GUI)

variability, 106, 108–109
vasculature
    morphology, 221–222, 260
    skeleton, 222, 246, 259
    topology, 318–323, 328–329
vein occlusion, 40
venous beading, 12, 35, 36, 38, 40, 70, 100, 344
venous dilatation, 12
vessel
    bifurcation, 188, 269, 272, 274, 306–312, 315, 317, 318, 328
    branching points, 187, 222, 223, 259
    crossing points, 222, 223, 259, 272, 274
    curvature, 312
    detection, 140
    detection using wavelets, 226, 229, 235, 237–238
    diameter, 70, 87, 100, 187–190, 193, 196–198, 200, 201, 222, 241, 257–260, 269, 271, 272, 275–278, 292–298, 312–315, 328
    edges, 270–273, 275, 277–280, 284, 285, 288–290, 313, 315
    extraction, 271–276
    graph, 274
    length, 222, 260
    length to diameter ratio, 188, 306, 311–312, 315, 317, 328
    lesions, 187
    manual segmentation, 223, 224, 229, 239–245, 249, 254, 257–260
    model, 270–271
    narrowing, 185–187, 190–193, 196, 200
    nicking, 185, 187, 191, 197, 198

segmentation, 11, 67, 71, 72, 271–276, 323
segmentation evaluation, 12, 241–245, 259–260
tortuosity, 12, 100, 188, 222, 275, 306, 312, 317, 318, 329
tracking, 11, 222, 259, 271–273, 275, 278, 279, 293
width, *see* vessel, diameter
video conferencing, 340
visual acuity, 49, 80, 94–96, 345
visual impairment, 29, 43, 46, 93–95
vitreoretinal surgery, 46
vitreous, 29

wavelets and wavelet transforms, 224–229
    analyzing wavelet, 225, 226, 229
    anisotropy, 228, 229, *see also* elongation
    basis, 225, 226
    compression, 343
    correction term, 225, 229, 259
    directional wavelets, 226, 228–229
    elongation, 228, 229, 237, 247
    Euclidean group, 226, 227
    frame, 228, 229
    Gabor wavelet, 228–229
    group, Euclidean, 226, 227
    Mexican hat wavelet, 229
    Morlet wavelet, 225, 228
    nonstationary signals, 224–225
    one-dimensional continuous transform, 224–225
    scale, 223, 225, 229, 235, 238, 241
    stationary signals, 224
    time-frequency uncertainty, 224–225, 228
    time-scale plane, 225
    two-dimensional continuous transform, 225–228
    two-dimensional discrete transform, 226
    vessel detection, 226, 229, 235, 237–238

width change, 269, 278, 292, 294–298
width, vessel, 222, 241, 257–260, *see also* vessel, diameter
Wilcoxon statistic, 243
Workbook 4.2, 84